CEREBROVASCULAR EVALUATION WITH DOPPLER ULTRASOUND

DEVELOPMENTS IN CARDIOVASCULAR MEDICINE

VOLUME 6

1. C.T. Lancée, *Echocardiology,* 1979. ISBN 90-247-2209-8.
2. J. Baan, A.C. Arntzenius, E.L. Yellin, *Cardiac Dynamics.* 1980. ISBN 90-247-2212-8.
3. H.J.Th. Thalen, C.C. Meere, *Fundamentals of Cardiac Pacing.* 1979. ISBN 90-247-2245-4.
4. H.E. Kulbertus, H.J.J. Wellens, *Sudden Death.* 1980. ISBN 90-247-2290-X.
5. L.S. Dreifus, A.N. Brest, *Clinical Applications of Cardiovascular Drugs.* 1980. ISBN 90-247-2295-0 (hardback), 90-247-2369-8 (paperback).
7. D.P. Zipes, J.C. Bailey, V. Elharrar (eds.), *The Slow Inward Current and Cardiac Arrhythmias.* 1980. ISBN 90-247-2380-9.
8. H. Kesteloot, J.V. Joossens (eds.), *Epidemiology of Arterial Blood Pressure.* 1980. ISBN 9-247-2386-8.

series ISBN 90-247-2336-1

CEREBROVASCULAR EVALUATION WITH DOPPLER ULTRASOUND

by

MERRILL P. SPENCER, M.D.

JOHN M. REID, Ph.D.

With contributions by

EDWIN C. BROCKENBROUGH, M.D.
ROBERT S. RENEMAN, M.D.
GEORGE I. THOMAS, M.D.
DONALD L. DAVIS, B.S.E.E.

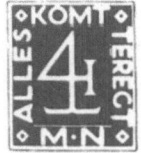

1981

MARTINUS NIJHOFF PUBLISHERS

THE HAGUE / BOSTON / LONDON

Distributors:

for the United States and Canada

Kluwer Boston, Inc.
190 Old Derby Street
Hingham, MA 02043
USA

for all other countries

Kluwer Academic Publishers Group
Distribution Center
P.O. Box 322
3300 AH Dordrecht
The Netherlands

Library of Congress Cataloging in Publication Data   CIP

Spencer, Merrill P
  Cerebrovascular evaluation with Doppler ultrasound.

  (Developments in cardiovascular medicine; v. 6)
  Includes bibliographical references and index.
  1. Cerebrovascular disease—Diagnosis.   2.   Diagnosis, Ultrasonic.
3.   Head—Blood-vessels—Examination.   4.   Doppler effect.
I.   Reid, John Mitchell, joint author.   II.   Brockenbrough, Edwin C.
III.   Title.   IV.   Series.
[DNLM: 1.   Cerebrovascular disorders—Diagnosis.   2.   Ultrasonics—Diagnostic use.
W1 DE997VME v. 6 / WL355 S745c]
RC388.5.S67   616.8'107543   80-23643

ISBN-13:978-94-009-8206-2   e-ISBN-13:978-94-009-8204-8
DOI: 10.1007/978-94-009-8204-8

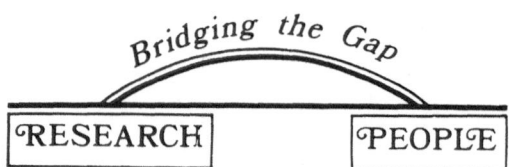

Bridging the Gap

RESEARCH   PEOPLE

Stroke Prevention
Heart Diseases
Cancer
Environment

The Institute of Applied Physiology and Medicine, 701 – 16th
Avenue, Seattle, WA, 98122 is a non-profit organization for medical research and education which extends itself beyond research to
bridge the critical gap between research and major health problems.

PREFACE

This book represents tangible results of the Institute of Applied Physiology and Medicine's objectives of bringing into clinical application the concepts and results of bioengineers and physiologists.

It has grown out of our experience in development of original Doppler diagnostic instrumentation and its application to more than 6,000 patients in non-invasive diagnosis of the extracranial cerebrovascular circulation. It gathers together bioengineering and physiological concepts which were initially developed for a graduate course for physicians and specialized medical technicians. It should be of particular interest to physicians and medical technologists whose specialties lie in the field of neurology, vascular surgery, and radiology.

The particular selection of techniques on our complete cerebrovascular non-invasive evaluation was chosen primarily to provide an integrated approach relying primarily on Doppler ultrasonic audio signals, but in addition utilizing a pertinent history and physical examination of the patient. The examination is performed by a specially trained physiology technician. Sufficient data is provided to the interpreting physician who develops a consultative report for the referring physician. The ultimate objective is prevention of stroke and symptoms of cerebrovascular insufficiency. The Doppler functional information supplements the angiography anatomical management decisions for angiography and surgery, anti-platelet or anti-coagulant medication, or to follow the patient with no special treatment.

As Doppler instrumentation and experience accumulates, the answer to many questions will come concerning the natural history of atherosclerosis and how it affects the cerebral circulation and patient management. As the instrumentation improves, both the speed and accuracy of the examination and reporting will improve. Of great potential is the new Infinite Gate Pulsed Doppler, as well as the advantages of real-time imaging of velocity profiles along the carotid and vertebral circulation.

ACKNOWLEDGEMENTS

We gratefully acknowledge the encouragement of the Medical Staff of The Providence Medical Center and the skill of physiology technicians Sheryl Clark, Wayne Ellsworth, Gail Glassen, Lou Granado, Jane Mayfield, David Moseley, John O'Brien and Karmann Titland. Josiane Petit-Tchoukaline provided much of the medical graphics for the text.

Many grants and contracts from the United States Department of Health and Social Services, the National Heart, Lung and Blood Institute, have supported research from which this book developed. These grants and contracts have included: HL 19341, HE 10248, H 4670, HE 08525, HE 09131, H 2630, HV 72926 and HL 15844.

TABLE OF CONTENTS

1. AN OVERVIEW OF NON-INVASIVE CEREBROVASCULAR EVALUATION USING DOPPLER ULTRASOUND

MERRILL P. SPENCER, M.D.

Approximately one-third of all strokes are caused by lesions developing in the cervical arteries supplying the brain. Doppler ultrasound provides the basis for the only non-invasive method of assessing local blood flow in individual arteries. When combined with other non-invasive techniques including the history and physical examination, many diagnostic interpretations, important in stroke prevention decisions, can be made concerning the extracranial blood supply to the brain (Table 1). Our present non-invasive system of cerebrovascular evaluation, shown in Table I, was developed from clinical experience with 6,000 patient examinations during a six-year period. They were referred to the laboratory because of symptoms of cerebrovascular insufficiency including TIA's and stroke or for non-symptomatic cervical bruits.

1. SUMMARY OF PRESENT CAPABILITY OF DOPPLER ULTRASOUND

Doppler ultrasonic detection of blood flow in the arteries was first utilized for extracranial cerebrovascular disease by Brockenbrough, 1956, to detect the changes in velocity of periorbital arterial signals. These techniques, refined and developed by others, have made an excellent contribution by detecting collateralization caused by hemodynamically significant carotid artery obstruction. They have a high sensitivity but have problems in specificity since the obstruction must be sufficient to produce collateralization. Also, intracranial collaterals from the opposite internal carotid or from the vertebral arteries, may diminish the apparent collateralization effect.

Other non-Doppler techniques for collateralization around the eye include indirect pressure measurements in the retinal artery, such as ophthalmodynamometry and cutaneous photoplethysmography. These techniques carry the same degree of accuracy as Doppler detection of collateralization and bear the same problems as Doppler. A serious disadvantage of all collateral techniques arises because they are indirect tests for obstruction and cannot separate a tight stenosis from total occlusion of the carotid artery.

Hand-held probing with the Doppler has also been applied successfully to detect obstructive disease of the vertebral artery and subclavian artery and a

Table 1. Doppler cerebrovascular evaluation. System of Spencer and Brockenbrough.

History:
>   Carotid insufficiency symptoms
>   Vertebrobasilar symptoms

Physical examination:
>   Neurological survey
>   Arterial palpation
>   Thoraco-cephalic ausculation
>   Arm pressures

Doppler examinations
>   Doppler imaging —
>>   Carotid bifurcation
>>   Subclavian-vertebral and low common
>   Hand-held probing —
>>   Ophthalmic artery signals
>>>   Posterior orbital
>>>   Periorbital
>>   External and internal carotid signals
>>   Vertebral artery signals
>>>   Base of skull
>>>   Anterior-supraclavicular
>>   Subclavian, axillary and brachial signals

Diagnostic interpretations
>   Carotid arteries —
>>   Bifurcation — stenosis and occlusion (of internal, external or common)
>>   Aneurysm
>>   Collateral evaluation
>>   Plaquing without stenosis
>   Vertebral arteries
>>   Stenosis
>>   Subclavian steal
>   Subclavian and innominate arteries
>>   Stenosis and occlusion
>   Cardiac —
>>   Low output
>>   Arrhythmias
>>   Miscellaneous

highly accurate test has been devised for vertebral to subclavian steal. Subclavian stenosis and vertebral-subclavian steal are frequently found when routine Doppler examination of these arteries is employed. Hand-held probing of the carotid arteries has also been developed by Gosling and by Pourcelot utilizing pulsatility characteristics to diagnose carotid obstruction. Rarely hand-held probing can detect abnormalities within the actual stenosis.

Direct Doppler imaging of the carotid arteries at the bifurcation has been developed with both continuous-wave (c-w) and pulsed Doppler ultrasound.

With c-w at least, it is possible to reliably and reproducibly detect high velocities up to 500 cm/sec. within a stenotic lesion as well as the secondary features of downstream turbulence, artery wall vibrations and changes in pulsatility. Common-Wave Doppler imaging can quantitate the degree of stenosis and can separate tight stenosis from total occlusion. The accuracy of c-w Doppler to detect stenosis is greater than 90% when compared with x-ray angiography.

A diagnosis of syphon stenosis can be made from the combination of findings of a bruit over the eye and a high pulsatility index in the internal carotid velocity pulse.

Non-stenotic plaques are also diagnosed because of the effect of calcium deposits in scattering the sound beam and producing abnormal Doppler signals. As the ultrasound beam traverses the arterial wall, scattering of the beam by calcium deposits or roughening of the lumenal surface produces recognizable features on the Doppler shifted signals. Recent in vitro studies of excised iliac arteries has confirmed that calcium deposits in atherosclerotic plaques can produce both asonic gaps in the Doppler image as well as inverted signal. In addition to these features, if fluttering caused by localized turbulence is detected without the high frequencies of stenosis, a diagnosis of nonstenotic plaque can also be made. A diagnosis of intimal ulceration cannot be made by Doppler ultrasound. Figure 1.

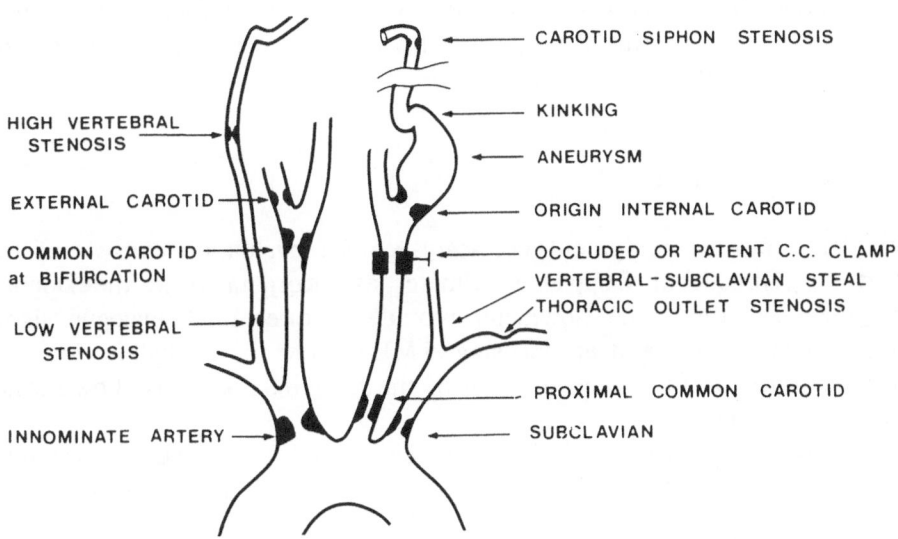

Figure 1. Obstructive lesions of the aorto-cerebral circulation diagnosed by Doppler.

The relative advantages of c-w and pulsed Doppler for extracranial cerebrovascular evaluation, are outlined as follows:

Advantages of c-w pulsed Doppler

1. Better signal/noise
   a. Cleaner signals
   b. Safer power levels
2. Higher frequency response
3. Easier vessel identification
4. Greater cost effectiveness

Advantages of pulsed Doppler

1. Separation of deep from superficial vessels
2. Higher resolution
3. Velocity profiles
4. Assists real-time pulse echo imaging

In our experience with both c-w and pulsed Doppler, the advantages of c-w outweigh the advantages of pulsed. As examples: the advantages of c-w allow a more accurate diagnosis of very tight stenosis and separation of this situation from total occlusion and the simpler procedure using c-w speeds the examination. The potential advantages of the pulsed Doppler in identifying deep lying vessels such as the vertebral are not material in the clinical setting because of the high accuracy and ease of c-w in detecting a vertebral artery signal at the base of the skull. The occasionally intervening occipital artery causes no confusion because firm pressure with the Doppler transducer obliterates this vessel. Currently, the advantages of pulsed Doppler exists in examination of the heart and the aorta where the separation of deep from superficial vessels is critical. It appears also to assist real-time ultrasonic echo imaging in identifying the carotid arteries.

2. DOPPLER IMAGING

Doppler ultrasonic equipment necessary for the evaluation consists of the Reid c-w Directional Doppler Flowmeter as incorporated in the Doppler imaging apparatus.* The flowmeter provides a directional analogue signal output using either a deep focusing 5 MHz probe or a shallow focusing 10 MHz probe. A functional diagram of the imaging system is shown schematically in Figure 2.

For bifurcation imaging the 5 MHz probe is fixed to the end of a scanning arm at an angle of 60° with the body axis and manually moved over the skin

* Available through Carolina Medical Electronics, P. O. Box 307, King, N.C., 27021, USA.

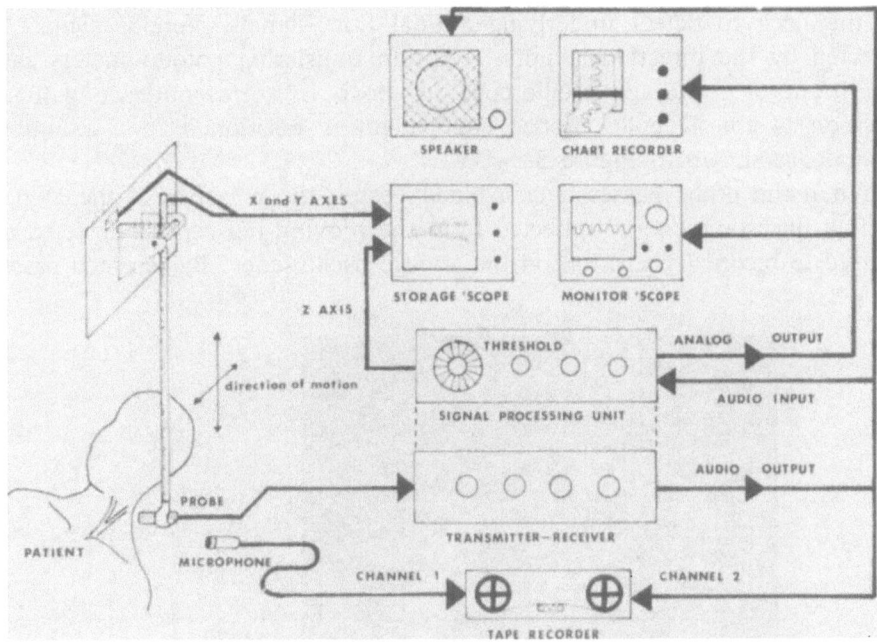

Figure 2. Functional diagram of the Doppler system for imaging of the carotid bifurcation.

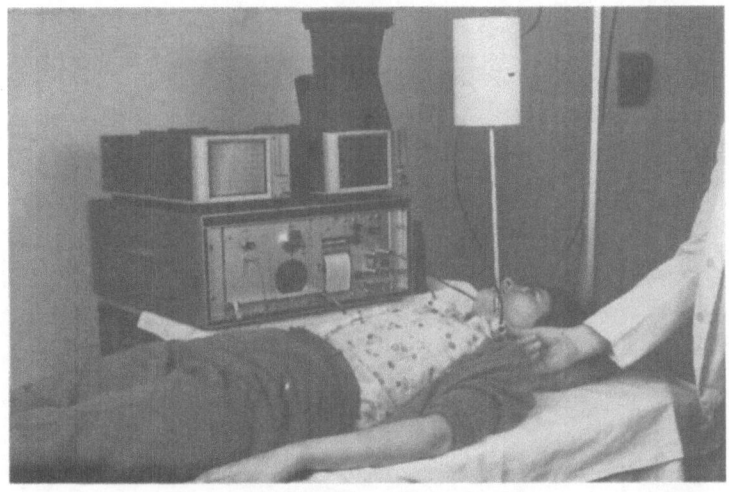

Figure 3. The imaging apparatus and position of the patient for carotid bifurcation imaging. The camera for photographing the stored image is shown to the right on top of the image scope. The X-Y trace scope is on the left with the Doppler electronics beneath. The Doppler probe is shown in the operator's hand, and the circuitry for position sensing is in the housing suspended above the patient.

of the neck to detect underlying arterial flow signals. Venous signals are rejected by the directional circuit. Position translating potentiometers cause the beam of a storage oscilloscope to move in correspondence with the position of the Doppler probe. The patient is positioned in a recumbent position as shown in Figure 3.

When the probe passes over a blood vessel, the presence of the Doppler shifted ultrasonic energy reflected from the moving red cells is detected and caused to record its position on the storage oscilloscope. By repeated passage

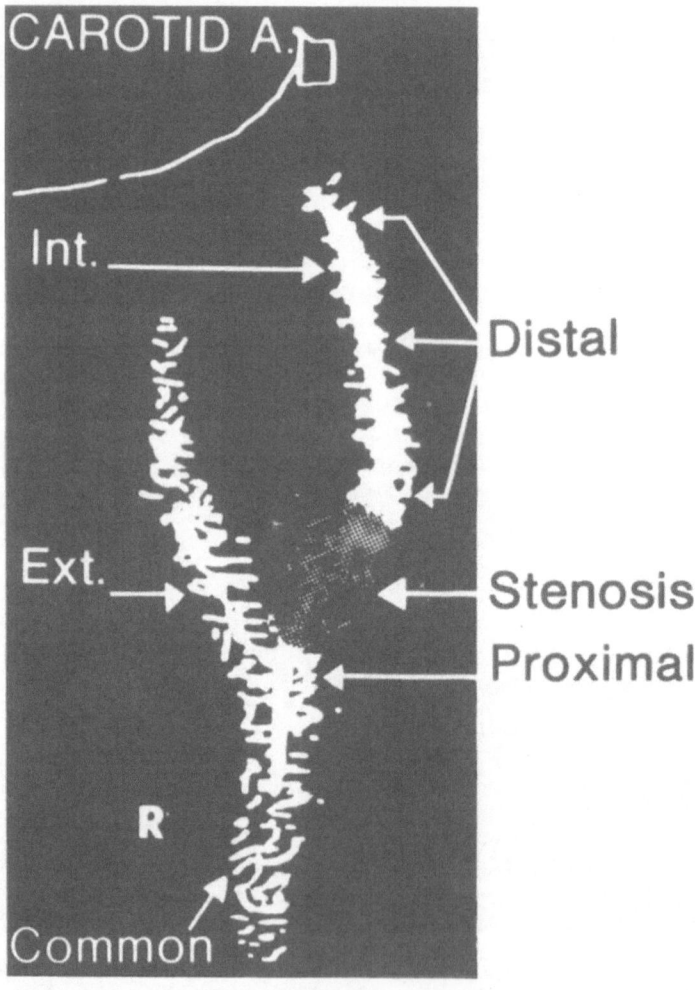

Figure 4a. Doppler image of the carotid bifurcation demonstrating points of selective audio recordings for stenosis at the origin of the internal carotid. The small square with the connecting line at the top represents the angle of the mandible.

over the carotid bifurcation, the technician gradually builds up and stores an image of the location of carotid blood flow signals. The image is similar to the lateral projection of the x-ray angiogram. Figure 4a.

A Doppler image of the carotid bifurcation of a patient is shown in Figure 4b. The image differs from the angiogram in that it presents additional information concerning the functional qualities of the blood flow which are represented in the audio Doppler signals. The Doppler sounds are available to

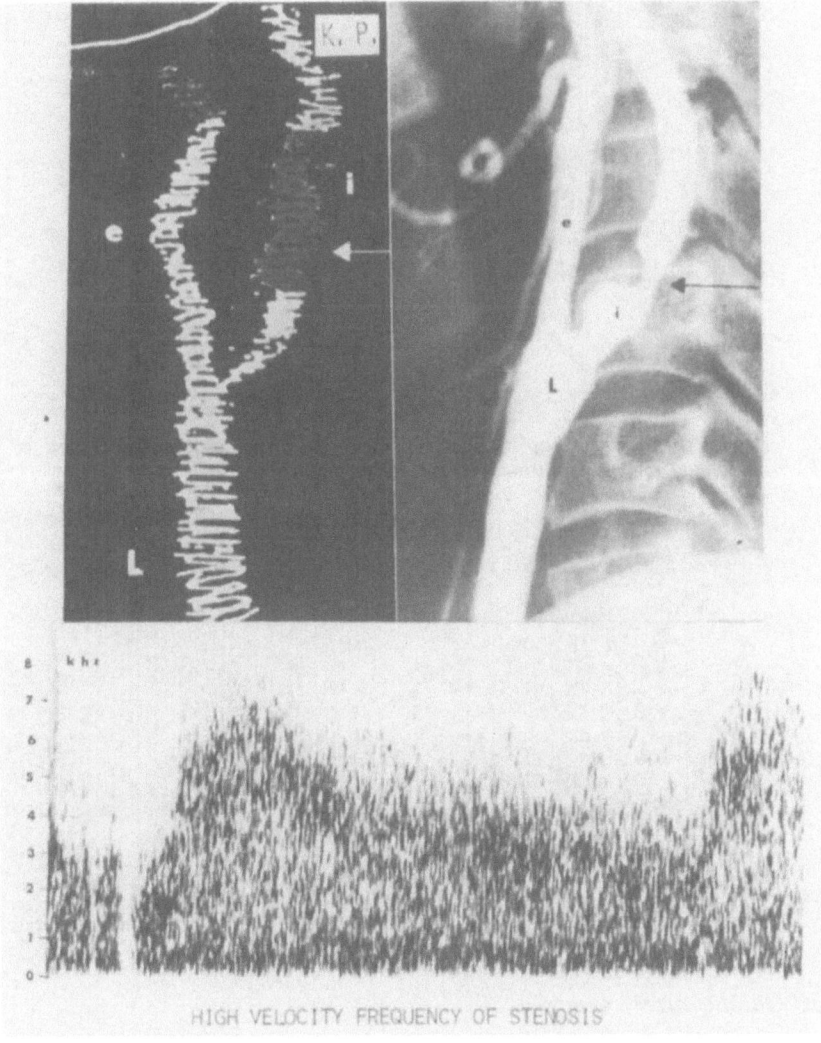

Figure 4b. Typical Doppler image of the carotid bifurcation. By convention, the internal carotid is pictured at the right-hand branch of the Doppler image. The arrow represents a region of high audio frequency at the origin of the internal carotid and represents a stenosis produced by atherosclerotic plaquing.

the operator throughout the examination and may be recorded at any point around the bifurcation. All data is stored in permanent files consisting of a photograph of the image, tape recordings of the sounds as well as a chart recording of the velocity waveforms.

The Doppler deep focusing probe consists of dual 5 MHz crystals providing for both transmitting and receiving and focused by means of a plastic lens to a beam width of 2 mm at a depth of 3.5 cm (Figures 5a and 5b).

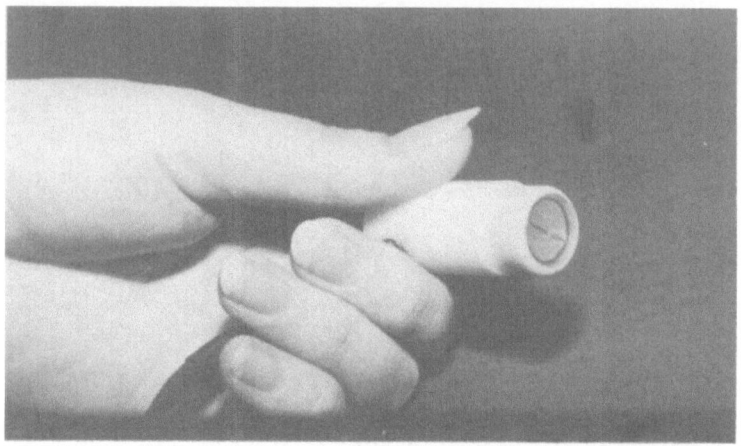

Figure 5a. The Doppler lens focusing probe. The 5 MHz crystal disc is divided into transmitting and receiving halves.

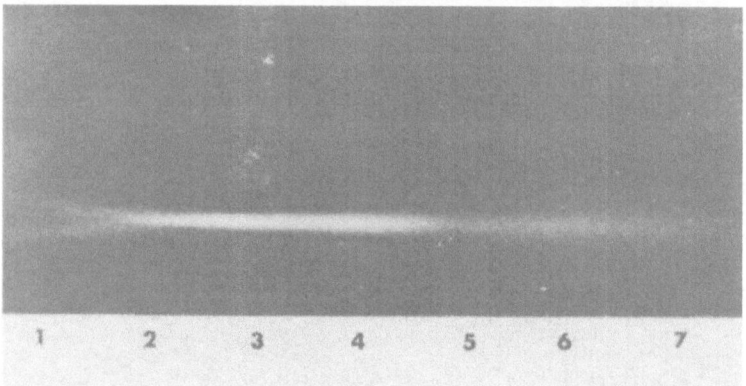

Figure 5b. Schilieren visualization of the ultrasound beam. The numerals represent centimeters from the crystal face.

2.1. Carotid artery stenosis

The Doppler imaging technique excels in localizing and quantitating carotid artery stenosis at the bifurcation and in establishing the hemodynamic significance. Characteristic audio signals are detected in and around the stenotic

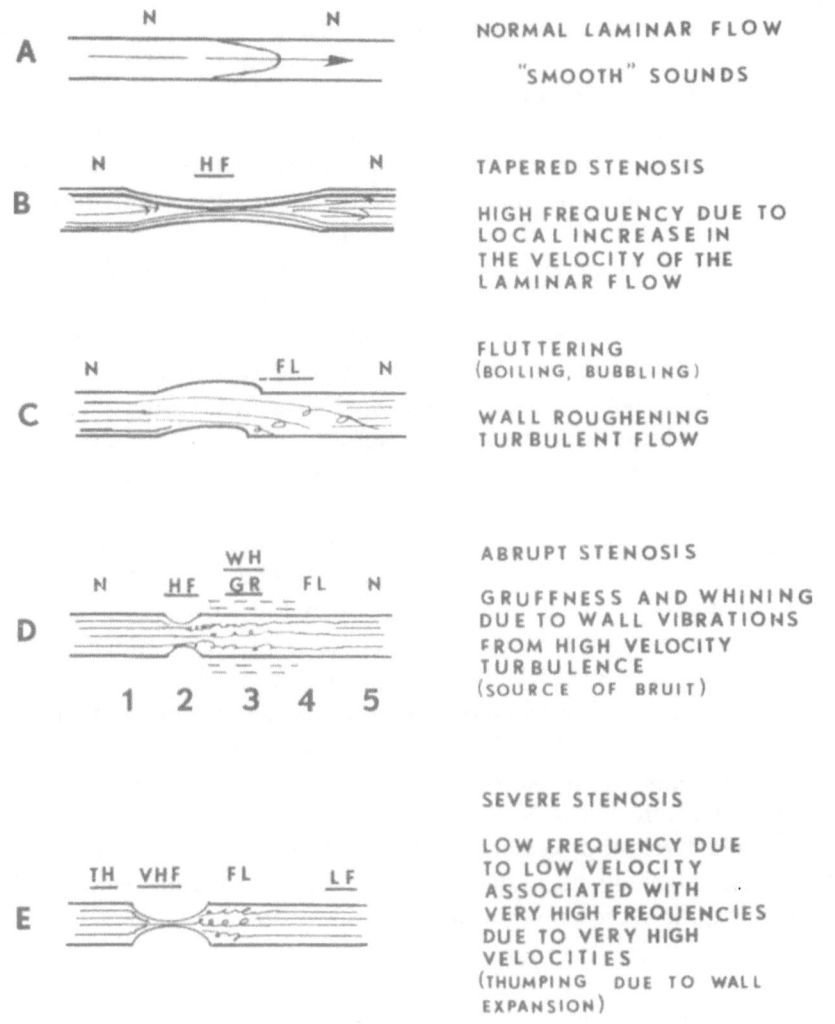

Figure 6. Local Doppler audio qualities in carotid artery stenosis.

segment. For descriptive purposes, five zones of signals may be identified (Figure 6, item D).

ZONE 1 — immediately upstream or proximal to the stenosis
ZONE 2 — within the stenosis itself
ZONE 3 — immediately downstream within 1-2 cm of the stenosis
ZONE 4 — further downstream 2-3 cm
ZONE 5 — far downstream beyond 4 cm

The most consistent diagnostic signal is an increase in Doppler audio frequency within the stenosis, Zone 2. This is caused by increased blood velocities within the stenosis. As the high velocity jet of segmental stenosis emerges into the downstream wider channel of Zone 3, a low frequency gruff or a moaning 'sea gull' quality is usually produced. A fluttering quality is often heard in Zone 4. The presence of high frequency combined with a gruff or fluttering quality is diagnostic of stenosis. The increase in frequency in Zone 2 is proportional to the increase in velocity within the stenosis. The degree of stenosis may be more accurately quantitated by comparing the frequencies in Zone 2 with those of Zone 4, 5, or Zone 1. If a severe (less than 1 mm diameter) stenosis is located beyond the origin of the internal carotid, a systolic thumping, produced by a water-hammer effect is heard in Zone 1. The frequencies are very low in Zones 1 and 5. The fluttering quality of Zone 4 is believed to represent lower velocity turbulence further down-stream and before laminar flow is regained. The gruff quality in Zone 3 sounds like the bruit heard with the stethoscope. It is produced by post stenotic wall vibrations driven by high velocity turbulence in the flow stream.

All diagnostic qualities of the Doppler image signal are not represented in a black and white (bistable) image presentation. The selected audio signals should be analyzed by ear or spectral analysis. A full color presentation of the physiologically important aspects of the signal is under development in our laboratories and may replace the necessity of listening to all the signals. In the meantime, a hand-coloring technique is useful to better represent the impor-tant diagnostic characteristics. In addition to the frequency qualities men-tioned above, important pulsatile wave patterns and directionality should be represented in future displays.

Figure 7 illustrates the bistable images produced in a patient with internal carotid stenosis beyond its origin from the common carotid along with the x-ray angiographic representation of the same region.

2.2. Non-stenosing plaques

The ability to diagnose calcified plaques was recognized during our first clinical use of the imaging technique by segments of weak or absent signals (Figure 8). Since then, experience has identified additional signals which represent non-stenosing plaques. The additional signals include segments with inverted and biphasic analogue tracings, as well as coarse, low frequency and systolic audio signals as well as fluttering signals not associated with frequen-cy increases. Non-sounding gaps in the Doppler image also occurred. The segments non-sounding or displaying inverted signals have been proven by surgery and pathological examination to be produced by densely calcified plaques. The mechanism of producing inversion in the analogue signal output is not known but believed to be produced by bending of the sound beam at

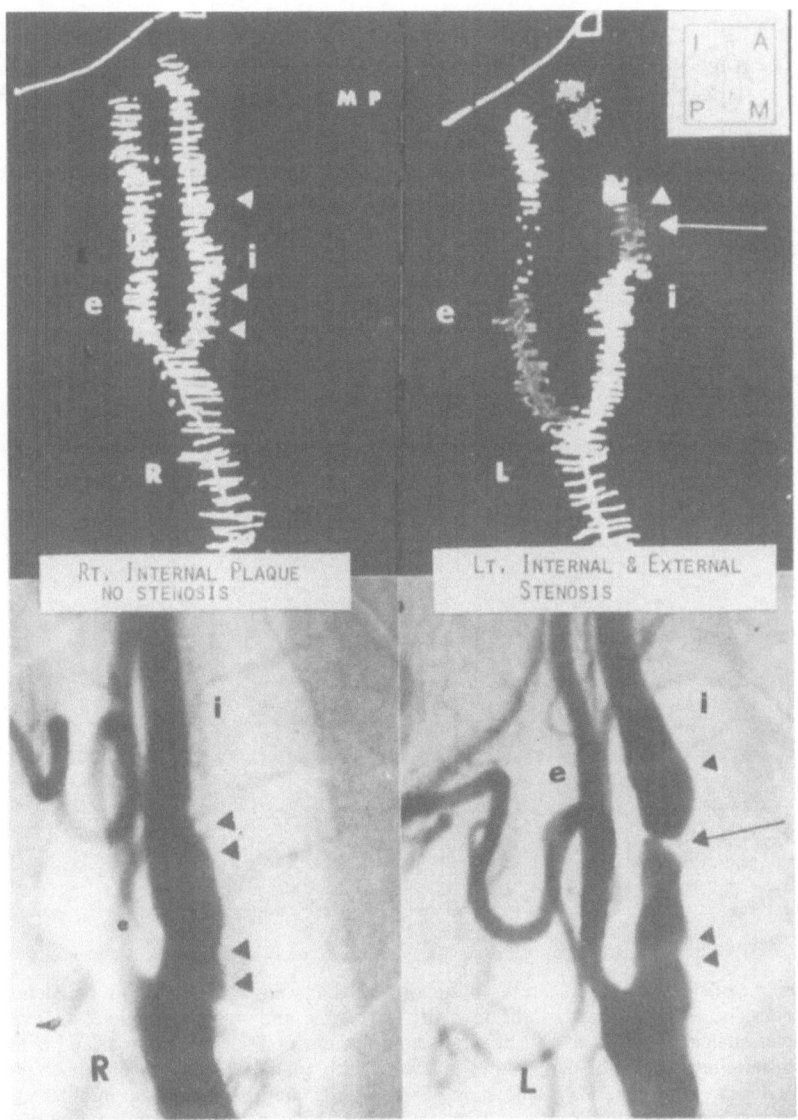

Figure 7. Internal carotid stenosis 3 cm above its origin. The arrows represent high frequencies occurring at the site of stenosis, and the gray scale represents a blue color coding for high frequency on the original image. In the left panel of the x-ray angiogram of this patient's bifurcation, the arrow indicates the stenotic segment. Zones 1, 2, 3, and 4 referred to in this text are well represented.

the edge of a calcium deposit. Xeroradiogram studies have proven useful in demonstrating calcium deposits in atherosclerotic plaques and have confirmed the Doppler diagnosis of non-stenosing plaques.

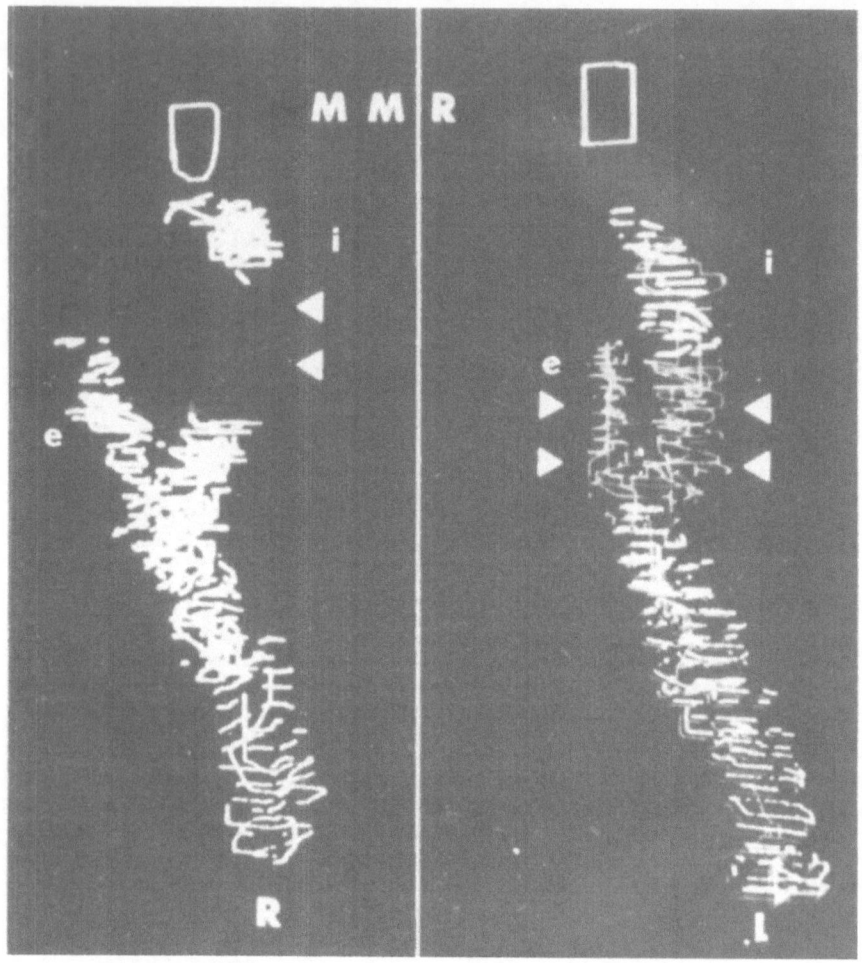

Figure 8. Bilateral Doppler carotid bifurcation imaging in a patient with nonstenosing plaques. The left-hand panel indicates, with gray scale and triangles, regions of inverted Doppler analogue signals at the bifurcation and origin of both the internal and external carotid arteries. The right-hand panel indicates, with triangles, a region of non-sounding segment representing dense calcification of the arterial channel. The distal internal signals of the internal carotid indicated no high frequency or downstream fluttering. Ophthalmic flow signals were normal, and no bruits were detected. The square figures above each image represent the position of the mandible angle.

2.3. Ophthalmic artery signals

Doppler examination of the periorbital and posterior orbital arteries is an important adjunct to bifurcation imaging to evaluate collateral carotid circulation. Use of the Doppler signals from the subcutaneous periorbital arteries was first developed by Brockenbrough. The periorbital arteries are examined with a shallow focusing Doppler probe. Circulation is considered normal if there is augmentation of the periorbital signals upon compression of the homolateral temporal or mandibular artery. It is considered negative if no compression response occurs and positive if temporal compression obliterates or reverses the direction of flow. A positive response indicates severe internal carotid obstruction. Our experience indicates the tests for collateral circulation are highly useful in a positive sense but cannot be relied upon if negative or normal.

The use of Doppler ophthalmic artery signals detected in the posterior orbit, behind the eyeball, was first reported by Spencer et al. and is considered to have some advantage over the periorbital signals because the retrobulbar signals represent arterial channels closer to the internal carotid and more consistently reflect the pressure dynamics between the Circle of Willis and external carotid branches. Posterior orbital signals are detected by placing the deep focusing lens probe over the closed eyelid and directing the ultrasonic beam through the globe (Figure 9). Normal audio signals are in the frequency range of 0.5-1.5 KHz, and the direction of flow is anterior from the Circle towards the probe producing a downward deflection in the analogue tracings. Interpretation of the posterior orbital signals is based on their direction, audio frequency, acceleration and amplitude.

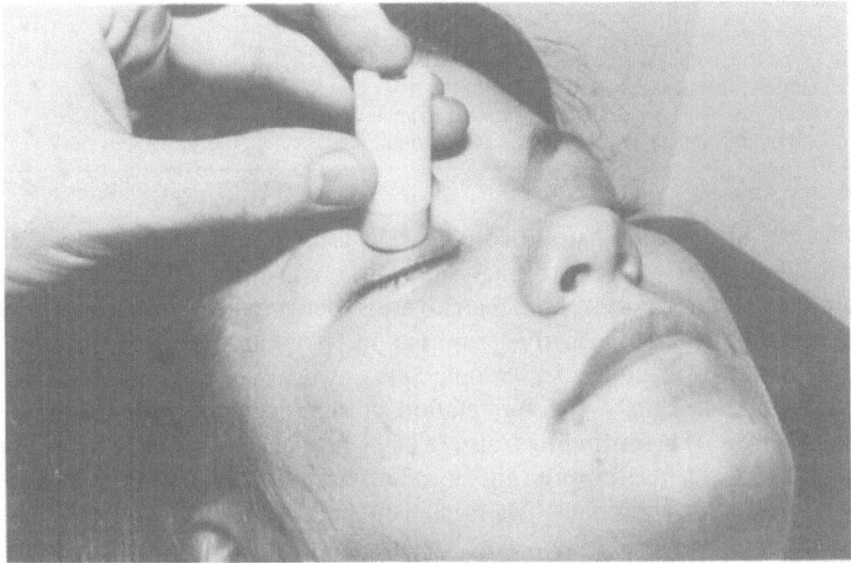

Figure 9. Position of the lens focusing probe over the closed eyelid for detection of the ophthalmic flow signals in the posterior orbit. The sound beam is directed through the lid and globe at an angle of 10° with the midline plane and rotated slowly until the strongest signal is found.

Of great importance is the finding of a reversal of direction of the ophthalmic artery flow (upward deflection in the tracing) and establishes that this pressure gradient is reversed from normal. An interpretation of lowered pressure in the Circle-of-Willis is made and that collateral circulation across the anterior communicating or from the posterior communicating arteries is insufficient. If the posterior orbital signal is of lower frequency than normal with low amplitude and damped characteristics, the same interpretation, as with reversal, may be made even if indicating flow is in the normal direction. Occasionally both normal and reversed directions are found. If the normally directed signal is of normal amplitude and frequency, the reversed signal is probably caused by a loop in an intraorbital artery and is not considered abnormal.

The correlation of ophthalmic Doppler flow characteristics with significant internal carotid stenosis, as judged from x-ray angiography, is shown in Table 2. The results indicate a high degree of correlation when posterior orbital signals are reversed or with abnormalities of low velocity, bidirectional and weak signals, but also show that completely normal ophthalmic flow signals do occur in the presence of severe stenosis or occlusion of the internal carotid.

Table 2. The correlation of ophthalmic Doppler signal direction with significant stenosis in the internal carotid.

89 patients with >50% stenosis from x-ray angiograms	
A. Ophthalmic signal reversed	25%
B. Ophthalmic signal bidirectional or weak with low velocity	37%
C. Ophthalmic signal normal direction and amplitude	38%

The use of common carotid compression is helpful in clarifying whether a normally-directed posterior orbital signal is arising from the homolateral or the contralateral carotid. The maneuver is performed if abnormal Doppler imaging is associated with the examination. If compression of the common carotid artery opposite the lesion obliterates, decreases or reverses the normal posterior orbital signal, an interpretation of significant stenosis by the lesion can be made. These findings also establish that considerable collateral is available to the Circle through the anterior communicating artery. If homolateral compression obliterates a normally directed signal, an interpretation can be made that no hemodynamically significant stenosis exists in the homolateral common internal channel.

2.4. X-ray angiographic comparisons

The advantages of x-ray angiography over Doppler ultrasound is its superior morphology and the intracranial information which it provides. The advantages of Doppler over x-ray angiography are that it is safe and painless, is less costly and requires a shorter examination time and provides superior functional information. In one sense its morphology may actually be superior to x-ray. This is because the c-w Doppler signal represents the blood velocities within the entire cross section of stenotic arteries unlike x-ray which is limited to a few projected diameters, at best not accurate through ±0.5 mm since plaques are usually asymmetrical Doppler accuracy in skilled hands probably exceeds x-ray angiography.

Table 3 represents the results of comparisons of the complete Doppler cerebrovascular evaluation with bilateral x-ray angiography in 148 bifurcations examined during 1975 at the Providence Medical Center in Seattle, Washington. The 74 patients represent all those studied by both Doppler and x-ray techniques. A 98% overall agreement was found for lumen stenosis greater than 50%. False-negatives exceeded false-positives. The false-positives consisted of patients in which the internal carotid failed to image but was, in fact, patent by x-ray examination. False-negatives generally consisted of Doppler stenosis indicated as less than 50% whereas by x-ray they were more severe.

Table 3. Doppler imaging of carotid bifurcation vs. x-ray angiography (74 patients undergoing both procedures).

Vessel	No. arteries x-rayed	False neg.	False pos.	% correct diagnosis
Internal	148	5	1	96
External	148	3	1	97
Common	148	1	0	99
All Vessels	444	9	2	98

Davis and Gingery * more recently published results of their comparisons between the complete Doppler cerebrovascular evaluation and x-ray angiography. Table 4 represents their findings over a 16 month period. They evaluated results from different subroutines. They found imaging alone to be the most accurate of the subroutines.

It is not apparent from our experience that special recordings or analysis of the carotid bruits adds significantly to the diagnostic accuracy over auscultation alone.

---

* Robert C. Davis, M.D. and Robert O. Gingery, M.D., Vascular Surgeons, Vascular Laboratory, 2940 Webster Street, Oakland, CA 94609.

Table 4. Non-invasive CVE vs. X-ray angios. Experience of Davis and Gingery (1977-78): 16 months, 133 patients, 257 carotids.

Test	% Stenosis	Sensitivity	Specificity	Accuracy
Ophthalmic	≥ 70	26	80	66
Phonoangio	≥ 50	59	82	74
Periorbitals	≥ 70	49	90	83
Imaging	≥ 50	90	84	86
Combination	≥ 60	94	94	94

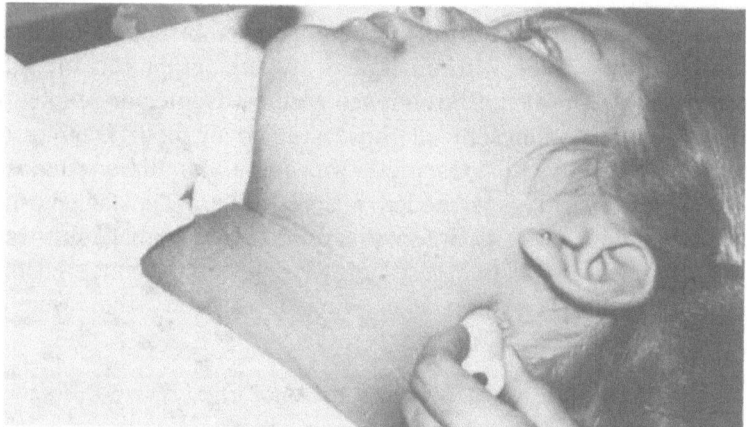

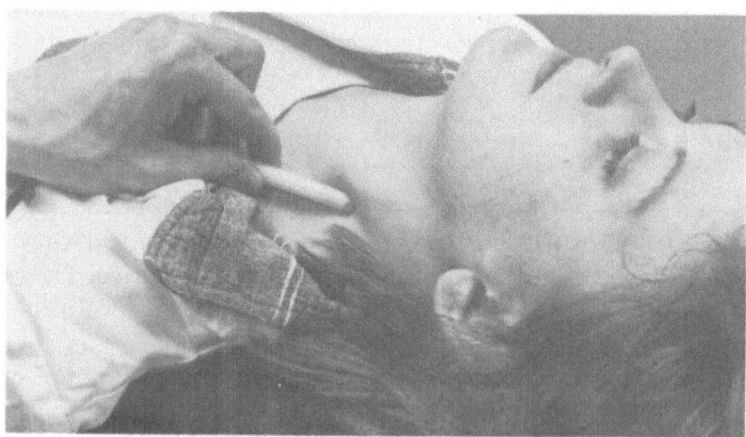

Figure 10a. (Upper Panel) Proper probe placement for detecting the posterior vertebral at the base of the skull. *Figure 10b.* (Lower Panel) The position of the Doppler probe for examining the anterior vertebral in the supraclavicular region.

2.5. Vertebral artery signals

Vertebral artery signals at the base of the skull are detected transcutaneously by placing the Doppler probe behind the mastoid bone and directing the sound beam lateral and slightly anterior toward the vertebral artery as it loops before entering the foramen magnum (Figure 10a). The normal vertebral sounds at the base of the skull represent a high diastolic flow pattern and low pulsatility similar to the internal carotid. The vertebral artery signals lower in the neck can be detected just above the medial end of the clavicle as it enters the ostium of the sixth lateral process (Figure 10b). At this point, pulsatility varies considerably from subject to subject and may be highly pulsatile with no diastolic runoff or may have a low pulsatility with high diastolic flow. The direction of flow in the posterior position is unreliable because of looping of the vertebral at this position.

2.6. Down imaging technique

The vertebral artery can also be delineated at the time of carotid bifurcation imaging searching posterior to the carotids. Segments of the vertebral in the

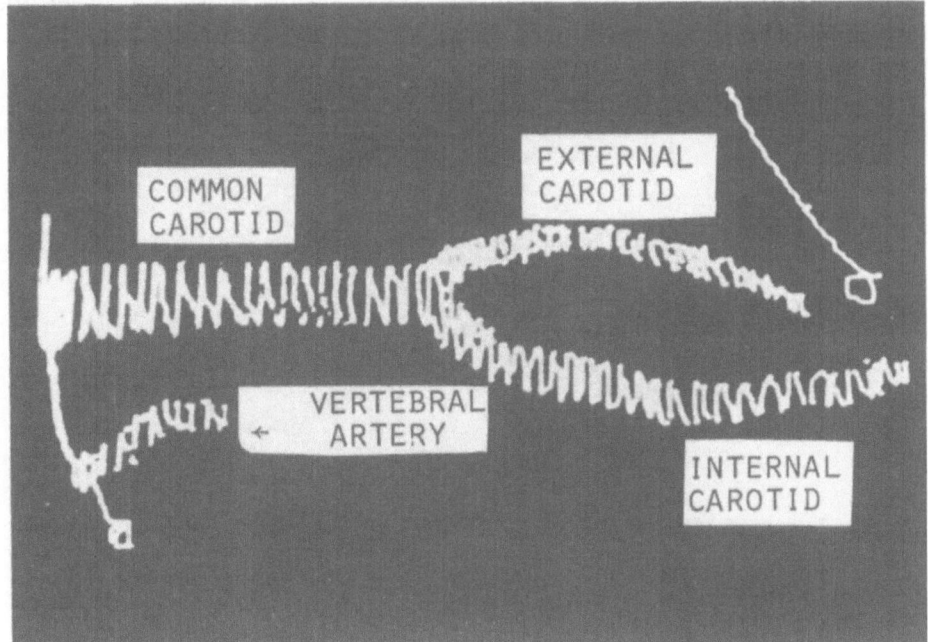

Figure 11. By reversing the Doppler probe disection and the imaging polarity switch, the proximal segments of the common carotid and vertebral can also be imaged.

mid-neck can sometimes be found as they pass between the lateral vertebral processes. It can also be imaged along with the lower common carotid behind the clavicle if the probe direction is rotated on the machine arm to direct the sound beam inferior instead of the standard superior direction. By reversing the polarity switch, the common carotid can be traced downward until the probe reaches the clavicle. By moving the probe 2–3 cm in a posterior direction, the sound beam will intersect the lower vertebral artery and an image of it can be made while recording Doppler audio qualities. This process is referred to as 'down imaging' (Figure 11).

Vertebral artery stenosis frequently occurs near its origin from the subclavian artery. This diagnosis can be made based on high frequency Doppler signals and other secondary characteristics found downstream to carotid stenosis.

2.7. Vertebral-to-subclavian steal test

In the presence of vertebral-to-subclavian steal, 'down imaging' indicates a reversal in flow. The diagnosis can be confirmed by means of a reactive hyperemia response in the homolateral arm. It is performed in patients with more than 10 mm of Hg pressure differences in systolic pressure between the two arms. The test consists of inflating a blood pressure cuff on the upper arm on the side of decreased pressure and holding the cuff pressure above systolic level for 3–5 minutes (Figure 12). At the end of the 3–5 minute

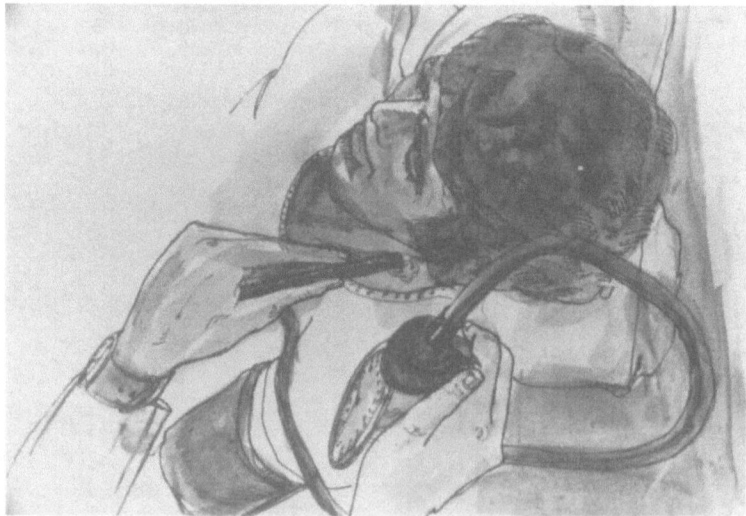

Figure 12. The subclavian-vertebral steal test as described in the text. The blood pressure cuff is on the arm and the Doppler probe is on the position indicated by Figure 10A, or 10B.

interval, the patient is asked to exercise his arm by opening and closing his hand. This maneuver further lowers the pressure in the arm. If a steal is present, the frequency of the vertebral Doppler signal will reverse or increase following release of the cuff. Reactive hyperemia may also be used to determine how symptomatic the steal is because cerebrovascular insufficiency symptoms such as vertigo may develop when they sit-up immediately following release of the cuff. This test may be performed with a non-directional Doppler instrument; however, the use of a directional Doppler allows a more subtle diagnosis of latent steal when the vertebral artery signal during control is in the normal direction and is reversed by hyperemia in the arm. Figure 13 represents typical analogue signals produced upon release of the cuff pressure in a patient with vertebral-subclavian artery steal.

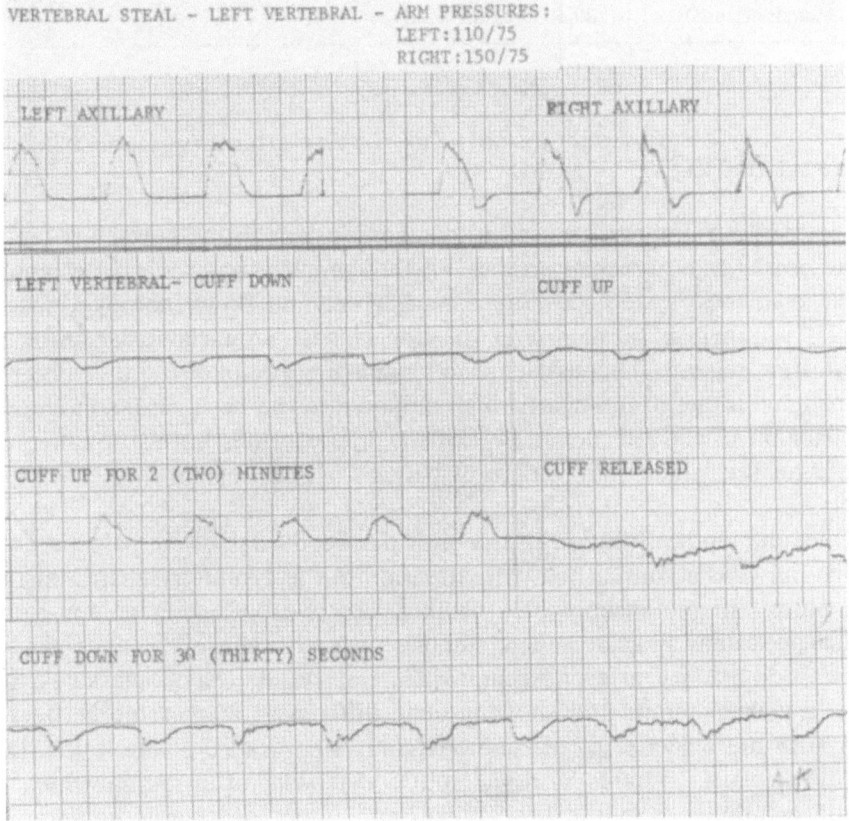

Figure 13. Doppler analogue signals in a patient with vertebral-to-subclavian artery steal. The upper left panel indicates abnormal absence of backflow signals in the left axillary artery, and the upper right panel indicates normal right axillary artery flow showing early diastolic backflow. The 3 lower panels represent the sequence of analogue signals during the reactive hyperemia test. The inflation of the cuff changes the direction from reverse to headward and release of the cuff returns the signal to the abnormal reverse direction at a higher velocity.

Table 5 lists the findings in 23 consecutive patients in whom the diagnosis of subclavian-vertebral steal has been made by use of the reactive hyperemia technique. Our experience indicates that the condition is more prevalent than originally thought but it usually does not produce symptoms of cerebrovascular insufficiency.

Table 5. 23 vertebral-to-subclavian steals as diagnosed by either x-ray angiography or the Doppler survey.

A.	Symptomatic	7 or 32%
B.	Asymptomatic	16 or 68%
C.	Left Vertebral Steals	15 or 65%
D.	Right Vertebral Steals	5 or 22%
E.	Kinking	1 or 4%
F.	Neg. Reactive Hyperemia Test with 22 mm of Hg	2 or 9%
G.	Symptoms produced by Blood Pressure Cuff	1 or 4%

3. EVALUATION OF DOPPLER SIGNALS OF THE SUBCLAVIAN AND INNOMINATE ARTERIES

Doppler ultrasound can be used to diagnose lesions in the subclavian, innominate, axillary and brachial arteries. In the complete non-invasive cerebrovascular evaluation system developed by Spencer and Brockenbrough, auscultation is routinely performed over the upper chest, supraclavicular and carotid bifurcation regions. This assists in distinguishing bruits of the brachiocephalic trunks and bruits in the heart which radiate into the neck. Bruits produced by obstruction of the subclavian or axillary arteries often have a low-frequency harsh quality which may radiate widely across the upper chest and up the neck.

Once the loudest location of the bruit has been established, palpation of the radial pulses is accomplished with attention to the symmetry characteristics of the pulses. In the absence of a bruit, a very weak, lagging or non-palpable radial pulse may indicate severe stenosis or total occlusion of the subclavian, axillary or brachial artery. Accurate bilateral systolic blood pressures, taken with a Doppler probe and showing large differences of pressure between the two arms are evidence of the hemodynamic significance of the lesion. Doppler flow signals provide a more subtle diagnosis of plaquing which may produce turbulence in the flow stream and is not necessarily compromising blood flow to the arm. In order to recognize abnormalities which may be present in a Doppler audio signal, it is necessary to understand what constitutes a normal Doppler signal in the subclavian artery (Figure 14).

With the 5 MHz probe in hand, the subclavian arterial signal is located by 'flashlighting' the probe just above the medial end of the clavicle. A normal

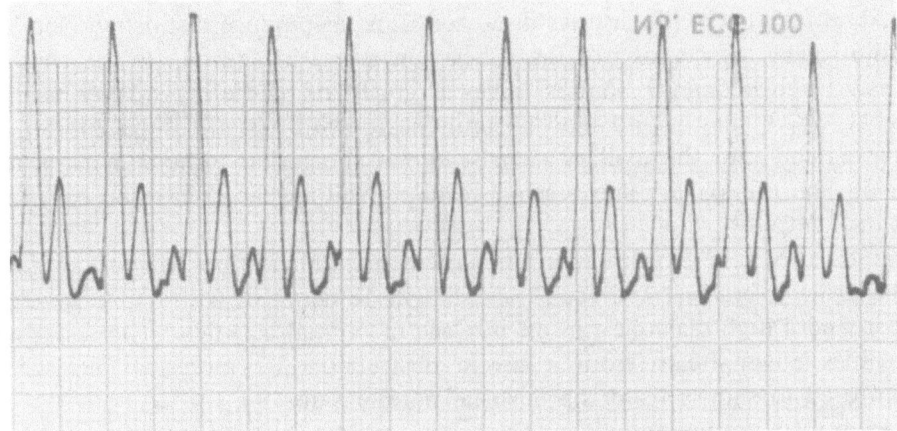

Figure 14. Analogue trace from normal subclavian artery illustrating velocity changes with characteristic backflow component generally associated with signals from resting extremities.

subclavian arterial signal with no significant disease will produce a crisp signal with sharp acceleration and a noticeable backflow component.

In young people with relatively elastic arteries, the signal may in fact have two or three backflow components, which gives a 'bouncing' quality to the analogue readout.

The axillary signal can be found by using the same technique used for the subclavian, that is, searching for the notch formed by the clavicle just medial to the head of the humerus. This signal should be similar in quality to that of the subclavian. The brachial artery signal is more useful in determining the hemodynamic significance of subclavian lesions. As with the subclavian and axillary arteries, the high peripheral resistance downstream to this vessel produces a signal with sharp acceleration and a backflow component which is audible as well as visible on the analogue tracing (Figure 15).

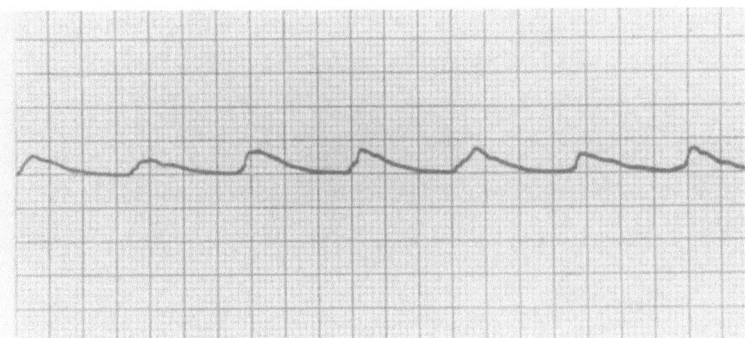

Figure 15. Abnormal velocity signals in the brachial artery. Progressively increasing obstructive stenosis eliminates the backflow phase, and increases diastolic runoff.

Abnormalities in the arteries discussed thus far produce distinctive Doppler audio signals. A stenosis of the subclavian artery in addition to the characteristic high-frequency sounds, gives a gruff and fluttering quality to the signal, which may sound like the bruit heard with a stethoscope. Fluttering may extend into the axillary signals, and if the lesion is hemodynamically significant, the axillary and brachial readouts will appear to have no backflow component.

In cases of severe obstruction, the downstream blood flow will be modified. The axillary, brachial and radial signals will be damped, with slower acceleration and a high diastolic run off in place of normal backflow. The abnormal qualities down-stream from a severe obstruction are more obvious when compared to signals from the opposite normal side.

Hemodynamically significant obstruction of the innominate artery reduces blood flow and Doppler velocity-frequencies in the right subclavian, vertebral, and carotid arteries. Vertebral flow may be reversed on the side of obstruction.

2. SOUND AND ULTRASOUND

JOHN M. REID, PH.D.

This unit is intended to introduce you to ultrasonic waves and to give you a background on how these waves travel in biological tissues so that you can better apply Doppler diagnostic instruments to clinical problems.

1. BASIC PROPERTIES

Ultrasonic waves are mechanical vibratory waves which basically are no different from audible sound waves. The only difference between ultrasound and sound is in the frequency of the vibrations. Middle-C on the piano is a note caused by the vibrations of the piano string 262 times per second. This frequency of vibration is usually just called the frequency and the unit is the Hertz, or cycles per second. As you know, each octave on the piano represents a doubling in frequency and higher frequencies have a higher pitch. A frequency of 25,000 Hertz (25 KHz), approximately 100 times higher in frequency than middle-C, is the highest frequency which the human ear can hear. Sound waves having frequencies higher than this are called ultrasound. If we go to frequencies which are 100 times higher in frequency than this upper limit of human hearing, we reach 2.5 million Hertz, (MHz), the most commonly used frequency in medical diagnosis.

The principal result of this high frequency is that the sound waves have a short wavelength and travel with properties which we usually associate with light waves rather than with sound. That is, ultrasonic waves can be formed into narrow beams instead of spreading out in all directions. Since they are coherent waves, they can exhibit some of the properties of laser-generated light waves such as showing pronounced interference effects. They can also be used to form and to reconstruct holograms.

The wavelength is a particular dimension of the wave which helps to define many of its properties. Figure 1 shows a vibrating surface at the left in contact with a region of space which is represented by the rows of dots. These dots can be thought of as being the molecules in the region of space. As the source vibrates, it moves back and forth from left to right, pushing against and pulling apart the molecules. Each new push moves the compressed region

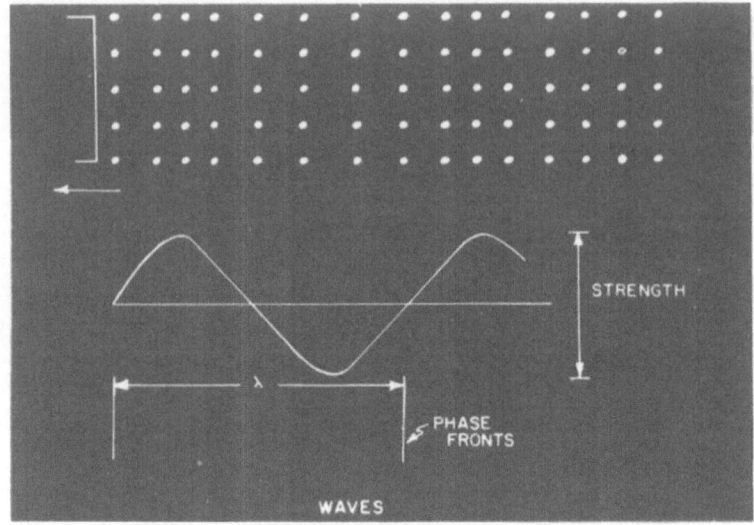

Figure 1. Definition of wavelengths. The wavelength is the physical distance between corresponding points of a repetitive wave form. At the upper left a transducer face is shown alternately compressing and spreading out the molecules of a medium. The wave is propagating from left to right.

to the right. This series of compressions is a *wave* and the distance between the compressed regions is the *wavelength*. The numerical value of the wavelength is found by dividing the velocity of the wave by its frequency. In equation form:

$$\lambda, \text{ wavelength} = \frac{\text{velocity}}{\text{frequency}}.$$

For average soft tissues in the body, we find:

$$\lambda \text{ (millimeters)} = \frac{1.5}{\text{frequency (MHz)}}.$$

When sound is formed into beams, we find that the minimum size of the beam is about one wavelength. A wavelength is, thus, an important parameter in setting the resolution of any diagnostic system using sound waves. To form such beams, it is necessary to use sources of sound which are large with respect to the wavelength. The probes which are applied to the skin are, therefore, usually 1 cm or greater in size.

2. INTERACTIONS OF SOUND WAVES AND TISSUES

Ultrasonic waves travel in nearly straight lines in most soft tissues of the body. They are absorbed or gradually weakened by the tissues and can be reflected or scattered back to the surface of the body. The average soft tissue of the body is a tissue of very high water content. Sound travels at the velocity characteristic of a saline solution containing proteins in these tissues. When sound waves encounter tissues which are not liquid-like, most of the energy is reflected. Such tissues are the hard mineralized tissues such as bone and teeth, in which the elastic properties are more nearly those of a solid, and tissues containing appreciable quantities of air. The principal organ which contains air in its natural state is the lung. Acoustic properties of this tissue are sufficiently different than those of average soft tissue, to cause nearly complete reflection of the sound at the surface of the lung. Air is encountered in other regions of the body as well, primarily the bronchi, trachea and folds in the bowel.

In average soft tissue sound is absorbed to a degree which is proportional to the frequency. In traveling into the body by 1 cm and back again, the power in the sound wave is reduced by 1/2 *for every MHz of frequency*. At a frequency of 5 MHz, sound waves which travel 1 cm into and 1 cm out of tissue will be reduced to 1/32 of the original power. Sound is absorbed by the same factor for each centimeter of depth. Therefore, lower frequencies are used for deep penetration.

These absorption figures are about average for muscle. They are less for fat and considerably less for blood, about 1/10 that for muscle. Absorption is caused primarily by the conversion of sound energy into heat by a process which appears to be specific for the macromolecules involved, primarily proteins.

Ultrasound waves can be bent, or refracted, by differences in velocity. The velocity in fat is about 10% lower than the velocity in other soft tissues. The bending effect can be calculated from Snell's law of optics. Because the velocities are very similar, the bending effect is small. Only if wedge-shaped pieces of fat of perhaps 1 cm maximum thickness are involved, can enough refraction result to displace a sound beam laterally by more than a few millimeters at a range of about 10 cm.

The reflection and scattering of sound is a much more pronounced and useful effect. These waves, which are sent back out to the examining probe from structures within the body, are used by a variety of medical ultrasonic diagnostic instruments. The strongest reflections arise from the greatest changes in the mechanical or elastic properties of tissue and hence are found at the boundary of soft tissue and bone or air-containing tissue such as the lung, as discussed above. Much smaller changes in elastic properties occur between and within many other organs of the body. Perhaps 1% of the incident energy can be reflected from smooth connective tissue sheets such as are found covering the kidney cortex, surrounding major muscle bundles, and in the walls of blood vessels. Smaller reflections, of the order of 1/10 to

1/100 of 1% occur between the muscle bundles in muscle and from smaller structures in kidney, liver, the fetus, uterine wall, placenta, and other organized tissues. The distribution of the echoes appears to follow from the distribution of connective tissues in these tissues.

Very small reflections can be observed, with special equipment, which arise from the red cells in blood. This special equipment has been used to measure the magnitude, angle dependence, and the dependence on frequency of these very weak ultrasonic reflections. Figure 2 shows the scattering cross-section as a function of hematocrit. When results for blood are extrapolated to low hematocrits, the value for the scattering of an individual red cell is obtained, which agrees with standard theory for scattering by compressible elastic spheres, to within better than 10%.

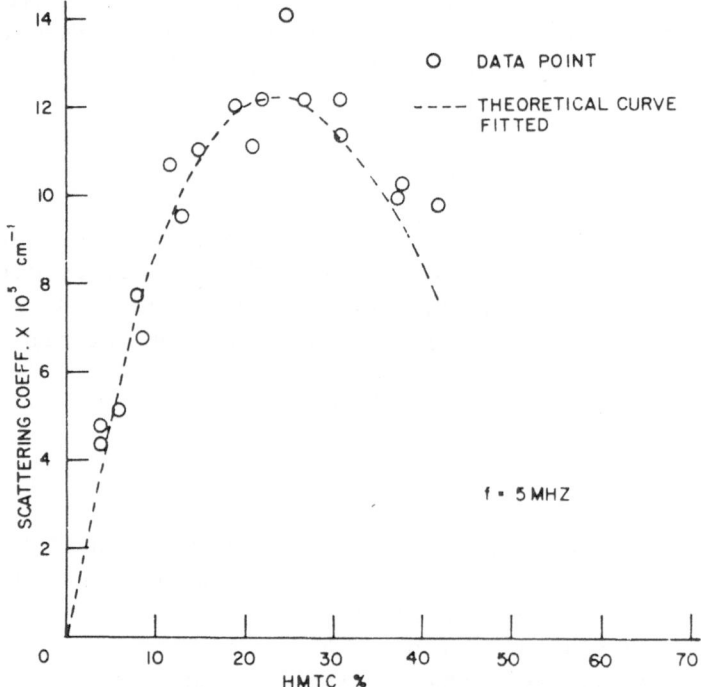

Figure 2. Measured values of back-scattering cross-section of human blood as a function of hematocrit. Data points show an increase with hematocrit up to 25% and a slight decrease thereafter.

The *Doppler effect* exists for ultrasonic waves. This effect is a change in the frequency of an ultrasonic wave when the transmitter, the receiver, or the scatterer are moving with respect to each other. Therefore, reflections from moving red cells have a different ultrasonic frequency from the transmitted frequency. This different frequency is a 'tag' by which reflections from the cells can be identified. Ultrasonic Doppler flowmeters respond only to reflections which have experienced a Doppler shift and not at all to the reflections from stationary structures which have no Doppler shift.

The amount of the Doppler shift, when the scatterer is moving with a particular velocity can be calculated from the rate of change of phase experienced by the wave as it travels from the transmitter to the scatterer and back to the receiver. The result is:

$$f_d \text{ (Doppler shift in Hertz)} = \frac{2 \begin{pmatrix} \text{velocity of} \\ \text{scatterer with} \\ \text{respect to probe} \end{pmatrix} \begin{pmatrix} \text{ultrasonic} \\ \text{frequency} \\ \text{in Hertz} \end{pmatrix}}{\text{(velocity of the ultrasound)}}$$

When the flowmeter probe makes an angle to the vessel, as shown in Figure 3, this equation can be modified. If we put in the actual value of the velocity and straighten out the units, we obtain:

$$f_d \text{ (Hertz)} = 13v \text{ (cm per sec.) } f \text{ (MHz)} \cos \theta.$$

In a practical case with an ultrasonic frequency of 5 MHz and an angle, θ, of 60°, the result is:

$$f_d = 32.5v \text{ (Hertz per cm per sec)}$$

A fortunate result of these numbers is that the Doppler shift frequency is usually within the range of human hearing. A velocity of 16 cm per second

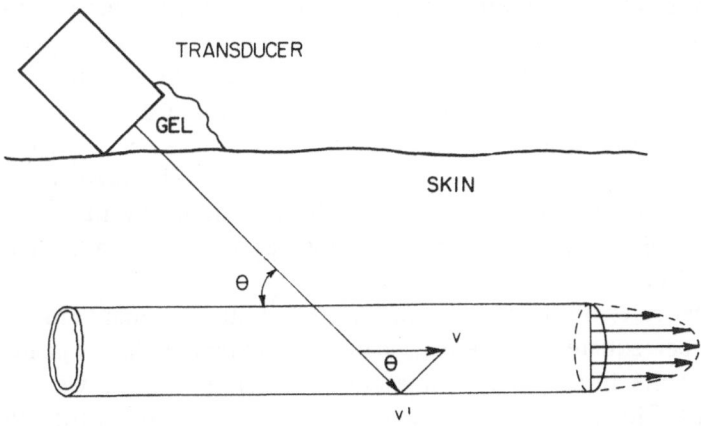

Figure 3. Sketch of transducer and soundbeam determining Doppler shift from a blood vessel.
    θ = angle between sound beam and blood vessel
    v = velocity of a red cell within the blood vessel
Arrows to the right show distribution of velocities within the vessel at an instant of time.

gives rise to a note about one octave in pitch above middle-C on the piano. Higher velocities give higher frequencies. Simply listening to the Doppler frequencies and using the discriminating abilities of the human ear and brain is a useful technique for interpreting many points in the dynamics of flow, as will be explained later. Another important point which is sometimes over-looked is that the Doppler shift is proportional to the ultrasonic frequency. The pitch from a 10 MHz flowmeter is, thus, twice that from a 5 MHz flowmeter. If the velocity is very high, due, for example, to the jet through a constricted stenosis, the resulting pitch may be too high for faithful reproduction or recording, or for some persons to hear.

3. SAFETY CONSIDERATIONS

High-power sound waves can affect tissues by several mechanisms. No observable effects have been demonstrated on intact mammalian tissues from the amounts of power used with medical diagnostic apparatus.

To discuss the damage question, we must define the units of exposure. For historical reasons, the rate of power transfer in Watts has been used. A Watt is a measurement of power and the warming or heating effect of ultrasound is proportional to the power density, expressed usually as Watts per square cm. This power density figure is termed the *intensity* of sound waves.

The intensity of most diagnostic ultrasonic equipment ranges between 10 and 100 Milliwatts per square cm. As a standard of comparison, the average power output of heat due to metabolic processes of the human body is about 10 Milliwatts per square cm. At intensity levels of 1–3 Watts per square cm, the conversion of ultrasonic energy to heat by absorption of the tissues becomes noticeable. The heat flow is greater than that due to metabolism and a distinct warming effect is noted. This effect has been used in physical medicine in ultrasonic therapy equipment. It has become very useful in athletics because the sound waves are absorbed more by muscle and tissues of high protein content than by fat, whereas for microwave diathermy the reverse is true.

At higher intensity levels, ranging from 1 Watt per square cm to thousands of Watts per square cm, damage can be obtained in liquid solutions. This damage results from the low-pressure areas in the sound wave tearing the liquid apart. This phenomenon, called 'cavitation', results in the production of small cavities in the fluid. This is a high-energy process and results in free radical formation and a variety of chemical and biological effects. Cavitation has not been demonstrated in highly viscous materials, nor at frequencies much over 5 MHz. The effect may be of some importance because the peak power of pulse ultrasonic apparatus, such as conventional pulse-echo clinical diagnostic machines and pulse-Doppler flowmeters, may reach into the 10 to 100 Watts per square cm range. Operation at high frequencies, where higher power levels are required to cause cavitation, and in bursts of extremely short time duration, one to five-millionths of a second, apparently prevents cavitation from occurring even in lower viscosity materials, such as blood.

Considerable interest in these tissue-altering effects of ultrasound has been maintained for many years. Currently investigations are under way on the use of ultrasonic heating for potentiating the effects of radiotherapy in tumors. These studies, and several studies directed specifically toward the possible hazards of diagnostic equipment, have not to this date been able to verify that any hazard exists from the use of ultrasonic diagnostic equipment at current power levels.

4. GENERATION AND DETECTION

Ultrasonic diagnostic equipment consists of transmitters to generate the ultrasonic frequency, transducers to convert the ultrasonic waves to electrical energy and vice versa, receivers to amplify the weak scattered wave, and display devices to present them to the human operator. The basic characteristics of these devices are determined by the interactions between tissues and sound waves mentioned above. The frequencies of ultrasound are very high and require electronic apparatus for generation and amplification. One MHz, for example, is a frequency found in the middle of the broadcast band when it is in the form of radio frequency energy. Higher frequencies up to 10 MHz are in the shortwave bands used by the military and a variety of land and mobile services. The basic arrangement is shown in Figure 4. The *transmitter*, thus, is an electronic oscillator producing electrical waves. These waves are converted into mechanical form by a transducer. The word *'transducer'* means to lead between, and refers to converting the energy from electrical form to acoustic form. The types of transducers commonly used in medical diagnosis are reciprocal and function equally well in converting reflected waves into electrical energy. The voltages from these reflected waves are

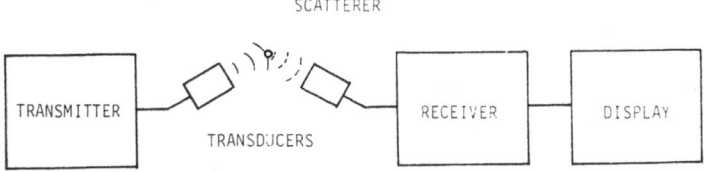

Figure 4. Block diagram of basic ultrasound system showing electronic components connected to transducer.

usually very small and require amplification to the level required to affect display apparatus. Display apparatus usually consists of cathode ray tubes similar to those used in a television set for displaying dimensions and coordinates, loudspeakers for listening to Doppler sounds, and various types of spectrum analyzers and strip chart recorders for reproducing flow waveforms and motion curves. These will all be discussed further in the next chapter.

The transducer is the most critical element in the entire Doppler flowmeter system. The choice of transducer determines the operating frequency, depth of penetration, size of the ultrasonic beam, and the frequency of the Doppler shift which is recorded from a blood vessel. In multiple crystal transducers, which are commonly used with Doppler flowmeters, separation of the transmitting and receiving elements can further localize the regions from which flow can be recorded.

The 'heart' of a transducer is a material which will change its dimensions when an electric field is applied to it or which will generate an electrical field when it is deformed by a vibration as sketched in Figure 5. This element, termed the *crystal,* is usually a single or a poly-crystalline material in which the crystal structure is aligned suitably with the field produced by electrodes applied to the surfaces of the material. Practically all medical transducers use a poly-crystalline ceramic which has the property of being electrostrictive. That is, it will change its shape in response to an electrical field. These ceramics are a poly-crystalline lead zirconate titanate.

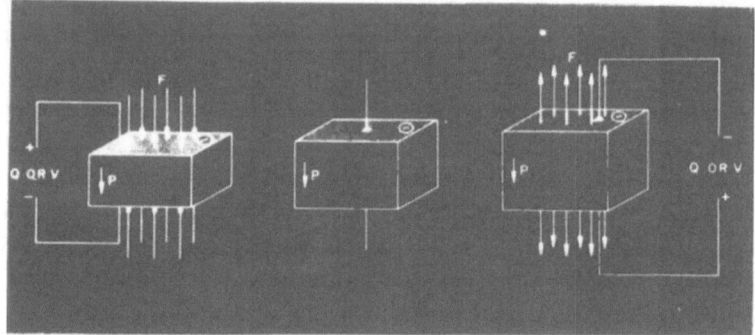

Figure 5. The center shows a biased ceramic material with electrodes on the major faces. Application of a voltage results in a change in thickness depending on the polarity. Application of pressure results in generation of a charge on the surfaces.

The components of the transducer (see Figure 6) besides the ceramic are the protective case, the lead wires connecting it to the electronic apparatus, and internal connections. Optional elements are backing materials used to provide isolation, greater strength, or to widen the bandwidth of the transducer for pulse operation; and a lens which may be used to focus the sound

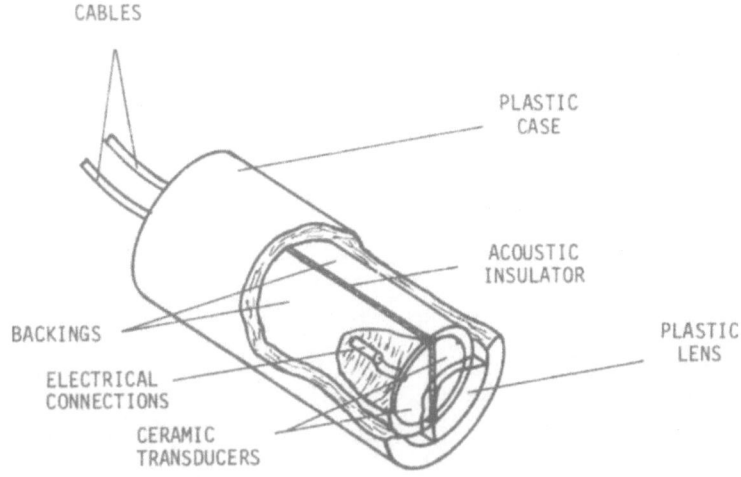

CABLES

PLASTIC
CASE

ACOUSTIC
INSULATOR

BACKINGS

PLASTIC
LENS

ELECTRICAL
CONNECTIONS

CERAMIC
TRANSDUCERS

Figure 6. Cut-away view of ultrasound transducer. Two elements are shown for Doppler operation, although only one is used for pulse-echo operation. Backing material adjusts pulse length of transducer, the lens focuses the field to produce narrow beams. (See Figures 8 and 10.)

beam. The shape of the sound field depends on the operating frequency and size of the elements.

The most sensitive frequency for operation of a transducer is the fundamental resonance frequency of the ceramic crystal element. The frequency at which the electronics operate is usually adjusted to coincide with the resonant frequency of the transducer. Although low frequencies penetrate more deeply into tissues, they also result in low Doppler shift frequencies, in longer wavelengths, and hence, wider beamwidths. Too high a frequency cannot be used, since the penetration will be too small or the Doppler frequency too high to hear. A compromise frequency is usually used. Most Doppler systems use frequencies between three and ten MHz. A chart of the frequency giving the theoretically best echo strength is shown in Figure 7. The low frequencies are preferred for penetration into the abdomen and heart and the higher frequencies for vessels in the extremities.

The outlines of the width of the field for two sizes of unfocused transducers shown in Figure 8 illustrate three major points.

1. The field consists of two different regions. The near-field, close to the transducer, is approximately cylindrical. The far-field, at greater ranges, diverges.
2. The minimum field width occurs at the range where the nearfield changes to the far-field, and this minimum width is approximately equal to the radius of the transducer. (The distance between the transducer and this

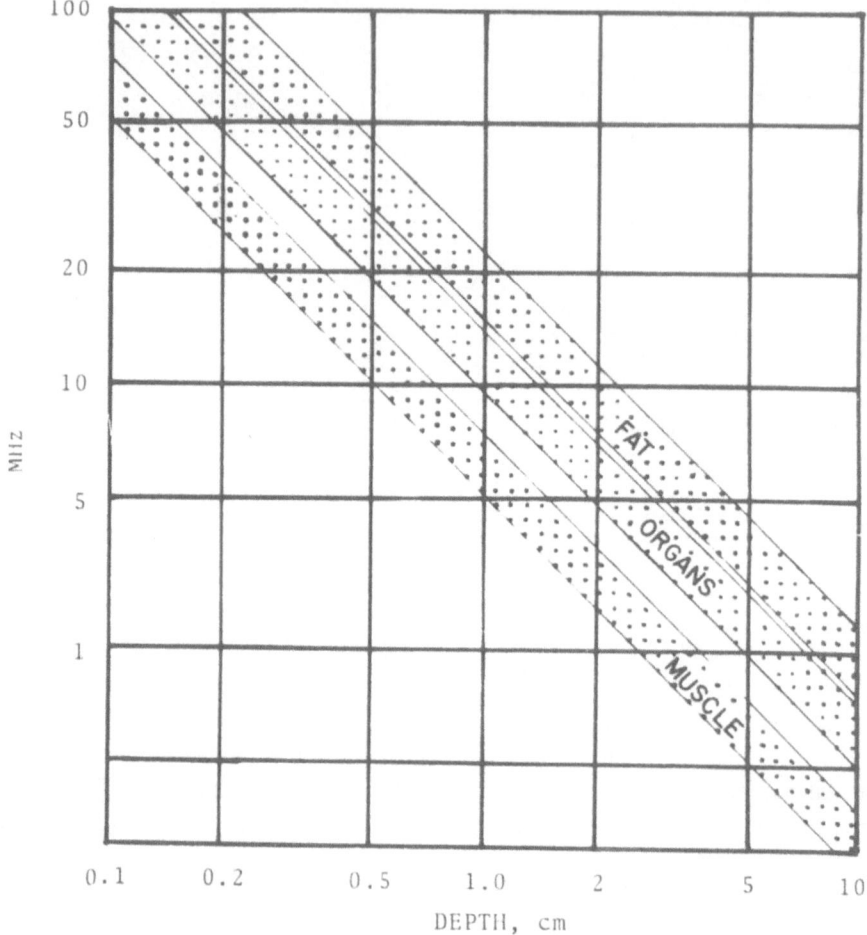

Figure 7. Chart of ultrasound frequency giving maximum echo strength from small scatterers (red cells). Theoretically determined frequency for depths of three intervening tissues, based on measured attenuation.

narrow point in the field is found by dividing the square of the radius by the wavelength, see Figure 9).

3. In the near-field, the width of the beam is *directly* proportional to the size of the transducer and in the far-field the width is *inversely* proportional to the size of the transducer.

The approximate appearance of the fields from focused transducers are shown at C and D, Figure 7. The four major points for focussed fields are:

1. The width of the field is determined by·the same divergence angle that governs the far-field region of the *unfocused* transducer.

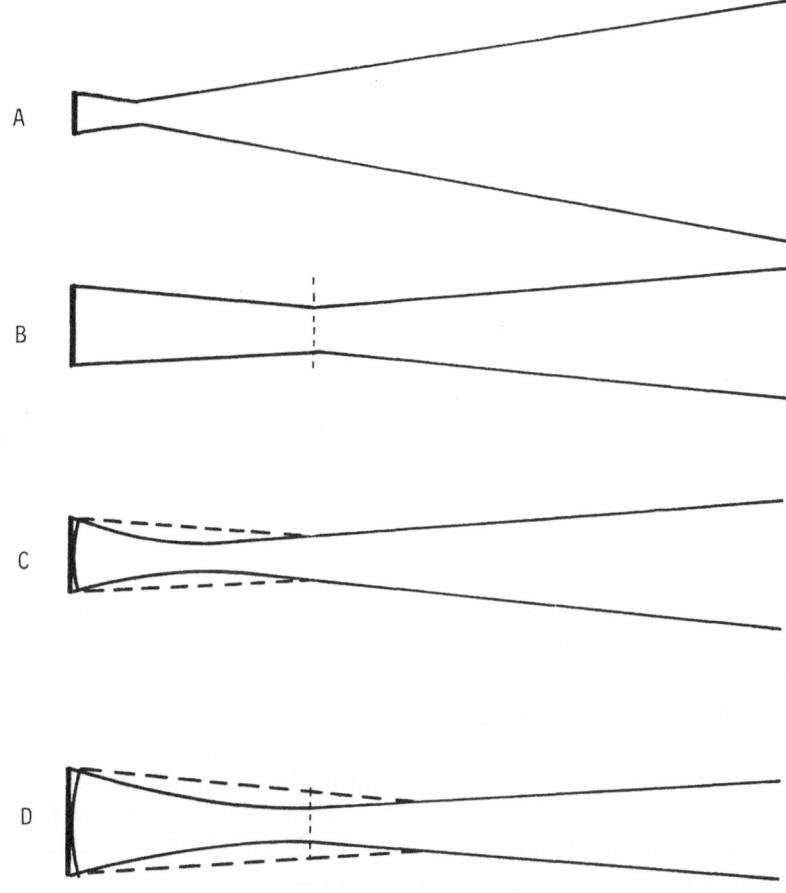

Figure 8. Outline of approximate field shape from focused and unfocused transducers.

A — small unfocused transducer.

B — larger unfocused transducer having a smaller field width at the range shown by the dotted line.

C — Effect of focusing transducer shown at 'B'. Field can be narrowed only at the near-field region.

D — Effect of increasing the size of the focused transducer at 'C'. A smaller field is obtained at the range shown by the dotted line.

2. A narrow field is produced only at distances that were previously within the wide near-field of the unfocused transducer. The far-field is not affected by focussing.

3. The width of the field at and beyond the focus is inversely proportional to the diameter of the transducer.

4. The intensity of the field drops off quite rapidly after the focal region is reached, so that the length of the focused field is limited.

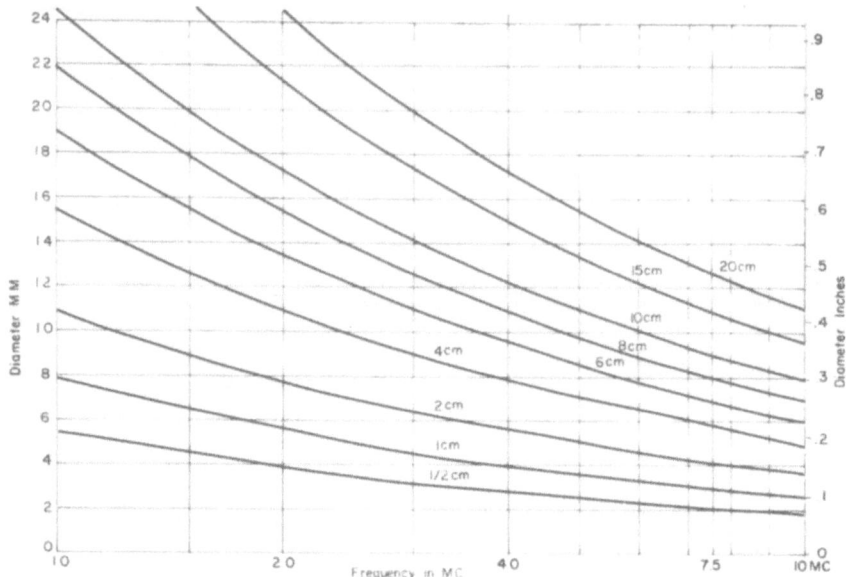

Figure 9. Chart of near-field extent as a function of transducer diameter and ultrasound frequency. Near-field extent is the parameter on the curves.

Focusing is accomplished by using plastic lenses (see Figure 6) or phased-array elements. Plastic lenses are relatively inexpensive and produce excellent results. Photographs of actual focused acoustic fields are shown in Figure 10. These were taken with a Schlieren optical system which makes the waves visible. For very strong focusing, bottom Figure 10, the field is concentrated at the focus and does not reach to long ranges.

In many Doppler transducers, the sending and receiving elements are separated. The region of space from which Doppler shifted signals can be

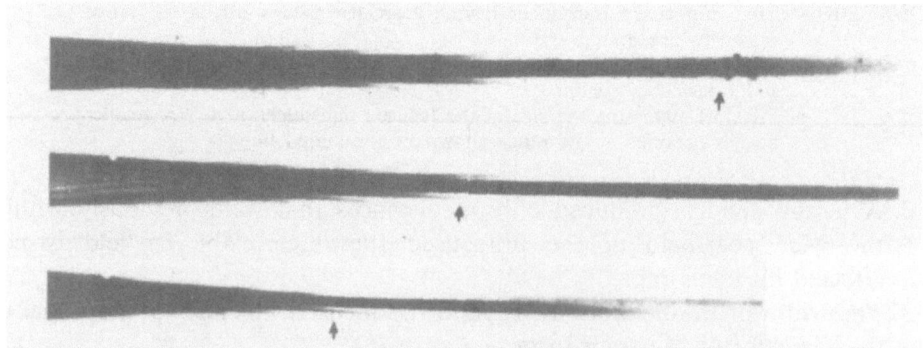

Figure 10. Schlieren photograph of actual sound field shapes for three different lenses applied to the same diameter transducer. Arrow marks focal length.

received is that region which is common to the ultrasonic field sent out by the transmitting transducer and the sensitive area of the receiving transducer. Since the receiving transducer has a sensitive area which is identical in shape to its beam pattern as a transmitter, it is possible to sketch the approximate location of the sensitive region. Such a construction is illustrated in Figure 11, which assumes that the near-field region of both elements extends across the entire sketch.

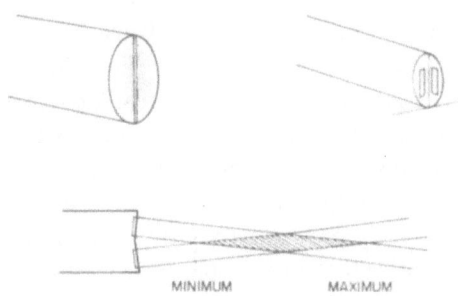

MINIMUM   MAXIMUM

Figure 11. Top cross-hatched areas show radiating faces for typical Doppler transducers. Bottom, the transmitted field and receiving sensitive areas overlap to define the region in space from which flow can be detected.

Usually the transmitter and receiver elements are placed closely together so that the sensitive region will cover as great a range in tissue as possible. In other cases, it is desirable to separate them to localize the sensitive region. An extreme example of such a transducer is the precordial probe developed by this Institute for its bubble detector. This probe is designed to be placed on the chest and receive signals scattered from blood and air emboli in the pulmonary artery only.

It is possible to use the same ceramic element for simultaneous transmission and reception in a continuous-wave system. Such a system has been developed by the Institute for use with its catheter flowmeter. These catheter flowmeter probes are about 1 mm in diameter and do not provide sufficient room for separate sending and receiving elements. This technique can be used with larger probes with the advantage that the sensitive region extends from the transducer face to a depth which is set by absorption in the tissues.

5. BASIC MEDICAL DIAGNOSTIC SYSTEMS

Different medical diagnostic systems have arisen because of the different methods used to separate the scattered or reflected waves from the transmitted wave. In the simplest system, the scattered waves may not be used at all, and a *through-transmission mode* can be used just like x-ray images. This type of system has not been successful in any clinical applications to date. The problem appears to be more one of anatomy than technology. Through-transmission paths free of lung, gas and bone are difficult to obtain except, perhaps, for the study of tendons, muscles and peripheral blood vessels in the extremities.

The first successful ultrasonic diagnostic systems used the principle of echo-ranging used in sonar and in radar. The basic echo-ranging system turns on the transmitter for only a very short time. This wave travels through the tissues sending back reflections at every change of elastic properties. These echoes are received, usually by the same transducer which is now quiescent, and amplified by the receiver. A typical oscilloscope display of the echoes is shown in Figure 12, top. The line on top represents a graph of the voltage on the horizontal scale which represents the time which has elapsed from the transmission of the pulse. This time is proportional to the distance between the transducer and the reflecting structure. Because sound waves travel at

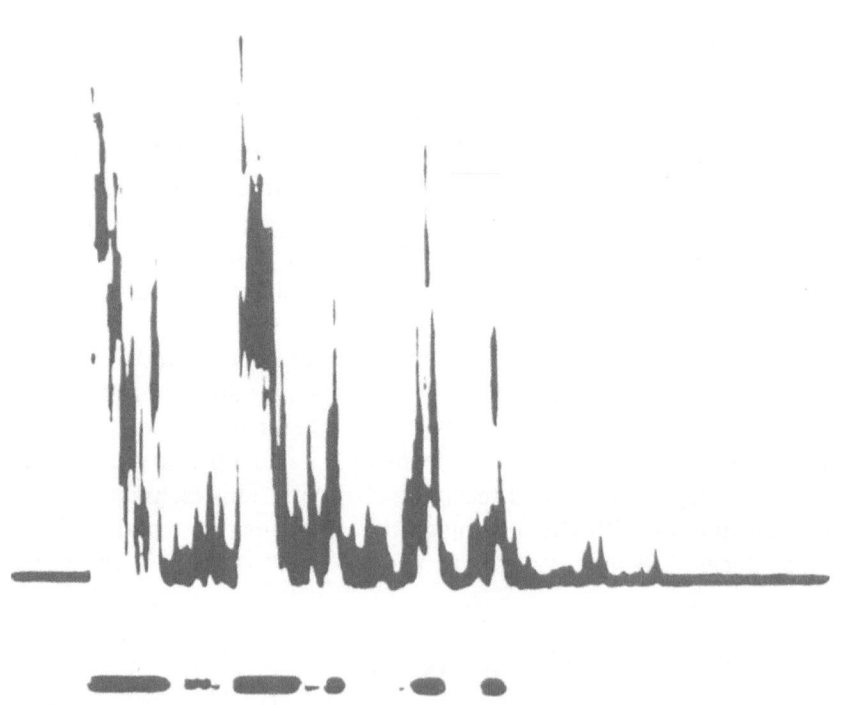

Figure 12. Top A-mode display of tissue echoes as a function of time or distance into the tissue. Bottom: Intensity modulated B-mode presentation of same echoes.

such a high speed in soft tissues (approximately one mile per second), they return in a rather short time. This is the principal reason for the use of television-type display tubes. The time which elapses between transmission of a pulse and the reception of an echo from a structure 1 cm away is 13.3 millionths of a second (microseconds). Recording pens or other mechanical objects cannot move rapidly enough to plot out this type of wave. This short time also means that the transmitting pulse cannot last for very long, or it would occupy several centimeters in space. Pulse-lengths the order of microseconds occupy distances in space in the order of millimeters. It was noted above that the resolving power of any system involving waves cannot be smaller than the wavelength. This restriction also applies to pulsed diagnostic systems. Modern diagnostic apparatus is within a factor of two of reaching the wave-length limit, in depth.

The information from a pulse-echo system is usually displayed in the form shown at the bottom of Figure 12. The voltages corresponding to the echoes of different strength are converted to spots of different brightness on the face of the display tube, just as a television picture is composed of regions of different brightness. These brightness areas are displayed in two distinctly different ways.

Pulse-echo echocardiography displays the position of the heart structures, which move. If the positions of the dots in Figure 12 were to be recorded on film moving vertically down the page, the recordings would trace out the time course of the motion of heart structures. Figure 13 shows the result for a typical echocardiographic examination. The structure which moves over the greatest distance range is the mitral valve and a curve of stenotic valve motion is shown. This type of display is called a *Time-Motion* or TM-*mode* display.

The other type of display of pulse-echo information is used in the clinical scanning equipment which is widely used in obstetrics and for the examination of the abdomen. In a scanner the transducer is moved by rotation or translation so that the sound beam sweeps through the tissues. If the line of spots of varying brightness on the face of a cathode-ray tube is moved so that it always corresponds to the sound beam in both position and direction, the spots on the face of the tube will trace out a map of the location of the reflecting structures. These ultrasonic scanning pictures are called *B-mode* scans. (Figure 14.)

Doppler flowmeters separate the scattered wave from the transmitted wave by arranging to be sensitive only to waves which have undergone a Doppler shift. For this reason, they can simultaneously transmit and receive continuously. These devices are called C-W, or *continuous-wave* flowmeters. The Doppler effect will exist for any wave scattered from moving structures and is also present on the frequencies contained in the pulse of pulse-echo systems.

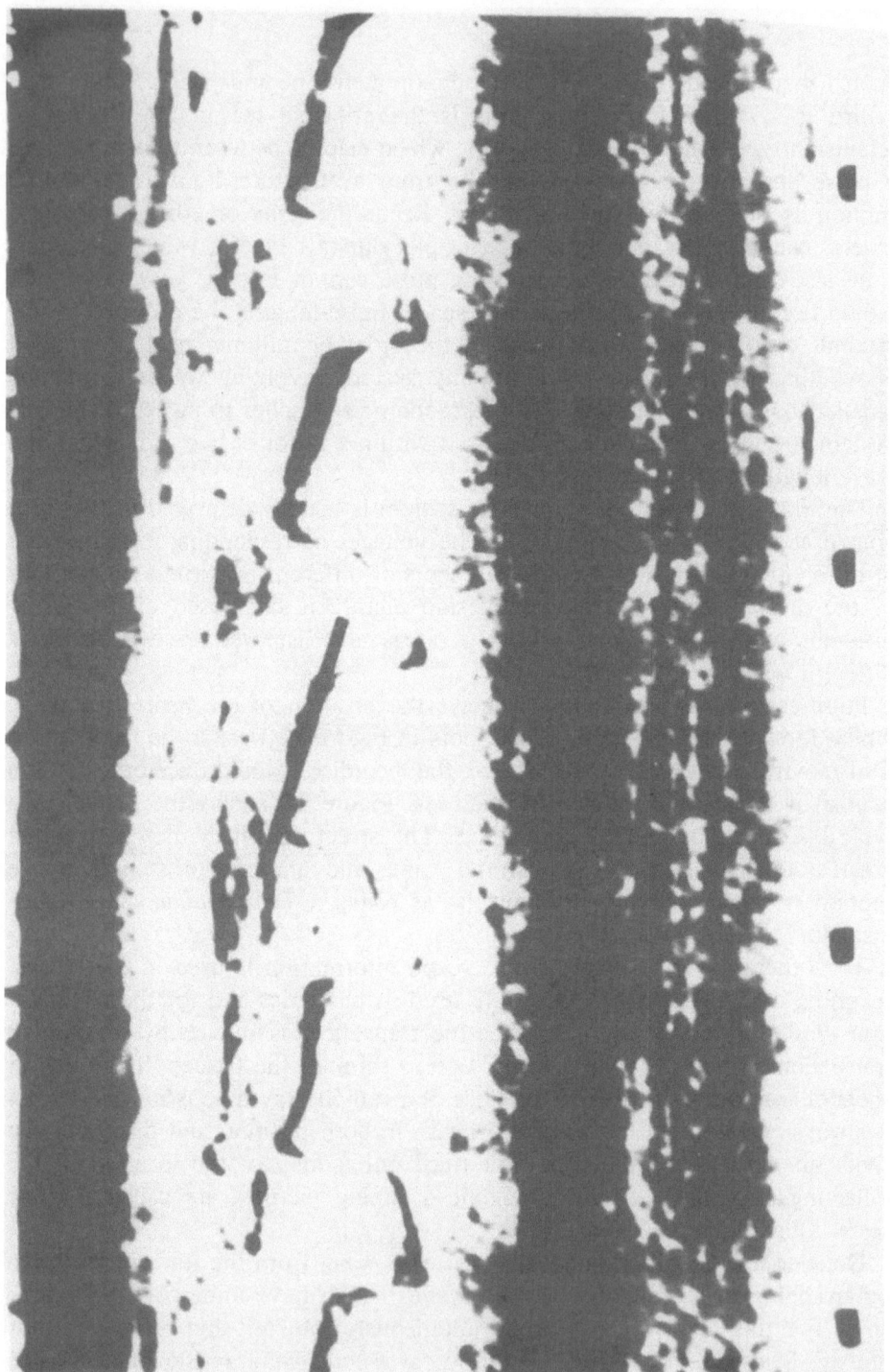

Figure 13. TM-mode recording of motion of mitral valve echoes as a function of time. Straight line marks slow posterior motion of anterior leaflet of mitral valve.

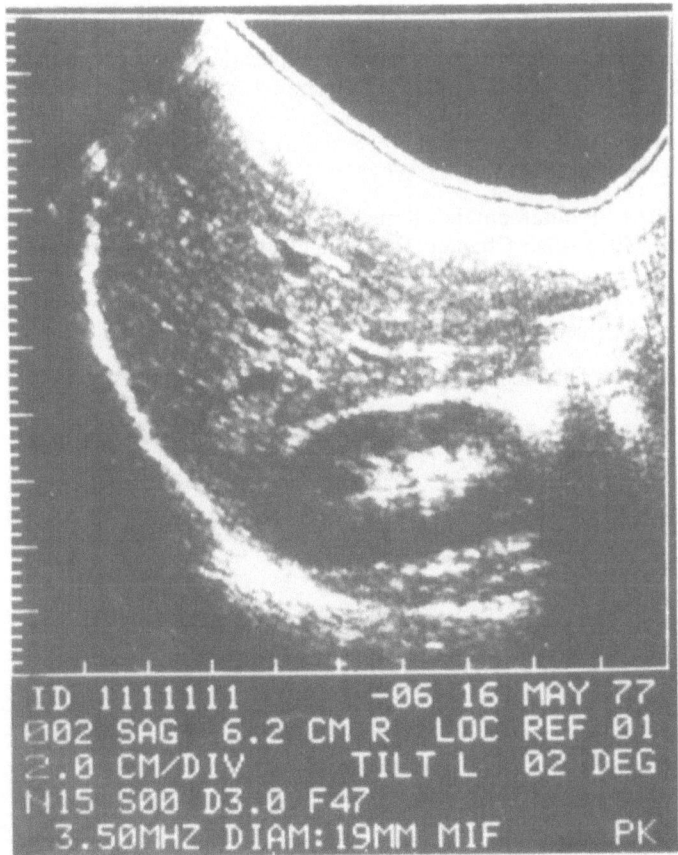

Figure 14. B-mode longitudinal scan of liver with kidney posteriorly.

A pulse-echo system which is arranged to respond to Doppler-shifted pulses is called a *pulse-Doppler*. Both cw and pulsed Dopplers will be described further in the next chapter.

REFERENCES

The best general references on all aspects of ultrasonic diagnostic systems currently available are:

1. Wells, Peter NT: Physical principles of ultrasonic diagnostics. London/New York: Academic Press, 1969.
2. Wells, Peter NT: Biomedical ultrasonics. London/New York: Academic Press, 1977.

The best general reference on all aspects of Doppler systems is:

3. Reneman, Robert S (ed): Cardiovascular applications of ultrasound. Amsterdam, London/New York: North Holland/American Elsevier Publishing, 1974.

General considerations in design and selection of Doppler instruments have been covered in the generally available text:

4. Baum, Gilbert: Fundamentals of medical ultrasonography. New York: G.P. Putnam's Sons, 1975. (See Chapter 27, 'Principles of Doppler Ultrasound'.)

General review of principles of application and interpretation of pulse-Doppler examination of the heart can be reviewed in:

5. King, Donald L: Diagnostic ultrasound. C.V. Mosby Company, 1974. (See Chapter by Donald W. Baker.)

3. DOPPLER FLOWMETER SYSTEMS

JOHN M. REID, PH.D.

This unit covers the operation of Doppler flowmeter systems in enough detail to assist the user in the selection of appropriate frequencies and transducers. The interfering effect of extraneous signals will be considered as they affect the choice of operating parameters. The choices available for processing and display of the Doppler information will be assessed from the viewpoint of their ability to extract meaningful flow information in the presence of interfering signals. The role of transducer selection in obtaining optimum results is examined in some detail as is the use of pulse-Doppler systems for obtaining depth information.

A block diagram of the basic Doppler system is shown in Figure 1. The functions shown in this diagram are carried out for either continuous-wave or pulse-Doppler systems. The transmitter excites a transducer to send out ultrasonic waves of a particular frequency. Another, or the same transducer can receive these waves which are fed to a receiver. A special property of

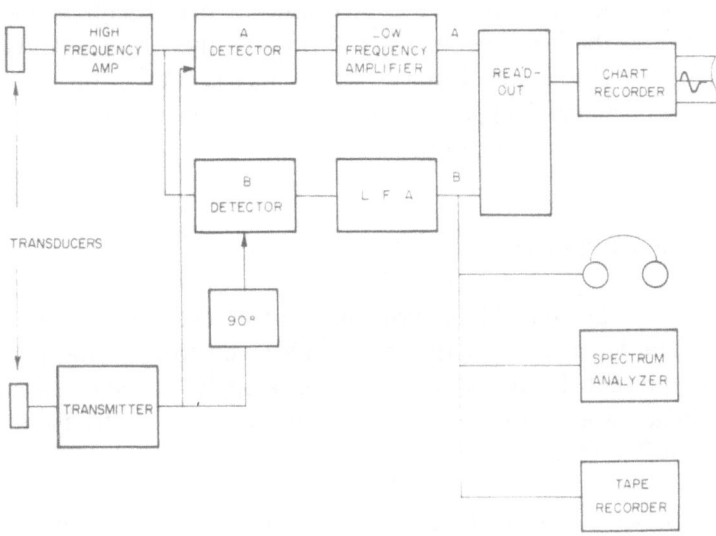

Figure 1. Block diagram of Directional Doppler flowmeter system. Functions are described in text.

Doppler systems is that the receiver has two inputs, the received wave, and the frequency of the transmitted wave. The output frequency of the receiver is the difference between the two inputs. This means that there is an output only for the reflections from moving structures. The low-frequency amplifier response covers the range of frequencies between roughly 200 Hz and 20,000 Hz or more. The choice of these pass-band frequencies for the Doppler receiver is extremely important in managing interference or artifact signals. A further step can be taken with the Doppler frequency signals coming from the receiver. If these are to be displayed in the form of flow velocity waveforms, the Doppler frequencies must be converted to a voltage. This is done by a readout, or analysis circuit which is a part of the Doppler flowmeter as shown in Figure 1. The signals can also be further analyzed and recorded.

Doppler systems can determine the direction of motion of flow because the direction of the Doppler shift depends upon the flow direction. If the moving blood is approaching the transducer, the Doppler shift is in the direction to increase the frequency of the scattered wave. The opposite is true if the flow is going away from the transducer. Special receiver circuits can detect the direction of the Doppler shift. Processing of the frequencies to indicate whether a particular Doppler frequency indicates flow toward or away from the transducer will be covered in Chapter 4.

As far as we are concerned in this unit, the effect of using a Directional Doppler receiver and readout system will be to make the polarity of the output voltage indicate the direction of flow. This means that a flow tracing which is above the baseline represents flow in one direction and a tracing which is below the baseline represents flow in the opposite direction. This characteristic of Directional Doppler flowmeters is missing in the much simplified non-directional Doppler flowmeters that have become useful for indicating only the presence of flow.

1. THE DOPPLER SPECTRUM

In dealing with Doppler blood flowmeters, we must deal with the Doppler spectrum. The Doppler spectrum is a name given to the band of frequencies which are present in the output of the Doppler receiver. A number of different frequencies are present because the red cells in the blood vessel are moving at different velocities.

The cells near the wall are nearly stationary and the cells in the center of the blood vessel are moving at a speed which, on the average, is twice the average velocity. Also, because the flow is not steady in time, the extent of the Doppler spectrum is continuously changing. Two representative Doppler frequency spectra are shown in Figure 2. These spectral plots are graphs of

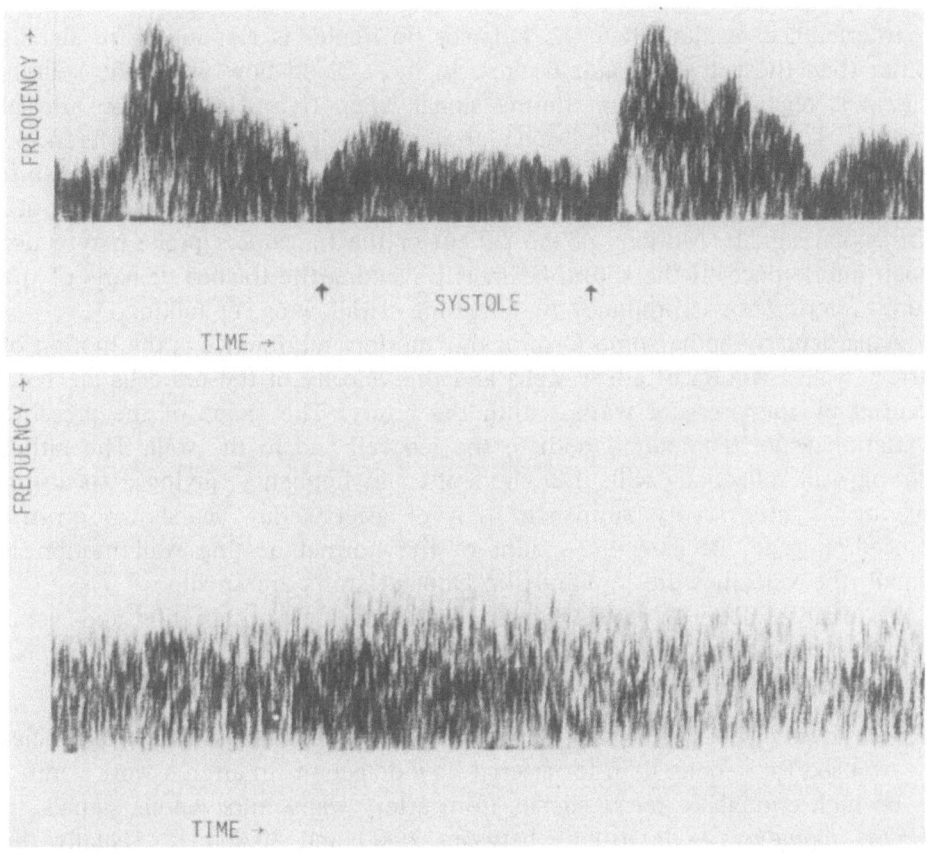

Figure 2. Spectrum analysis records of Doppler signals recorded from normal artery, top, and vein, bottom.

the Doppler frequency vertically as a function of time horizontally. The density or darkness of the plot is meant to indicate the strength of the Doppler signal having that particular frequency. Note that the pulsations in arterial flow due to the beating of the heart show clearly (Figure 2). As the heart beats, the blood is moved in the arteries at first very rapidly, and then more slowly. The exact shape of the maximum velocity waveform can indicate quite a bit about the state of the blood vessel and of the peripheral resistance bed which it is feeding. These matters will be discussed in the physiology chapter. In contrast to the flow in arteries, the flow in veins is both lower in frequency and more continuous with time. The cross-sectional area of the veins is several times that of the arterial vessels, hence the flow is slower. Variations in venous flow usually are caused by variation in pressure inside the chest cavity and, thus, synchronize with the breathing cycle rather than heart rate.

Interference results when the Doppler flowmeter is responding to signals other than those the operator desires. In most blood flow work, the venous signal is regarded as an interfering signal when trying to diagnose arterial disease. To the vein man, however, the arterial signals are an interference.

Any motion of otherwise stationary structures which causes Doppler shift frequencies within the pass-band of the Doppler flowmeter will produce artifactual signals. Motions of the patient or the transducer probe may cause such interference. If the sound beam is traversing the trachea or parts of the lung, interference is produced by coughing, swallowing, or talking.

A particularly bothersome form of this motion interference is the motion of artery walls. Motion of artery walls and the velocity of the red cells are both caused by the pressure wave within the artery. The shape of the pressure variation wave is imparted both to the red cell and to the wall. The rather strong wall reflections will, thus, be shifted in frequency, giving a spectrum having a pattern very similar to that of arterial flow as shown on the preceding page. Because the extent of the normal, resting wall motion is small, the velocities are low and the Doppler shifts are small.

To analyze Doppler shifts caused by blood flow in arteries and veins requires equipment whose low frequency amplifiers (Figure 1) have appropriate lower pass-band frequencies. These are set as follows:

Lower frequency — Is usually between 20 and 1,000 Hz. Lower frequencies are used for venous than for arterial flow detection. In arterial work it must be high enough to reject signals from artery walls, and venous signals.

Higher frequency — Is usually between 2,000 and 80,000 Hz. Usually the lowest value required is used to minimize noise and increase sensitivity in vein diagnosis.

2. PROCESSING AND DISPLAY

Each of the processing or display techniques available has its own set of advantages and disadvantages. This discussion will cover all of the major processing types in widespread use. Those processing techniques which are not generally available or in widespread use, but which may be important in the future, will be discussed in Chapter 5.

The three types of processing and display to be discussed here are 1) the direct spectral display, 2) processing circuits for recorder display, and 3) scanning for the display of anatomical relationships.

2.1. Direct spectral display

The human ear is an excellent processing and display means for many types of Doppler flow spectra. With very little training the listener can appreciate the correlation between pitch of the wave and flow velocity. Listening to pulsatile flow of arteries is particularly easy. It is even possible to sketch out the approximate shape of the blood flow waveform while listening to the Doppler sounds.

The ear is also amazingly good at rejecting interference in separating the flow from veins and arteries. The characteristic sounds of coughing, breathing, and moving are soon learned and the ear can wait and follow the flow sounds as soon as they can be discerned after such events take place. More surprising is the ability of the ear to separate arterial and venous flow. This ability apparently comes about because the spectra are additive. When the sound beam crosses both an artery and a vein, each vessel produces a set of independent Doppler sounds. While listening to the two distinctly different sets, the ear can appreciate the pulsatile nature of the arterial flow while being aware of a more steady low-frequency background due to venous flow. With a little more difficulty, the listener can listen for the venous flow and ignore the higher pitched sounds of arterial flow.

The principal drawback to using the ear to analyze Doppler sounds is that no permanent records are produced and the ranges of human hearing may not be sufficiently wide. Permanent records are displayed by the circuitry to be discussed later in this section. The restricted frequency range of the human ear or of the sound reproduction apparatus used in connection with the Doppler equipment is a most serious restriction.

Human beings can hear Doppler frequencies down to 20 Hz if they are reproduced on high-quality headphones or expensive speakers. Otherwise, frequencies much below 200 Hz will not be heard.

If Doppler frequencies in excess of 10,000 Hz are to be analyzed by the ear, high-quality speakers or headphones again are required. The high frequency hearing of persons who are operating or interpreting Doppler sounds should be checked because of the possible impairment in the high frequency range which can occur in individuals over thirty years of age.

Spectrum analysis can also provide a permanent record as shown in Figure 2. On-line spectrum analyzers also can be purchased which will print out the spectrum. This display has most of the advantages of the ear-listening method. It misses very little and can simultaneously display flows from arteries and veins. In addition, the eye, by looking at the maximum frequency, can deduce the waveform of the pulsatile flow in arteries, independent from nearby venous flow. It also provides a permanent record for storage.

The principal disadvantages of the spectrum analysis approach are size and cost. Spectrum analyzers range from $ 10,000 upwards and real-time analyzers usually start around $ 25,000. The future world of micro-processors may allow the spectrum analysis to be done by the fast-Fourier transform method at much reduced cost.

Directional spectral analysis can be obtained without the necessity of using two analyzers. Special circuits are used which offset the frequency corresponding to zero flow to some convenient value. This offset frequency then represents zero flow and the spectra for flows in both directions will be represented above and below the new zero flow baseline.

2.2. Processing circuits

Processing, or readout, circuits function to convert a Doppler spectrum into a flow waveform. They are basically frequency-to-voltage converters whose output is a voltage that can be recorded on an ordinary strip chart recorder. The principal advantage of such circuits has been to provide an interpretable flow waveform at minimum cost. Two types of readout circuits are known, and they differ radically in their performance.

The most common form of readout circuit has been the zero-crossing frequency meter. Such a meter attempts to count the number of cycles in the Doppler spectrum and derive a voltage proportional to the frequency. These circuits work well when the signal strength is large, interference is at a minimum, and the spectrum has a constant shape. They are widely used in multi-channel flowmeters in physiological studies involving animals, where the transducer can be placed directly on the blood vessels. The principal drawback in zero-crossing meters is that they are essentially a pulse device, generating an output pulse whenever input is sufficiently large. They are, thus, subject to being triggered by random electronic noise, power supply hum, and transducer probe motion artifacts.

The other type of readout circuit has been developed primarily at the Institute of Applied Physiology and Medicine and in Holland. This circuit, described in Chapter 4, uses analog multiplying elements to construct what is really a small analog computer. The function of this computer is to develop an output voltage which is proportional to the average frequency of the Doppler spectrum, *independent of the shape of the spectrum.*

An unexpected advantage of this analog computer circuit is that it does not respond to random noise voltages or power supply hum. It appears to be remarkably insensitive to probe motion artifacts, as long as these artifacts do not produce voltages too large for the electronics to handle. This circuit is much more expensive than the zero-crossing circuit, but its insensitivity to interference artifacts helps make the entire concept of Doppler scanning practical.

The analog computer circuit exists in two forms at the present time. The basic circuit was designed originally to calculate volume flow with implanted transducers. When used transcutaneously, the amplitude of the output waveform depends upon the depth of the blood vessel. This has not been found to be a problem while operating in the scanning mode, although it is somewhat of a drawback when trying to compare waveforms. A circuit which removes this amplitude dependence is under development. It is called an automatic gain control readout circuit, and is currently being tested. Since the readout is only a portion of the Doppler receiver channel, this newer type of circuit can be added to existing directional Doppler systems.

All readout circuits constructed to date have the disadvantage, when they attempt to record Doppler-shifted signals arising from arteries and a nearby vein simultaneously, of producing 'mixed' waveforms. It has been demonstrated that it is possible to separate these simultaneous signals on the basis of their flow direction. Phase shift circuits added to the Doppler receiver between the basic receiver section and the readout circuit (A and B, Figure 1) can separate the spectrum from flow toward the transducer from the spectrum due to flow away from the transducer. We are currently constructing phase shift networks suitable for addition to our scanners.

2.3. Scanning displays

Doppler scanning systems use motion of the probe combined with a narrow ultrasonic beam to map the regions from which Doppler-shifted signals are received. In continuous-wave Doppler scanning, the transducer can be passed back and forth over the surface of the skin to build up a map of the major blood vessels as if they were all squashed down flat on a plane. Such a flat projection of blood vessels results when x-ray arteriograms are taken so that the interpretation is similar. This system is described further in Chapter 4.

4. DOPPLER IMAGING SYSTEMS

JOHN M. REID, PH.D.; MERRILL P. SPENCER, M.D.;
and DONALD L. DAVIS, B.S.E.E.

The search for a practical, clinically applicable system for non-invasive detection and diagnosis of atherosclerosis followed early demonstrations that ultrasound could be used. Pulse-echo systems were the first to be investigated and showed that, although plaque could be visualized or its absorption properties made apparent in vivo, some types of plaque would not be visualizable [1]. Apparently, fatty plaque or plaque whose blood tissue interface was not at right angles to the sound beam could not be differentiated from blood. Interest was then focused on imaging of the blood itself through various types of imaging systems based on the ultrasonic Doppler effect. The first of these was a pulse-Doppler system which produced cross-section flow images [2]. The present authors developed a continuous wave (c-w) Doppler system which, by ignoring the depth coordinate, produced a plan view geometrically similar to an arteriogram [3]. The c-w system to be described here was devised as a clinically-applicable screening tool for diagnosis of surgically correctable flow disturbance in large arteries. It has been applied to the carotid and vertebral arteries of the neck and evaluated on more than 3,000 patients in our clinics alone. Other centers have reported active use of this equipment [4, 5].

A detection or screening technique suitable for use in a hospital or small clinic must meet a number of requirements. The requirements for non-invasive, in vivo application are met by all of the ultrasonic diagnostic instruments. Further requirements for accuracy and sensitivity as well as the overall requirement of cost-effectiveness have been met by the c-w imaging system. Study of etiology and epidemiology requires a variety of instruments capable of presenting different types of information.

A sensitive and accurate system must respond to the actual flow in a vessel and not simply picture a lumen diameter. X-ray arteriography itself is limited by the fact that only a linear dimension of the vessel rather than its area is shown and no indication is given of the interference to flow caused by a specific lesion. To provide accurate information on the condition of the patient, assessment of the collateral circulation around the lesion is necessary. A clinical system must be able to be used in connection with various compression maneuvers to evaluate the amount and source of this collateral circulation, particularly when dealing with blood flow to a critical organ such as the brain.

We have found that in 20–30% of patients, absorption by atherosclerotic plaque will prevent imaging of arterial lumen directly under the plaque. In these cases the assessment of flow interference from this plaque must be done on the downstream flow.

Cost effective screening generally requires that the system must be useable by a trained paramedical individual. An absolute minimum of tuning and similar adjustment controls are necessary to minimize the technical component of this training. The medical component of the training can be minimized if the system does not act in a highly interactive mode, that is, a detailed knowledge of anatomy and physiology should not be required of the operator. If blood flow channels must be recognized by location and shape or function, then more highly trained medical professionals are required. Fortunately, devices based on the Doppler effect can easily be set to image only flow in arteries or veins and minimize the training required. A basic requirement of systems operated by a paramedical individual is the production of adequate documentation for the patient's record and for later medical interpretation. The c-w system produces one picture per blood vessel rather that a series of cross-sectional photographs, and, together with tape recordings and chart records giving the Doppler sounds and flow waveforms at a limited number of specific sites within the vessel, comprises a cost-effective battery of records. Interpretation of the Doppler sounds does involve a certain amount of training or the use of spectrum analysis at the present time. Current work involves coding these audible features into a color image.

1. THE CONTINUOUS-WAVE DOPPLER IMAGING SYSTEM

1.1. Basic imaging system

The basic system is shown schematically in Figure 1. The Doppler transducer is held in a scanning arm at a fixed angle with respect to the skin and manually moved over the skin surface. Arm position-translating circuits cause the beam in a storage oscilloscope to move in correspondence with the position of the Doppler probe. The transducer is focused to an effective sensitive region with minimum diameter and with length suitable for the anatomy being studied. When the probe passes over a blood vessel the presence of the Doppler-shifted wave scattered from the moving red cells is detected by an ultrasonic flowmeter and the output is processed to brighten the display on the oscilloscope. System outputs are: first, a lateral projection view of the artery which is photographed for storage; second, the Doppler

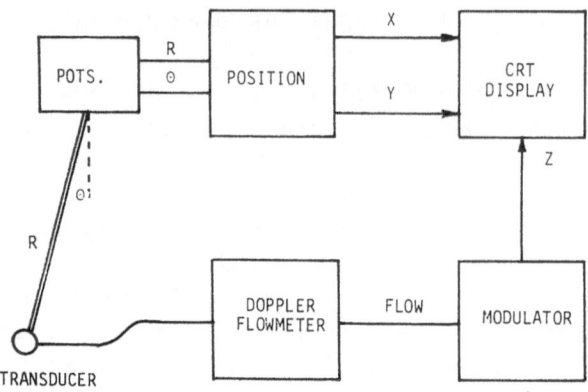

Figure 1. Block diagram of continuous-wave Doppler imaging system using a manually-scanned arm. Arm is positioned to move transducer over skin surface.

sounds recorded on a standard tape recorder for spectrum analysis or later listening; and third, chart recordings of the flow waveform to document direction of flow and identification of blood vessels. Not shown in Figure 1 is the ear-pulse detector used for operator guidance in performing compression maneuvers.

In addition to the use in the basic imaging mode shown in Figure 1, the highly-focused probe of the Doppler flowmeter is used hand-held for flow assessment in arteries where imaging is not required. In our application, imaging is used to identify the common carotid and the internal and external carotid branches in the neck. Some experience has been gained with imaging the subclavian-vertebral junction as well. Hand-held applications involve the detection of vertebral flow in the neck and thn direction of flow in the ophthalmic artery and its branches behind the eye.

2. TRANSDUCER

A transducer with excellent lateral resolution is fundamental to the operation of the system. We have developed a 5 MHz Doppler transducer, using separate elements for sending and receiving the sound, which is mounted behind an epoxy plastic lens focusing the sound field to a narrow beam at a nominal 2.5 cm from the transducer. The narrow beam exists between approximately 1.5 and 3.5 cm from the face of the transducer. A plot of equal Doppler return voltage contours from this transducer is shown in Figure 2. This figure was obtained by scanning across a plastic tube of 1 mm inside diameter containing very small moving air bubbles. The resulting contours of equal

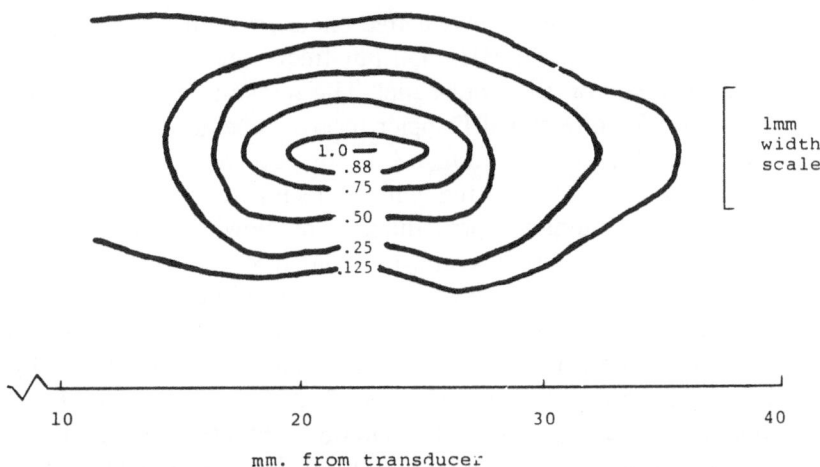

1mm
width
scale

10   20   30   40

mm. from transducer

Figure 2. Equal Doppler signal contours, lens focusing. Flow in 1 mm I.D. tube.

Doppler return voltage are plotted in the figure. The figure shows that, if we image all flow above 1/8 of full scale, the 1 mm wide flow stream will image as being 2 mm wide and thus 1 mm is the basic resolution of the system under best conditions.

3. SCANNING ARM

The scanning arm performs the dual function of positioning the transducer with respect to the patient and indicating the position of the transducer on the surface of the skin. Any mechanical assembly restricts access to the patient and is awkward to some extent. The present arm has the advantage of being light enough to be supported by a single post of standard orthopedic framing which can be clamped to hospital stretchers and cots in a variety of ways. The arm can be readily repositioned for scanning of vertebrals low in the neck and the femorals and popliteals in the leg. The primary bearing surfaces in our present design are composed of commercially available elements using hardened steel surfaces in the shape of balls and cylinders. This semi-kinematic design provides for exceptional smoothness and freedom from wear and lubrication problems. Linear transducers are used to feed spot-positioning voltages to the display oscilloscope.

4. CIRCUITS

The electronics console houses the basic ultrasonic Doppler flowmeter circuit and a number of auxiliary units which are necessary for efficient clinical use.

The basic Doppler flowmeter allows a free choice of transducers at operating frequencies between 2 and 11 MHz. Output frequency is controlled by plugging in a quartz crystal on the front panel. The transmitted frequency and 90° quadrature signals for directional Doppler receiver operation are derived from the crystal oscillator [7, 8]. No transmitter or receiver tuning controls are needed either for operation by the clinical technician or as a part of the manufacturing or maintenance procedures. The flow waveform voltage for control of the imaging oscilloscope and for chart recording is derived from the Doppler spectrum by an analog circuit [7, 8]. This circuit has been realized by using off-the-shelf integrated circuits as shown in Figure 3. This circuit has the advantage over the zero-crossing detector that it is not disturbed by brief noise pulses. Noise pulses cause false triggering of the input Schmitt Trigger used in most zero-crossing meters. The circuit of Figure 3, however, operates as a correlator and produces an output only for frequencies which are simultaneously present at both inputs and which have the proper phase relationship. The ability of the circuit to function with noisy signals was tested by applying a phase-quadrature 1 KHz audio signal and the normal circuit noise from the flowmeter. An RMS voltmeter was used to measure the RMS noise level at the input terminals (see Figure 3) and the audio signal adjusted to double the RMS voltmeter reading. This procedure assures a signal power equal to the noise power, that is, a signal-to-noise ratio of unity. It was found that the direct voltage output of the circuit was 10 times the random fluctuations produced by the noise alone, or present when the audio signal was applied. Expressed in dB's, this means that a 0 dB input signal-to-noise ratio produced a 20 dB signal-to-noise ratio at the output. To achieve this performance it is essential to use the balanced circuit rather than the original unbalanced form [9]. The low-pass filters shown in Figure 3 are essential to

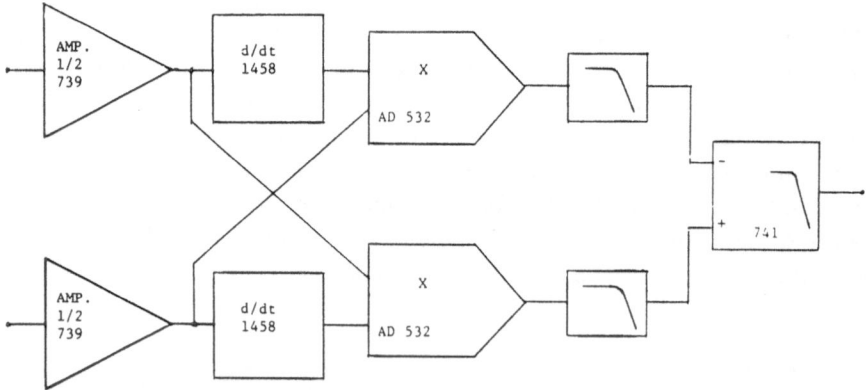

Figure 3. Doppler signal processing circuit. Difference-frequency, phase quadrature, input signals from directional Doppler receiver are processed to derive an output voltage proportional to Doppler frequency shift.

prevent over-driving of the output difference-taking amplifier, which is required to balance out noise-generated potentials.

Auxiliary circuits consist of the spot-positioning circuits already mentioned, an ear-pulse detector and recording circuits. The ear-pulse detector used a light-emitting diode and photocell to measure the pulsatile blood component in the ear lobe. When the common carotid on the monitored side is compressed, cessation of ear pulses shows that complete occlusion has been obtained. The Doppler system is usually being used to observe the direction of flow in the ophthalmic arteries at this time. The combination allows determination of the source of flow in a portion of the Circle of Willis while occluding the circulation for only 1 to 2 heartbeats.

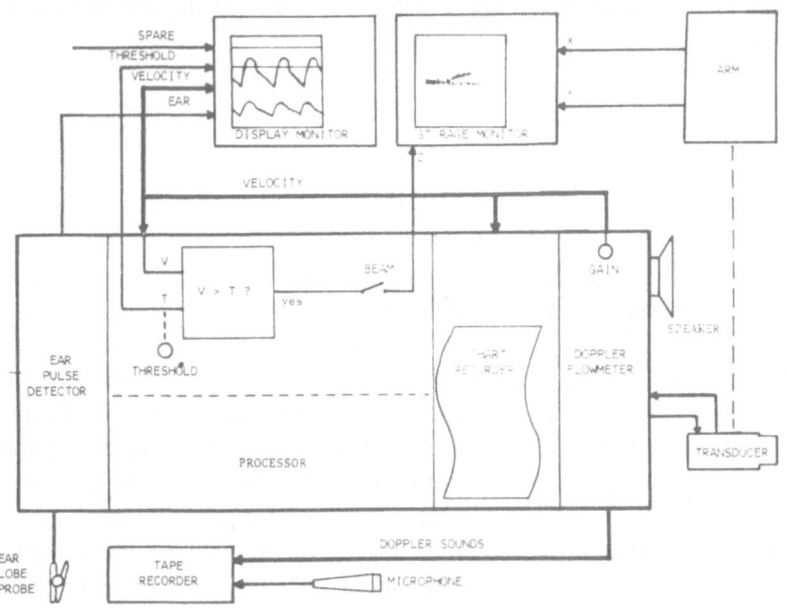

Figure 4. Doppler Scanning System.

5. THE RECORDING SYSTEM

The recording system, as diagramed in Figure 4, consists of a chart recorder and tape recorder controlled together with a footswitch so that the operator can gather all of the records which are required for medical interpretation without generating any unneeded records. Foot switch control is used to keep the chart recorder and tape recorder running together to record flow at selected sites. The operator identifies the site by observation of the previously made image map. The bright spot on the display indicates position of the sound beam relative to the vessel. Operator comments identifying the location of the recording are spoken into the microphone connected to one channel of our stereo tape recorder. Each record is thus identified as to the branch of the artery, as well as whether it is at the site of a suspected stenosis or upstream or downstream from the site.

Valuable operator guidance is provided by an auxiliary oscilloscope connected to a four-channel multiplexer. This oscilloscope displays the pulsatile flow waveform output for operator guidance without wasting chart paper. The oscilloscope also displays simultaneously the position of a threshold voltage setting. Only flow signals which come above this threshold are used to modulate the storage oscilloscope. The other display channels are the ear-pulse detector output and a spare which can be used for electrocardiogram or other input.

6. CLINICAL EXPERIENCE

Clinical experience has been obtained which relates directly to the engineering design of the system and is being used to guide our future plans. A most significant clinical finding is the high rate of incidence of plaque which absorbs the sound beams sufficiently to produce an isolated 'hole' in the records. When this occurs, the nature of the flow upstream and downstream of the hole must be assessed to determine if a hemodynamically significant lesion is present. Current efforts with spectrum analysis indicate that if stenosis is present within the non-sounding segment, characteristic sounds are produced by the turbulent downstream flow. These include a low-frequency component and a simultaneous, random, high-frequency component. Further downstream it appears that either eddying or wall vibrations contribute to a low-frequency 'fluttering' type of signal. Analysis of these records is still being conducted.

It appears that it could be extremely valuable to eliminate the interpretive step of listening to such recordings or of making spectrum analysis to detect flow interference. An effective way of presenting the data would be to code the occurrence of the specific types of signals onto the image by the use of appropriate colors. This work begins with the technician using felt pens to code our clinical images. As experience is gathered with the particular types of sounds, we plan to instrument the entire processing using a color display system. This would give a single record per side containing all of the basic flow information.

When the c-w system was initially planned, it was considered to be a feasibility study, because we felt that manual scanning would produce relatively crude images and that the entire procedure, although valuable, might be unacceptably slow. We found, however, that the procedure is relatively fast. About 15 minutes are required to make a scan from each side of the neck. The rest of the procedure, ranging from history-taking to collateral flow assessment, getting the patient on and off the cot, etc., takes about one hour. The final physician interpretation of the complete battery of tests requires an additional 15 minutes on the average. It appears presently that the c-w imaging is quite acceptably fast and moreover, none of the current developmental systems offer much promise of speeding up the assessment. The basic restriction to the speed of Doppler imaging systems is set by the heart rate. Maximum blood velocity is reached for only about 1/3 of the cardiac cycle, recurring at a rate of about once per second. Whether the c-w system is used to produce a single line across the vessel or a so-called real-time Doppler scanner is used to produce a complete cross-sectional picture in this length of time is relatively immaterial. Both must wait for the heart to beat again to take the next record, and the same number of heartbeats will be required to do a complete assessment. Velocity profile methods require a great deal of averaging and may require up to ten or more profiles to be taken at any one position to average random fluctuations. In some pulse-Doppler systems the range gate position must be monitored by the operator and adjusted to the region of the vessel. A pulse-Doppler with enough gates to eliminate the need for position adjustment could perform relatively fast imaging in the depth dimension, but this image could not be directly compared to the angiogram. A 20–30 gate system remains an attractive addition to the present c-w system for rapid data gathering.

Eventually the c-w system could be used for screening of stroke-prone populations if the operator skill and training required could be reduced by use of the color display and some form of automatic scanning added. Our efforts are proceeding in these directions.

REFERENCES

1. Reid JM, Barber FE, Nation AW, Mozerski DJ, Strandness DE: Ultrasonic rotational fast scanner. 24th Annual Conference on Engineering in Med and Biol, Las Vegas, 1971.
2. Hokanson DE, Mozersky D, Sumner DS, Strandness DE: Ultrasonic arteriography: a new approach to arterial visualization. Biomed Engng 6:420, 1971.
3. Reid JM, Spencer MP: Ultrasonic Doppler technique for imaging blood vessels. Science, 176:1235-1236, 1972.
4. Blackwell E, Merory J, McKinney WM, Toole JF: Evaluation of carotid and vertebrobasilar insufficiency by Doppler ultrasound scanning. Joint Mtg on Stroke & Cerebral Circulation, Dallas, TX, Feb 1976.
5. Turnipseed WD, Lubow M, Vasko JS: Surgical repair of the occluded carotid artery. Joint Mtg on Stroke & Cerebral Circulation, Dallas, TX, Feb 1976.

6. Spencer MP, Brockenbrough EC, Davis DL, Reid JM: Cerebrovascular evaluation using Doppler c-w ultrasound. Ultrasound in medecine. Proc of World Fed of Ultrasound in Med and Biol, San Francisco, August 1976.
7. Reid JM, Davis DL, Ricketts HJ, Spencer MP: A new Doppler Flowmeter system and its operation with catheter mounted transducers. Symp on cardiovascular applications of ultrasound, Amsterdam/London: North Holland/American Elsevier Publishing, New York, 1974.
8. Reid JM, Davis DL, Phillips JB, Spencer MP: Transcutaneous flow mapping with continuous wave Doppler. Symp on cardiovascular applications of ultrasound, Amsterdam/London: North Holland/American Elsevier Publishing, New York, 1974.
9. Arts MGJ, Roevros JMJG: On the instantaneous measurement of blood-flow by ultrasonic means. Med Biol Engng 10:23-35, 1972.

5. OTHER ULTRASONIC TECHNIQUES AND CURRENT RESEARCH

JOHN M. REID, PH.D.

New developments are always of interest to anyone in a diagnostic field. This chapter is designed to bring you up-to-date with the current research which is being done in alternative systems of arterial imaging and to acquaint you with the research direction being followed at the Institute of Applied Physiology and Medicine.

The two techniques which are currently being developed in other laboratories, pulse-echo arterial wall imaging and pulse-Doppler two or three-dimensional flow geometry imaging, were developed by or in close collaboration with our engineering group many years ago. The pulse-echo artery wall visualization system was abandoned by us, since it is not capable of visualizing flow obstruction caused by plaque containing primarily fatty material. The pulse-Doppler flow imaging system is considerably more complex technologically, and is limited in its maximum Doppler frequency range. The provision of the depth coordinate would be useful in some cases where the internal and external branches of the carotid appear to overlie each other in our straight, lateral projection. The ability might, thus, be valuable as an addition to the continuous-wave imaging system. At the same time, the pulse-Doppler range information requires an additionalsearching step in range and appears to be so much slower than continuous-wave imaging that it is not suitable for routine clinical use as the sole system in the present (1979) commercial instruments.

The Institute's future research program is directed toward the solution of clinically important problems with new or additional equipment *which is compatible with* the scanner systems currently being used in our clinics and available from Carolina Medical Electronics, Inc. These include engineering developments to increase the speed of imaging and ease of use as well as the gathering and presentation of additional diagnostic information to improve the accuracy of the results. These efforts are described in more detail below.

1. THE INSTITUTE RESEARCH PROGRAM

The Institute research program is designed to improve the speed and accuracy of examination by means which will be compatible with the present instrumentation and which appear to be justified on the basis of our extensive clinical experience. Our primary effort is directed on lines which are somewhat different from the lines followed by the developers of the advanced systems discussed in the following pages. We have found that the most meaningful diagnostic information is the physiological information on flow. Our major effort, therefore, is directed toward getting better physiological, that is, functional information. We are trying to get it more accurately, more rapidly, and in a form which requires less operator training. Systems being developed elsewhere appear to be concentrating on improving the geometrical (morphological) information in the image. Our experience indicates that this is not the most desirable direction in which to proceed. The geometry of the flow channel is of lesser importance.

The basic engineering rationale for improving the physiological information before the geometrical is that in many cases highly absorbing plaque will prevent the cross-section geometrical imaging systems from obtaining any useful output. In cases of soft, fatty plaque the obstruction will not be seen at all! They, therefore, cannot be used as the *sole* examining instrument. The continuous-wave system, with its emphasis on high-quality Doppler information, is capable of determining the character of flow downstream from such plaque. Pulse-Doppler, on the other hand, will miss the high-frequency jet flow from stenosis. The continuous-wave system has more subtle advantage. It produces one image per side. Real-time systems produce hundreds of images every minute and require considerable operator judgement as to which image is to be saved for medical interpretation.

It would appear to be a real advantage to combine the flow characterization information from the Doppler sounds with the present geometrical information on the flow maps. This can be done by gray-scale or color-coding the flow information onto our present image. Our general plan is to encode the maximum Doppler velocity, spectral broadening, fluttering, thumping, and inversion of flow direction onto the image. We plan to do this in a way which will allow visual interpretation of the picture image in an efficient manner.

We believe this to be a fruitful direction to follow since a rudimentary form of a color-coding system has already been described by D.N. White of Kingston Hospital in Ontario. This system encodes only the peak velocity as one of three distinct colors. It is made by Diagnostic Electronics, Inc.

The problem of imaging bifurcations whose plane is not parallel to the skin is one of the most troublesome clinical problems encountered. There are two basic ways of attacking this problem and we are planning to explore both ways before deciding on the technique to be instrumented. The first way is to provide a real-time Doppler scanning capability by attaching a scanning head to our present scan arm. This system would automatically scan across a vessel diameter and should be capable of making one picture line per heartbeat. The operator would then draw this scanning head along the course of the vessel and 'paint' out a picture in our present format. With such a rapid scanning system it would be relatively simple to reposition the scanning arm to scan at a slightly different direction in case the bifurcation is not parallel to the skin.

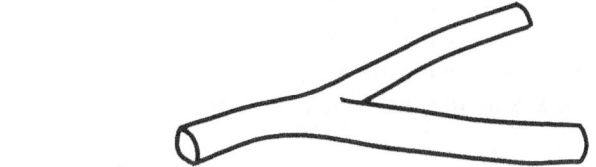

Figure 1. Plane view of bifurcation.

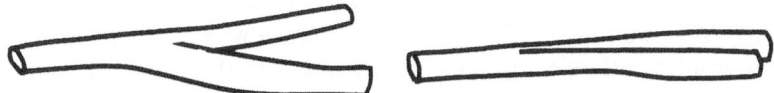

Figure 2. Rotated views of bifurcation.

Fortunately, most peripheral vessels occur in round appendages, and it is possible to shift the scanning plane around the neck or leg until a better image of the bifurcation is obtained. See Figures 1 and 2. The femoral-profundus junction in the leg is rather difficult to scan from the direct A/P view, but by shifting the scanning head inside of the thigh an acceptable scan has resulted. The carotid bifurcation is highly variable in orientation, but fortunately seems to be parallel to the skin in most cases. It is clear that a desirable improvement in the system would be provision for obtaining scans more rapidly so that several scans could be taken to present different views.

Because of many questions on the feasibility of constructing a real-time Doppler scanner, we are also following an alternative approach to the bifurcation imaging problem. This approach is to use a pulse-Doppler to obtain range information, but guide its application with the continuous-wave scan map. With this ability, the pulse-Doppler could drawn along the course of the vessel and a second map of flow velocity as a function of depth along all or part of the course of the vessel would be obtained. We have built a unique form of pulse-Doppler for this purpose. This pulse-Doppler does not require separate circuitry for each range gate, but rather derives a voltage proportional to velocity at each range of the system. It, thus, operates as if it had an infinite number of range gates and should require considerably less operator attention. It is described further below.

The Institute is and can be involved in many other smaller programs than the above. These major development programs are the subject of a research contract from the National Institutes of Health to fund the development and testing of these systems. In addition, the Institute is able to provide specialized transducers for scanning other sites, and performing other types of diagnosis. We are able to design and fabricate transducers calculated to provide specified field shapes, at particular distances and directions form the transducer housing. Direct contact with us is generally necessary to establish the medical requirements and the acceptability of the final design.

2. B-MODE PULSE ECHO SCANNERS

B-mode pulse echo scanners are really miniaturized versions of clinical B-mode scanning equipment. They operate by emitting a short pulse and timing the delay until a reflection is returned to measure the range of the reflecting structure. These systems were described in more detail in Chapter 2. The scan format is that of a cross-section. Transducer motion is used to provide one coordinate and depth into the patient is the other coordinate. These cross-section views for arteries can be arranged in either of two ways as shown in Figure 3. To the left we have the cross-section representation in

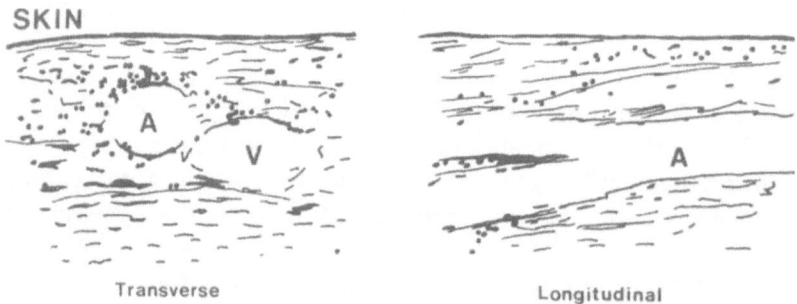

Figure 3. B-mode Scans.

which the artery or vein appears roughly as a circle and at the right a longitudinal section. At least short sections of artery can be shown in longitudinal cross-section which makes the identification of the blood-filled space generally easier.

A particular advantage of these small B-scanners is that they can scan very rapidly by either electrical or mechanical means. They also have a self-contained water coupling bag built into the instrument to provide optimum resolution. Because of the rapid scanning, they have come to be known as 'real-time' scanners. By 'real-time' we mean that the operator sees the picture that is being taken instantaneously.

In terms of historical development, the first artery scanner of this type was developed under the direction of Dr. Reid at the University of Washington and reported by Tomey and Reid in 1969. An early clinical finding from the operation of this instrument was that it *could not* detect build-up of fatty plaque. We obtained excellent images of the carotid bifurcation in patients who had no flow! It appears that these instruments are the best in picturing the arterial walls.

In research into the causes and management of atherosclerosis the wall position information may well be quite valuable. A number of other groups are pursuing the development of this type of scanner primarily for these purposes. The Institute made a conscious choice in developing its arterial scanning system because of the previously bad clinical experience with the pulse-echo scanners. The B-mode pulse-echo scanners have an additional disadvantage in routine clinical use. They share the disadvantage of all ultrasound B-mode imaging systems in operating in an interactive mode. The operator must recognize the anatomy of the structures and position the transducer accordingly. Since it is generally impossible to make individual pictures of the dozens or hundreds of scans made by such a rapid scanner, considerable judgement is required in selecting a particular scan to be saved for medical interpretation. The technologist, thus, does the diagnosis or the doctor is required to manipulate the instrument. There appears to be a role for such a device in certain critical cases, but it appears not to be well adapted to the clinic.

Continuing research is being done primarily by three groups in this country. The original Reid scanner at the University of Washington was adapted by Barber and Baker to operate in connection with a pulse-Doppler which will be the next system described in this chapter. This system seeks to add the Doppler information about flow to the pulse-echo system and obtain a simultaneous display of where the blood is flowing and its relationship to the walls of the artery. Further discussion of this system really belongs under the next section.

About two to three years ago the National Institutes of Health awarded contracts to encourage the development of atherosclerosis imaging systems. One approach was to combine a pulse-echo real-time fast scanner and a pulse-Doppler. This contract was awarded to Green at Stanford Research Institute with clinical evaluation to be conducted at the Mayo Clinic in

Minnesota. The Doppler does not attempt to image the flow, but rather to measure the velocity profile within the blood vessel. This system will also be discussed in more detail below.

Another contract was awarded to Dr. Olinger of Case Western Reserve. The group doing the technical development is from the old CBS Laboratory and led by Dr. Nigam. They have produced a pulse-echo fast scanner which has produced images of plaque within a vessel wall. A commercial version, based on a design by Glenn, is available from Biodynamics, Inc.

The preliminary research results from these instruments indicate that certain types of plaque, probably calcified, will produce strong echoes at least when they are oriented so the surface of the plaque is at right angles to the soundbeam and shadows cast on normal structures when they are not. We expect that *these systems will fail to find obstruction caused by uncalcified fatty plaque* as we demonstrated in several cases with the first system at the University of Washington. Detailed images of some non-occluding plaques are very good.

3. PULSE-DOPPLER

Pulse-Doppler systems are basically similar to the familiar pulse-echo ultrasonic diagnostic systems. The systems function by selecting the echoes from a particular depth by turning on a 'gate' in the receiver when the echoes from this depth are returning to the transducer. This spectrum for listening and recording in the same manner as described previously for Doppler equipment. The principal additional circuitry required is that necessary to maintain coherence between the transmitted wave and the Doppler receiver reference voltage and the filtering required to remove the pulse repetition rate of the pulse-echo system. This restricts the maximum Doppler frequency that can be heard.

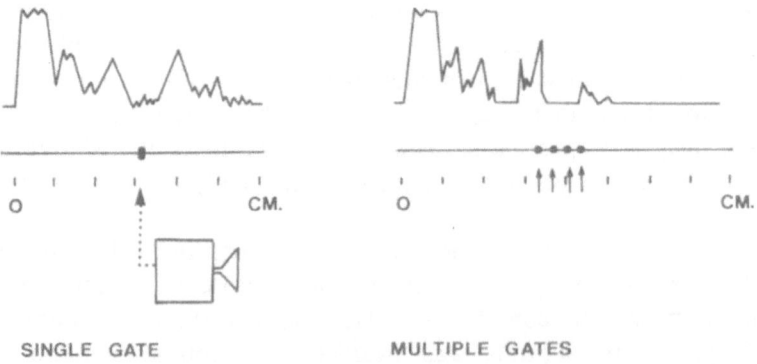

SINGLE GATE   MULTIPLE GATES

Figure 4. Pulse-Doppler A-mode Displays.

A pulse-Doppler determines Doppler frequencies as a function of depth as well as along the dimensions established by transducer motion over the skin surface. It has the distinct advantage of being able to listen to flow in a vessel which is behind another vessel and of separately listening to flows in more than one vessel at one time. A typical display format is shown in Figure 4.

At the top of the figure a regular A-mode trace shows the echoes as a function of depth for any one transducer position. On the trace below the occurrence of the Doppler gate is marked by a brightened spot. The depth of this spot is adjustable, and the Doppler sounds produced by moving structures *at this depth* are heard on a loud speaker, recorded on a chart recorder, etc. If the pulse-Doppler is connected to a scanner display, the presence of Doppler information can be indicated by brightening the display just as we do with the continuous-wave imaging system. In this case, the scan format will be basically similar to the format discussed in the previous section for B-mode pulse-echo scanners and looks something like the sketch in Figure 5.

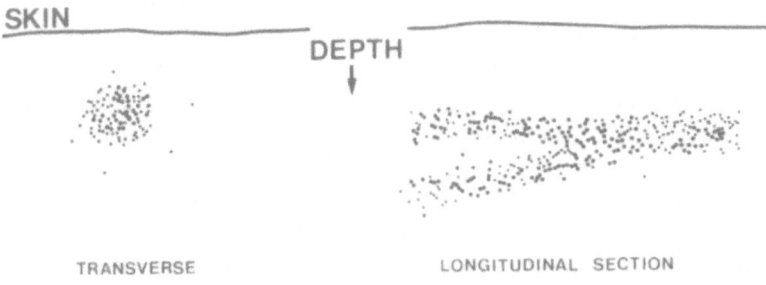

Figure 5. Pulse-Doppler B-mode Displays.

The display on the left is a cross-sectional image, and that on the right the corresponding longitudinal image.

Because of the slow picture build-up rate necessary if the listening depth has to be manually adjusted for each probe position to cover the depth ranges which encompass the blood vessel, it is an advantage to provide multiple gates in the pulse-Doppler, although this increases the complexity of the equipment. In a multiple gate system several gates are positioned quite close to each other in time and, hence, sample the Doppler flows at a number of positions in space. Five to twenty range gates are commonly used. With this small number of gates it is generally not possible to image flow at all depths, and a manual operator adjustment is still required to position the bank of gates over the general position of the artery.

An interesting type of pulse-Doppler display can be obtained when the various range gate positions span the diameter of an artery. Figure 6 shows

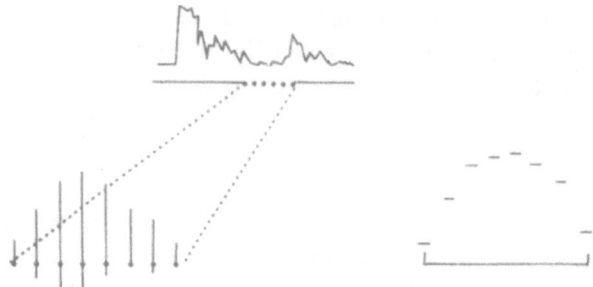

Figure 6. Velocity Profile Display.

the face of an oscilloscope with the various gate positions indicated on the X axis. This is really a small part of the range sweep illustrated in the first figure in the pulse-Doppler section. If the magnitude of the Doppler shift frequency is applied to the vertical axis of the oscilloscope, the display on the left results. The height of the bars is now proportional to the velocity, and the profile of the spectrum within the vessel can be seen both in systole and diastole. Such displays are very interesting for observing the flow distribution across the vessel at bifurcations and the presence in reversed flow in some phases of the cardiac cycle in some vessels. A more stable display for photographing can be obtained by gating these bars so they appear only at a particular phase of the flow cycle. A gated systolic profile appears as shown on the right of the figure.

The Institute of Applied Physiology and Medicine has developed and successfully demonstrated in vivo a unique type of pulse-Doppler. This system was described before by others, but had not previously been made to work in vivo. This system acts as if every point on the range axis, Figures 4 and 6, had a gate. The gates are very narrow and close together so that we

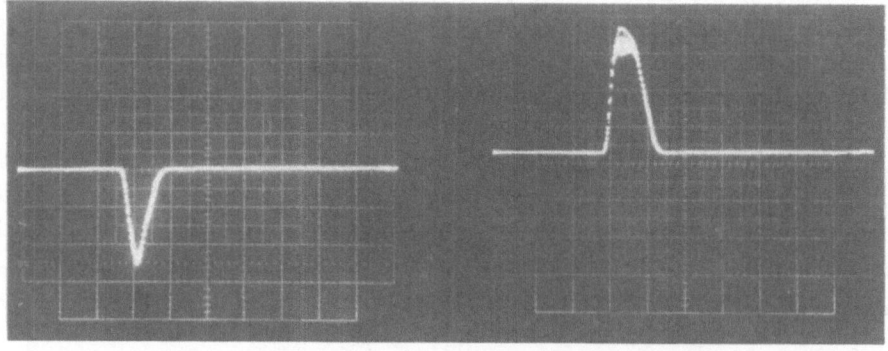

Figure 7. Infinite-Gate Pulse-Doppler Velocity Profile.

have termed the system the 'Infinite-Gate Pulse-Doppler.'. Velocity profiles from the system are shown in Figure 7. At the left we see the profile from the jugular vein; and, to the right, a profile from the common carotid. The vein appears to be small because the transducer was compressing it. This instrument can be used to make any of the types of Doppler scans shown in Figure 5 by intensity modulating an oscilloscope with the output voltage.

The Infinite-Gate Pulse-Doppler system can be used in a unique fashion in combination with the continuous-wave system to produce biplane images. Figure 8 shows the scan format. The c-w image is saved on the oscilloscope and used to guide te pulse-Doppler transducer along the vessel. The scan format of the pulse-Doppler thus presents a side view of the selected branch of the carotid. Conventional transverse sections (see Figure 5) are also possible as an aid in locating the bifurcation.

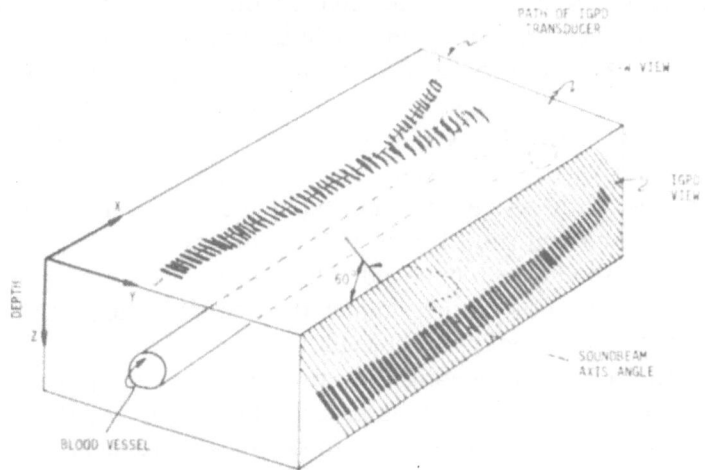

Figure 8. Shows the scan format of the Infinite-Gate Pulse-Doppler when combined with the continuous-wave system to produce bi-plane images.

The basic limitation of all pulse-Doppler systems is that the repetition frequency of the pulse-echo system must be higher than the highest Doppler frequency which can be recorded. This sets an upper limit on the maximum Doppler frequency that can be obtained from any particular depth. For propagation in average soft tissue this restriction can be stated:

$$\text{Doppler Frequency in KHz} = \frac{39}{\text{range, in cm}}$$

This absolute maximum Doppler frequency is not reached in most practical cases. Functioning pulse-Doppler flowmeters have a practical upper limit given by:

$$\text{Doppler Frequency in KHz} = \frac{13}{\text{range, in cm}}, \text{ approximately.}$$

This restriction is fairly severe. For a 2 cm range, 6.5 KHz is the maximum Doppler frequency and for 10 cm of range, 1.3 KHz. The only practical way to overcome the limitation on recordable flow velocity is to use a very low frequency ultrasonic wave which will lower the frequency of the spectrum, but with attendant loss of spatial resolution.

Pulse-Doppler flow measuring and imaging systems are fairly old. The first clinical results on imaging arteries by this means appeared in 1971 under the authorship of D.E. Strandness, Jr. and E. Hokanson, of the University of Washington and Seattle Veterans Hospital. This system used five range gates and used an unfocussed 4 mm diameter probe with a manual scan and manually set range gates. A group of about 70 patients was done in a pilot study, although this effort was not reported medically for almost two years afterwards. There has been no rush to clinical use of this system, although a second group at the University of Iowa under Dr. Barnes has been reporting results. A basically similar system with more than 20 gates was built by Peter Fish at Kings College Hospital in London. This system has been applied mainly to occlusive disease of the legs, and I am not aware of reports of clinical findings. Both systems are now commercially available, from Hokanson personally, and from the British G.E. Company.

A third group should be mentioned, whose focus is directed toward obtaining absolute volume flow figures, rather than simple detection and localization of stenosis. The group is directed by James Meindl of the Stanford University Electrical Engineering Department, with the project leadership provided by Hottinger. These efforts appear still to be in the laboratory stage. Finally, a single gate pulse-Doppler without imaging capability is obtainable from Advanced Technology Laboratories, Bellevue, Washington. They have 3 MHz units for listening to flow within the heart and a 5 MHz peripheral vascular unit. They provide the basic A-mode display with indication of the position of their single sampling gate.

4. B-MODE SCANNER/PULSE-DOPPLER COMBINATION

A number of combinations of these two advanced techniques have been proposed to overcome the limitation of B-mode scanners. These techniques all add the Doppler information to the output of the system. In all cases the Doppler system operates at a lower speed than the B-mode scanner. *Only the B-mode imaging is 'real-time.'* The step of adding the Doppler information requires a searching step to position the Doppler listening region within the vessels and produce a recordable output.

SKIN

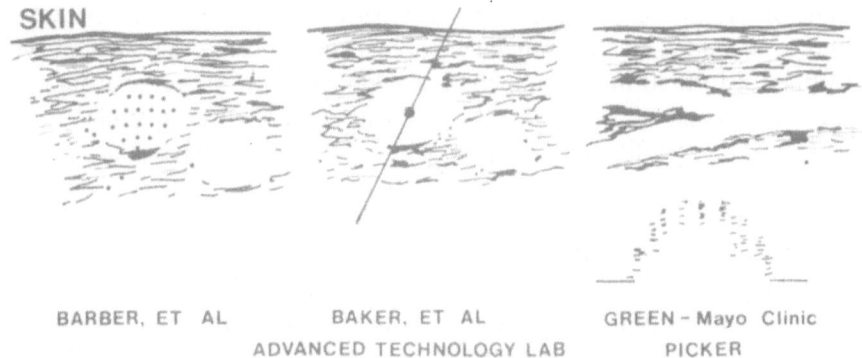

BARBER, ET AL   BAKER, ET AL   GREEN – Mayo Clinic
              ADVANCED TECHNOLOGY LAB   PICKER

Figure 9. Combined B-mode Pulse-Echo and Pulse-Doppler Systems.

Common features of these systems are the use of an automatic scanner to form the B-mode image and a manual setting of the range gates to obtain the Doppler information. The scan formats differ, and are sketched in Figure 9.

The first system was developed by Barber, using Reid and Tomey's basic scanner. A five gate pulse-Doppler transducer separate from the B-mode transducer was stepped across the scan field, producing a line of Doppler information every half second. The Doppler field was filled in with a series of rectangular dots in a small fraction of a minute. The system was built at the University of Washington, and did not receive any reported clinical trials.

The University of Washington system has been redesigned using digital circuitry by Dr. Brandestini. The result is to produce a duplex system which has 256 range gates. The research· system has been coupled with a color display for simultaneous presentation of fixed echoes and moving blood. The display appears similar to the left hand image of Figure 9, except that the Doppler dots are very close together.

A system built by Baker, Daigle and others of the University of Washington Bioengineering group is available as the ATL Duplex Scanner. Its scan format is shown at the center of the figure. A single gate pulse-Doppler is provided by a separate transducer fixed within the scanning housing. The whole scan unit must be positioned laterally to place the diagonal line indicating the axis of the Doppler beam over the structure of interest. The range gate can then be adjusted to be within the region of interest for listening to a single channel of flow information. Although manually positioning the whole scanning head appears to be awkward, they have an excellent mechanical design which is quite lightweight and easily manipulated.

The system which is close to use and commercial available (Picker) is that built at Stanford Research Institute by Green for clinical trials at the Mayo Clinic. This system has separate B-mode and Doppler outputs as shown on the right of the figure. Some marker such as the slant range line of Baker is planned to be added to the B-mode section to indicate the region from which the Doppler information is obtained. The Doppler information appears on the second oscilloscope in the form of a velocity profile display from 20 range gates. This is a systolic gated display which requires averaging of about ten heartbeats to obtain one velocity profile. It has not yet been reported exactly how the Doppler probe is moved with respect to the mechanical B-scanner if, indeed, this is the plan. Because of the size and weight of the mechanical scanning head, the present unit requires mounting on a dental x-ray arm to the wall of the examining room. Only the B-mode scanner has received extensive clinical trials and has shown that it can detect plaque under some conditions. The question of detectability of soft fatty plaques by this system has not been discussed.

5. CONCLUSIONS

It is clear from the experience of the many clinicians using Doppler systems that such systems are essential to obtaining complete physiological information on the extent and significance of cerebrovascular disease. The Institute development program is thus geared to improving the utility of Doppler information. We are trying to make it more accurate and more easily obtained. At the same time, some additional geometrical information would be very useful, primarily that showing the actual location of the bifurcation. Various pulse-Doppler systems under development by ourselves and others appear to be able to answer this question. Such instruments cannot be used *alone* to perform the Doppler evaluation because of their high-frequency limit which would miss many stenoses. A practical alternative is to switch a pulse-Doppler system to perform as a continuous-wave system to complete the examination. B-mode, real time imagers appear to have a real place in investigating research questions such as the reversibility of small plaques. Their applicability to present day clinical judgments is much less certain since minimal plaquing or cratering on the wall, even in the presence of symptoms, is generally not subject to operation. The rather high cost of these instruments also appears to limit their use in the average clinic.

The future holds many developments in the combined use of pulse- and continuous-wave Doppler, as well as B-mode imaging, together with color displays of the Doppler and waveform information. We believe the Institute of Applied Physiology and Medicine is in the forefront of these developments and plans to make all future devices completely compatible with the existing continuous-wave scanners.

6. TECHNIQUE OF DOPPLER EXAMINATION

MERRILL P. SPENCER, M.D.

A high level of expertise is required on the part of the technician to fully utilize the capability of Doppler ultrasound and to arrive at an accurate diagnosis. It is necessary that the interpreting physician have a thorough understanding of the hemodynamics of the circulation, in order to direct the technician to the information that is required for the interpretation. Close and frequent communication between the technician and the physician is necessary to develop a physician-technician team, so that the patient can benefit from the high level of skill of the technician and the broad and deep perception of the physician. The physician should gain sufficient familiarity with the techniques of Doppler examination, that he or she can perform the test and be aware of the difficulties that the technician encounters.

The purpose of this chapter is to disclose the technique for obtaining diagnostic Doppler signals from the extracranial cerebral circulation. The detailed explanation of the diagnostic qualities is discussed in other chapters throughout this text. The complete noninvasive cerebrovascular examination, as developed by Brockenbrough and Spencer, including pertinent history and physical examination, as well as a detailed Doppler examination, can be performed by skilled technicians in 30 to 60 minutes. The trainee should schedule 1½ hours, but should not detain the patient longer, because impatience and fatigue will deteriorate the quality of the information. Generally, experience with 100 patient examinations is required to develop confidence in how to handle and solve the many problems which will be met. The level of skill developed by the specialized Doppler technician often exceeds that of other medical technician specialties and the technician should be rewarded for learning to make the decisions which are required in a successful examination.

At the time that the patient's appointment is made, the patient should be advised that the examination requires no special preparation, that it will cause no pain and carries no special danger. At the time of the appointment, the technician should explain what will occur, and approach the examination with a positive attitude.

All Doppler examinations can be performed with the patient in the supine position, but many of the subroutines may be performed in the sitting

Table 1. Non-invasive cerebrovascular evaluation: patient examination routines and subroutines.

Routines	Key	Doppler subroutines
A. History		
Name, age & sex		
Chief complaint		
Previous stroke or TIA		
Aphasia, motor or concept		
Weakness, paresis		
Numbness or tingling	If amaurosis	(1)
Visual disturbance	If amaurosis	(1)
Dizzyness		
Vertigo, imbalance and syncope	If vertebro-basilar	(3)(4) and (5)
Confusion, loss of memory		
Diabetes, hypertension, smoking, heart disease		
Claudication	If claudication	(6)
Medications, angiograms		
Vascular surgery		
B. Physical Examination		
Speech		
Facial weakness		
Leg, arm and grip		
Pulses – radial	If weak or lag	(3)
Temporals and carotids	If unilateral weakness	(7)
Brachial artery	If difference	(3) (8) (4) and (5)
Pressures	or unobtainable	
Ascultation		
Carotid bifurcations		If bruit (1)
Low common carotid	If bruit	(5)
Supraclavicular	If bruit	(3) (4) and (5)
Upper chest	If bruit	(3) and (4)
Eyelids	If bruit	(1)
C. Doppler Routines Right and Left		
Hand-held vertebral artery		
Anterior supraclavicular	If Rv or biphasic	(4)
Base of skull	If Sy or biphasic	
Ophthalmic artery posterior orbit	If LF, BD, or SA	(1) and (9)
	If internal HF or NS	(1) and (9)
	If HF in CC	(1) (7) and (9)
	If Fl in CC	(5)
	If signals unclear	(1) (2) and (9)
Carotid imaging	or if incomplete image	

Legend

Sy = systolic (low diastolic runoff; LF = low frequency, HF = high frequency)
Rv = Reversed from normal direction; Biphasic = reversal of direction within each pulse
Bd = Bidirectional (either towards or away from probe)
SA = Slow acceleration (damped)
NS = Non sounding (no Doppler signal found)
CC = Common carotid artery

Table 2. Doppler subroutines.

1. Periorbital Doppler with compressions
2. Hand-held carotid signals
3. Subclavian, axillary and brachial signals
4. Vertebral steal reactive hyperemia test
5. 'Down imaging' of common and vertebral
6. Pedal systolic pressures
7. Temporal flow signals
8. Brachial systolic pressures
9. Common carotid compressions

position. The sequence of the examination is not critical, but in routine handling of patients and in transferring of the information to the interpreting physician, it is important that the test be performed in a consistent manner. Our experience has led us to begin with the hand-held Doppler techniques performing the imaging of the carotid bifurcations towards the end of the examination. The final few minutes should be used for subroutines, which may clarify and reconfirm the important findings. Tables 1 and 2 outline the routines and subroutines as well as indicate key findings which trigger the necessity for Doppler subroutines.

1. HAND-HELD DOPPLER TECHNIQUES

1.1. Examination of the vertebral arteries

The Doppler vertebral signals may be detected in three locations: posterior at the base of the skull, anterior in the supraclavicular position, and along the spine in the midspinal position. The midspinal postion is best utilized at the time of Doppler imaging. Signals from the anterior vertebral artery can be detected with a shallow focusing probe (10 MHz is a useful frequency) just above the clavicle as the artery enters the ostium of the sixth lateral process (Figure 1a). The patient's head is turned slightly to the opposite side and the probe pressed behind the sternocleidomastoide muscle, which is moved by medial pressure on the probe towards the midline and the probe pressed deeply into the neck. It is helpful to locate the position of the common carotid signal before deep probing for the vertebral in order to avoid confusion with the common carotid. The probe shaft should be directed at approximately a 45° angle with the axis of the body in a headward direction.

Confirmation of the source of the Doppler signal, being in fact from the low cervical vertebral, can be assured by a technique developed by Von Reutern (1980). While listening to the supposed lower vertebral artery, a series of rapid vibrations are made with the fingers of the free hand in the post-mastoid space at the base of the skull. This maneuver vibrates the

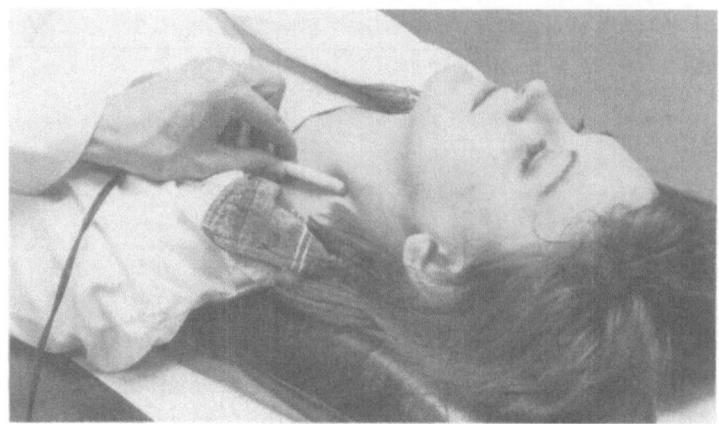

Figure 1a. Positioning of the 10 MHz probe for detecting anterior vertebral signals.

vertebral artery at the base of the skull and superimposes a series of slow oscillations which can be heard at the low neck position to confirm the signal in the low neck as in fact from the vertebral artery.

The quality of the vertebral Doppler signals at the anterior inferior position exhibits a pulsatile component which varies considerably from subject to subject. It may be highly pulsatile with no diastolic runoff similar to the external carotid signal. This difference is presumably because of the variation in muscular supply of branches of the vertebral artery above this position. The direction of the signal is not entirely reliable, but a reversed flow direction may represent a vertebral-to-subclavian artery steal.

The posterior vertebral artery velocity signal at the base of the skull can be located with the deep focusing 5 MHz probe placed behind the mastoid bone and directing the ultrasonic beam medially and slightly superior towards the foramen magnum (Figure 1b). The patient's head is turned slightly to the opposite side. With patience, slow rotation and 'flashlighting' of the probe beam, the signal from the vertebral artery as it courses through its loop before entering the foramen will be detected with a quality of low pulsatility and high diastolic flow very similar to the qualities of the internal carotid artery. At this point the vertebral artery flow is normally supplying only the basilar artery in parallel with the vertebral of the opposite side. Firm pressure should be applied in order to assure compression of the occipital artery which may lie more superficial in the path of the ultrasound beam. Qualities of the occipital artery display high pulsatility similar to an extracranial artery that supplies extracranial structures. If the quality of the signal detected in the base-of-the-skull position changes with probe pressure, the signal detected is prob-

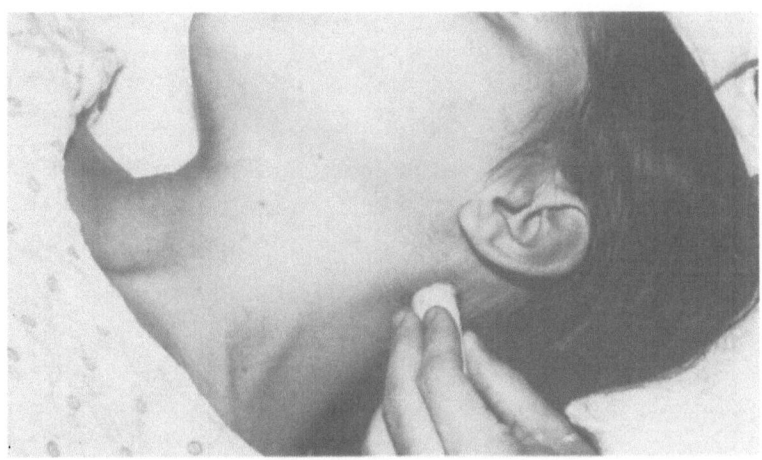

Figure 1b. Placement of the 5 MHz lens probe for detecting artery signal from the vertebral artery at the base of the skull.

ably that of the occipital artery and not the vertebral which is more difficult to occlude in its deep coursing position.

1.2. The subclavian, axillary, brachial and radial artery signals

These subroutines are performed when indicated by complaints of the patient suggestive of thoracic outlet syndrome, when there is a suspicion of subclavian or innominate artery obstruction generally indicated by a difference in systolic arm pressures of greater than 10 mm of mercury, by a bruit whose maximum intensity is in the supraclavicular region, or by symptoms of vertebral basilar insufficiency.

The subclavian artery signal is found behind the medial end of the clavicle by placing the probe in the supraclavicular position and directing the sound beam inferior and medial in direction (Figure 2a). Subclavian signals are characterized by strong and high degrees of pulsatility with a sharp acceleration, marked backflow phase and extremely small diastolic flow.

The axillary artery signal is detected below the clavicle in the notch between the clavicle and the head of the humerus (Figure 2b). The probe is directed posterior in a slightly lateral direction and after detecting the arterial pulsations should be maneuvered carefully to bring out the maximum backflow phase obtainable. The characteristics of the axillary are very similar to the subclavian artery signal. Abnormal characteristics to be observed here are fluttering qualities of turbulence during peak systolic flow, absent backflow and low frequency systolic components with elevated diastolic runoff.

The brachial artery signal can be detected at the elbow just above the antecubital fold and anterior to the medial condyle. The normal brachial

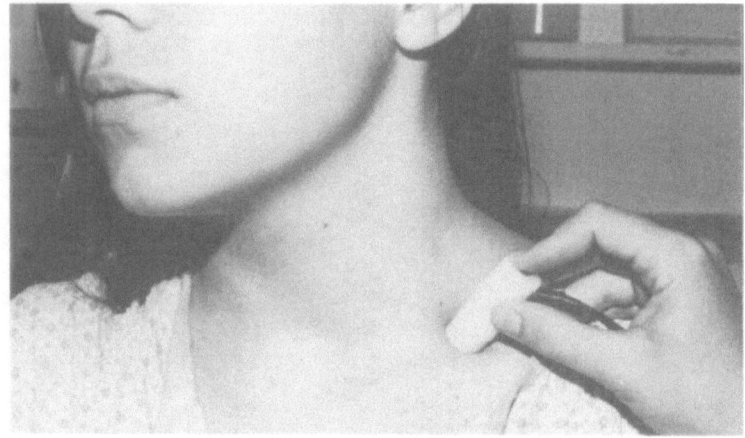

Figure 2 a. Position used to find the signal of the proximal subclavian artery.

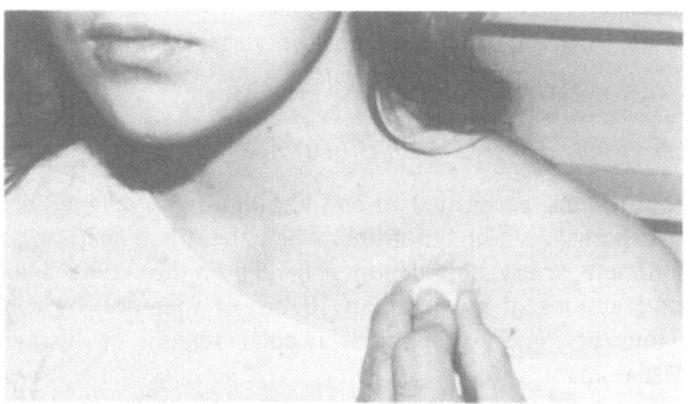

Figure 2b. Placement of 5 MHz probe for detecting the axillary artery signals below the clavical.

signal is similar to the subclavian and axillary with a high pulsatility, strong backflow phase in early diastole and low diastolic runoff in the resting arm. Hemodynamically significance obstruction of the subclavian or innominate artery will produce lower pulsatility, lower systolic velocities; reduction or elimination of the backflow phase, and elevation of the diastolic runoff to the end of the cardiac cycle. The direction of the probe is optional but it should be angled at approximately 30° with the axis of the artery. The choice of the direction here of course will influence the polarity indicated on the analog strip chart tracings. The radial artery signal is detected at the wrist and also displays characteristics similar to the brachial artery. A higher level of diastolic runoff in the radial artery is normal but the dicrotic notch at the time of the backflow phase is strong. The brachial and radial artery signals are best detected with the shallow focusing 10 MHz probe.

1.3. Vertebral-to-subclavian steal subroutine

This examination is performed if a steal is suspected, if there is more than 10 mm of mercury pressure difference between the two arms, or if there is a

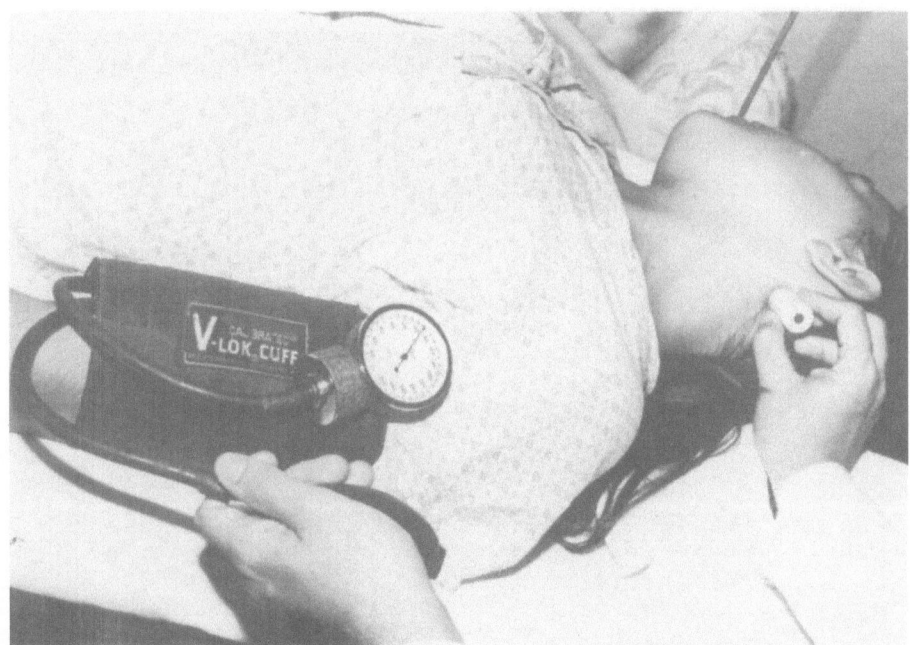

Figure 3. Technician demonstrating the technique used to perform the vertebral-to-subclavian subroutine.

bruit in the supraclavicular region (Figure 3). The test may be performed utilizing the Doppler signals from either the anterior, posterior or midneck positions, but the posterior position at the base of the skull is preferable because the vertebral signal there is generally more reliable in representing the vertebral artery. If the steal syndrome can be demonstrated to effect the flow at this position, it may be of greater clinical significance. Utilization of the anterior vertebral signal is least reliable because if the vertebral is in fact occluded on the side of the examination, collateral developments may provide a signal which is incorrectly assumed to represent the vertebral artery. Steal, of course, may be detected in any branch of the subclavian artery beyond an hemodynamically significant obstruction.

The principle of the test for vertebral steal depends on detecting a significant change in the vertebral artery velocity produced by a sudden drop in subclavian artery pressure. The pressure drop is produced by eliciting a reactive hyperemia response in the arm (Figure 4). The hyperemia is produced by ischemia resulting from occlusion of the subclavian artery and exercise of the forearm musculature. A standard blood pressure cuff is applied to the upper arm on the side suspected of vertebral steal or subclavian obstruction.

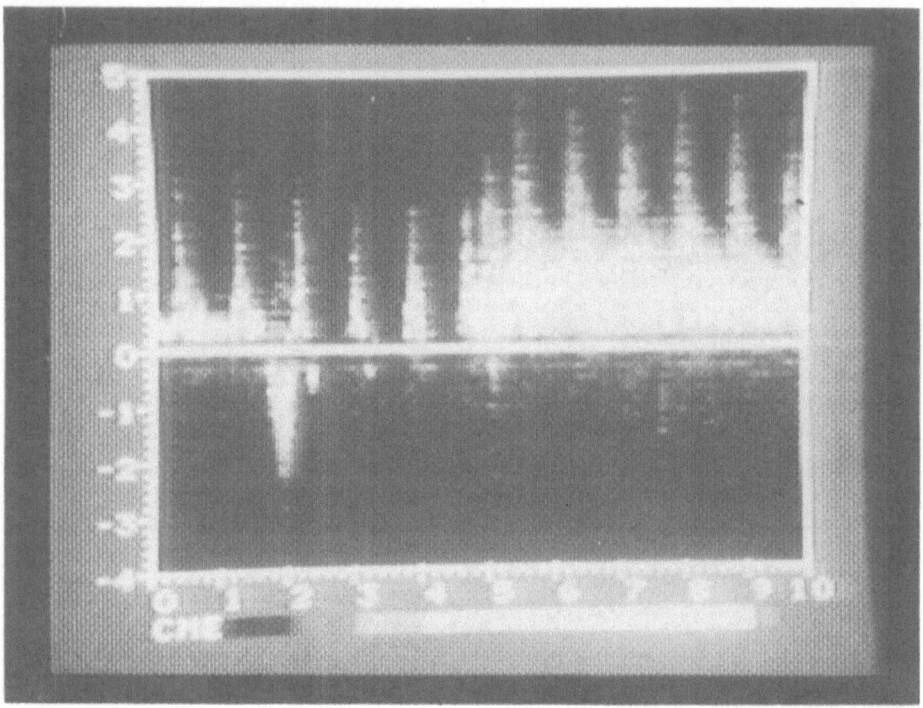

Figure 4. Bidirectional Doppler Spectrum of brachial artery signals and reactive hyperemia response following fist clenching. At 2 seconds a venous pulse produces a negative spectrum upon clenching. At 4.5 seconds the fist is released followed by high diastolic flow of hyperemia. (See chapter 15 for further details on the display).

The vertebral artery signal is located with the Doppler probe and a sample of that signal documented on the magnetic and strip chart recorders as a control. The cuff is then inflated to 10–20 mm above the systolic blood pressure and held in the inflated position for three to five minutes. During the final 30 seconds of the cuff inflation, the patient is asked to vigorously grip and release the fist on the side of examination. Periodic examinations, at one-minute intervals, during cuff inflation reconfirm the position of the Doppler signal, and provide further control for the deflation signals and also may indicate a meaningful change from the pre-inflation signal. The signals of most value are those which are recorded immediately prior, during and after rapid deflation of the cuff.

A subclavian steal from the interrogated artery may be diagnosed if the Doppler frequencies are increased at the time of the deflation maneuver. Any change in the signal, in form or direction, during cuff inflation or deflation indicates that a hemodynamically significant subclavian or innominate obstruction is present and affecting vertebral blood flow even though a steal may in fact not be present. Many subleties of vertebral flow aberrations caused by subclavian obstruction have been defined by Pourcelot and Von Reutern (1978).

The clinical and patient significance of vertebral steal should be ascertained at the time of this examination by eliciting the hyperemia response. Additional time, with the patient in the recumbent positon and sitting the patient up immediately following release of the cuff (Figure 4). If no symptoms are produced or if symptoms of vertebral basilar insufficiency are not exacerbated by this maneuver, the steal is probably not of clinical significance and surgical repair of the subclavian obstruction will probably not benefit the patient. If, however, the patient has symptoms prior to the test and these symptoms are exacerbated by cuff deflation and change when in the sitting position, the steal is probably significant and surgical repair by grafting or endarterectomy may ameliorate the symptoms.

1.4. Examination of the ophthalmic artery in the posterior orbit

The ophthalmic artery signals are detected in the posterior orbit by placing the deep focusing 5 MHz lens probe over the closed eyelid and directing the ultrasonic beam through the eyeball at an angle of 10 to 15 degrees from the midline plane (Figure 5). The patient is requested to direct their gaze towards the opposite side in order to remove the lens of the eye from the path of the sound beam. The lens is a strong acoustical absorber and weakens the returning Doppler signal. For additional safety, the jelly should be applied directly to the probe and not to the eyelid itself. The maximum signal can be elicited by slowly rotating the probe through small angular variations or by sliding the probe a few millimeters on the eyelid. If there is difficulty in obtaining an adequate signal, the probe should be angled in a superior position to find the ophthalmic artery as it may be coursing closer to the roof of the orbit. The signal should not be picked up with the probe angle greater than 30° from the midline plane as this wide angulation may lead to unreliable directional indications.

The qualities of the normal ophthalmic signal are very similar to those of the internal carotid artery with a low pulsatility and high diastolic runoff. The

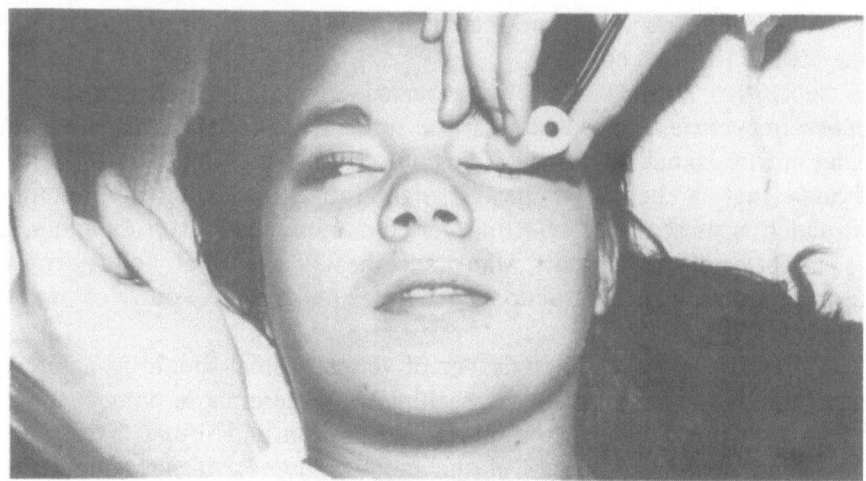

Figure 5. Placement of the 5 MHz probe for examination of the ophthalmic artery signal in the posterior orbit.

frequencies represent velocities similar to those in the internal carotid and the direction of the signal is anterior towards the probe. Other qualities of importance are the amplitude of the signal and the acceleration at the beginning of systole. A strong and high frequency signal in the reverse direction away from the probe is diagnostic of significant internal carotid obstruction. Internal carotid obstruction may also produce other abnormalities though the signal may be normally directed. The posterior orbital signal may be considered abnormal if normally directed signals display low frequencies and a slow rise demonstrating a 'damped' quality. Occasionally, two directions may be detected by different probe positions. In this situation the signals may be considered normal if the normally directed signal displays normal frequency amplitude and acceleration. Though a loop in the ophthalmic artery may be the cause for bidirectional signals, such signals may represent subtle changes in flow distribution. Occasionally internal carotid obstruction will by means of collaterals maintain anterior directed signals in the posterior orbit, while in the anterior orbit the external carotid provides retrograde flow. A careful search should be made for the best quality signals obtainable.

1.5. The periorbital examination

In Chapter 11, the periorbital collaterals are discussed in detail by Dr. Brockenbrough, who first conceived of the utilization of the Doppler probe for detecting evidence of collateral circulation to internal carotid obstruction. This

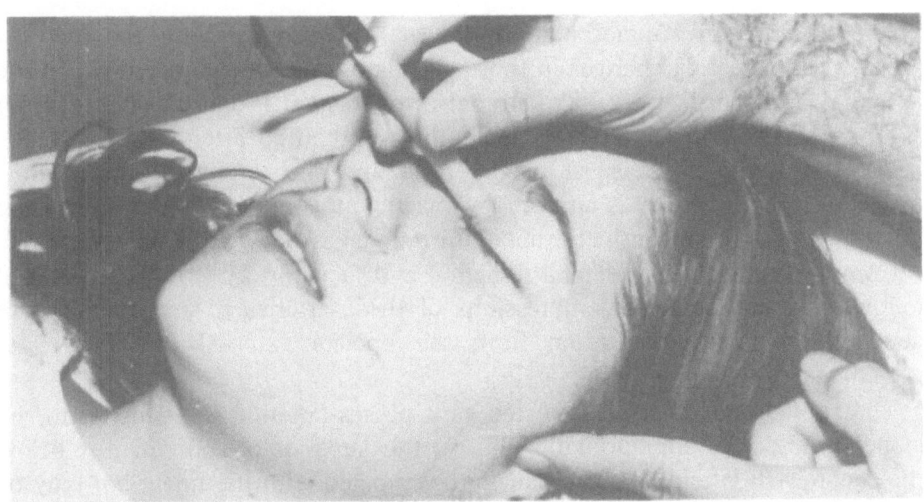

Figure 6a. Probe placement for examining the frontal artery. For this procedure it is necessary to use the shallow focusing probe.

section will discuss only the technical aspects of performing the periorbital examination. The periorbital examination is performed if there are abnormalities suggesting carotid obstruction in either the posterior orbital examination or in the carotid bifurcation image.

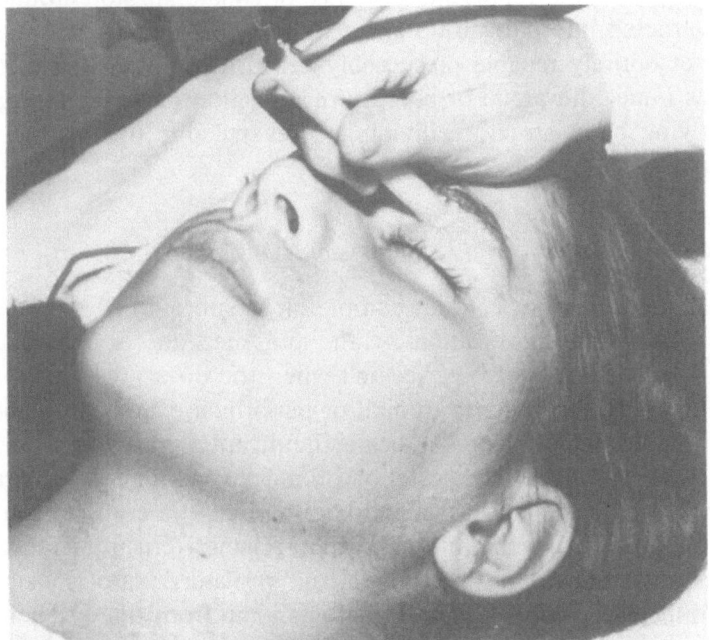

Figure 6b. Probe placement for examining the supraorbital artery.

The frontal and supraorbital arteries are interrogated with the Doppler probe while detecting changes in those signals by selective compression of the temporal and facial artery. The frontal artery signal is located at the inner canthus of the eye as it arises from the ophthalmic artery to supply the tissues on the medial aspect of the nose and the forehead. The shallow focusing 10 MHz probe is utilized by placing it gently over the artery and maneuvering slightly until the maximum signal is detected (Figure 6a).

Compression of the ipsilateral temporal and facial artery is then carried out followed by contralateral compressions of these arteries if abnormalities are detected or if collateralization from the oposite external carotid is suspected.

The supraorbital artery is detected as it passes anterior and superior to the globe through the supraorbital notch on the superior orbital rim just below the eyebrow (Figure 6b). It can usually be palpated with the finger but may be detected with the Doppler probe even if not palpable. The probe beam should be directed well under the orbital rim but taking care not to detect the palpebral artery signal in the eyelid. As is in the case with the frontal artery, compressions of the ipsilateral, temporal and facial artery will in the normal subject either produce no change in the signal or will cause an augmentation of the signal direction and frequency in normal anterior direction towards the probe. Obliteration, diminishment or a change in direction is considered an abnormal response and represents evidence of collateralizaton around a significantly obstructed internal carotid artery. The initial direction of the detected signal is not entirely reliable presumably because of angulation of the artery as it passes under the probe or because of reflection of the sound beam from the underlying bony structure dividing a reverse direction pathway for the sound beam.

1.6. Unilateral common carotid compression subroutines

The unilateral common carotid compression subroutine is performed in selected cases where clarification of the presence and source of collateral pathways is needed. It is also performed when the DOPSCAN findings appear to be in conflict with the posterior orbital or periorbital examination signals. For example, when Doppler signals indicate significant stenosis or total occlusion of the internal carotid while posterior orbital signals and periorbital signals appear normally directed, contralateral common carotid compression can confirm that the normal ophthalmic signals are arising from intracranial collaterals and that significant obstruction of the ipsilateral carotid exists. If the normally directed posterior orbital signal is arising from the ipsilateral carotid, it would be considerably diminished or obliterated by ipsilateral compression.

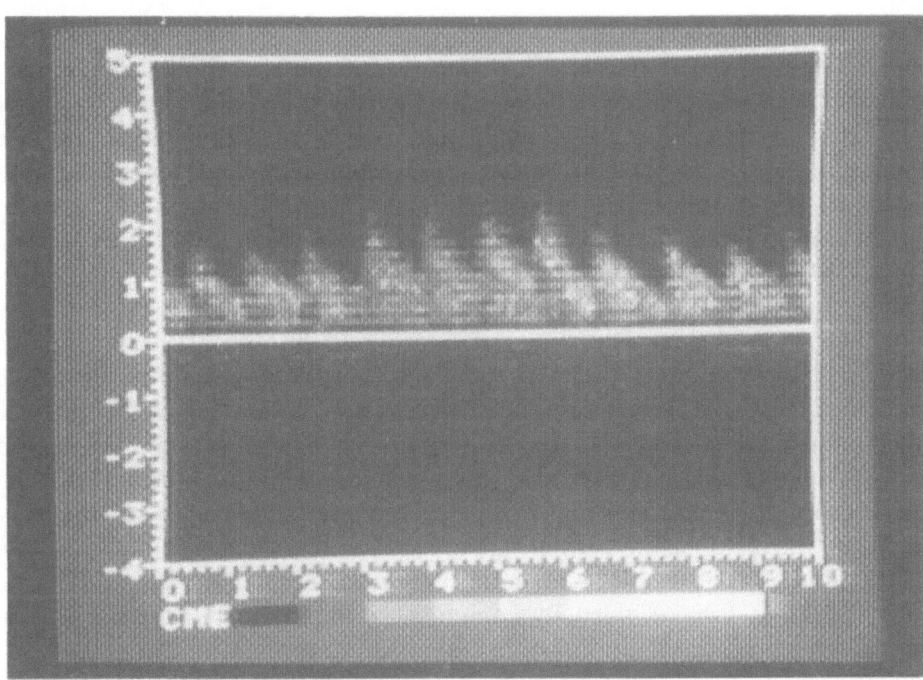

Figure 7. Spectral display of posterior vertebral artery signals augmented by common carotid compression in a normal 25-year-old female.

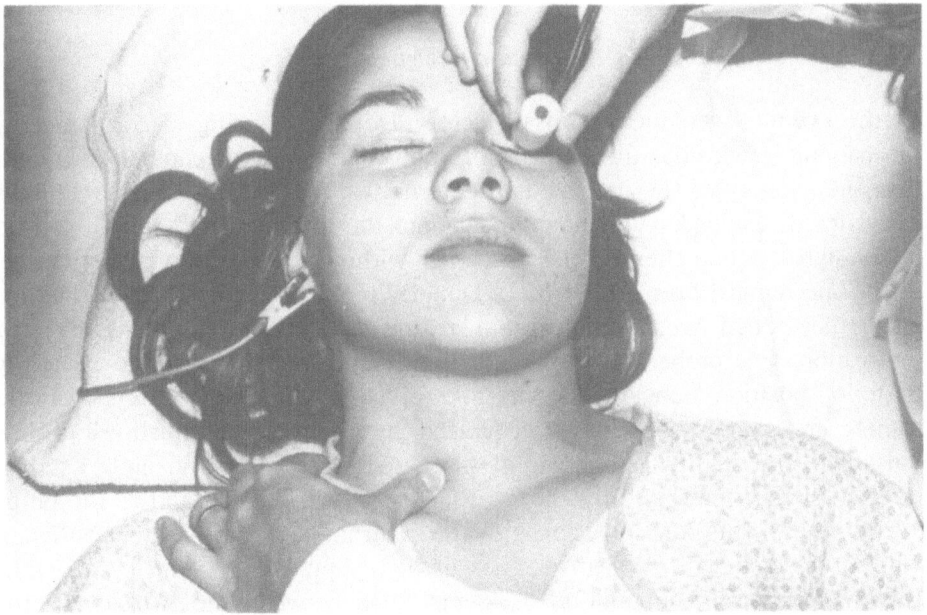

Figure 8. Technician demonstrating proper placement of 5 MHz lens probe, ear pulse detector, and hand placement for doing common carotid compression.

Carotid collateralization from the basilar artery can be established by Doppler probing of the vertebral artery at the base of the skull while compressing either carotid artery. Many subjects demonstrate augmentation of the vertebral artery signal upon carotid compression establishing the basilar artery as a collateral channel for carotid obstructions, establishing the presence of connections through the Circle of Willis (Figure 7).

The safest procedure for common carotid compression involves several important components. The carotid should never be compressed at the bifurcation but should be compressed low in the neck where it first becomes palpable above the clavicle (Figure 8). Compression and release should be performed slowly and held for two to four heartbeats while monitoring the ipsilateral ear pulse. When confronted with special cases such as low bifurcations and bilateral stenoses, it is recommended that no attempt at carotid compression be made by the technician until discussing the problem with the supervising physician. Persons should be carefully qualified by expert physicians in the field before authorization for carotid compression maneuvers. Utilization of the ear pulse monitor provides both confirmation that the carotid was in fact occluded by compression and decreases the number of compressions necessary to complete the examination. Compression may be utilized while interrogating either or both the posterior orbital signals or the periorbital signals.

1.7. Hand-held assessment of the carotid signals

In the event of technically unsatisfactory Doppler imaging or for screening the patient at bedside, the hand-held Doppler subroutines can serve to confirm the patency of the internal and external carotid arteries. It is sometimes easier for the skilled technicians to separate the internal and external carotid artery signals when they lie close together without the positioning limitations of the mechanical arm. The 5 MHz Doppler probe is removed from the arm and is positioned over the bifurcation region at a position slightly above the bifurcation. The probe is angled medial and superior and moved to a slightly posterior position beneath the mastoid process where the internal carotid signals are sought. They are recognized by their typical qualities of low pulsatility and high diastolic runoff discussed elsewhere. The probe is then directed slightly anterior and the internal signal will be lost, and as the probe is continued in its rotation signals of the external carotid or a branch thereof will be detected with typical qualities of higher pulsatility with low diastolic runoff. By repeated angulation back and forth between the two signals the operator can often assure himself that the internal signal is indeed patent. The hand-held examination of the external and internal is not recommended for a substitution for bifurcation imaging because such 'blind' probing does not allow a systematic search of the bifurcation and the all-important origin of the internal carotid artery (Figure 9a).

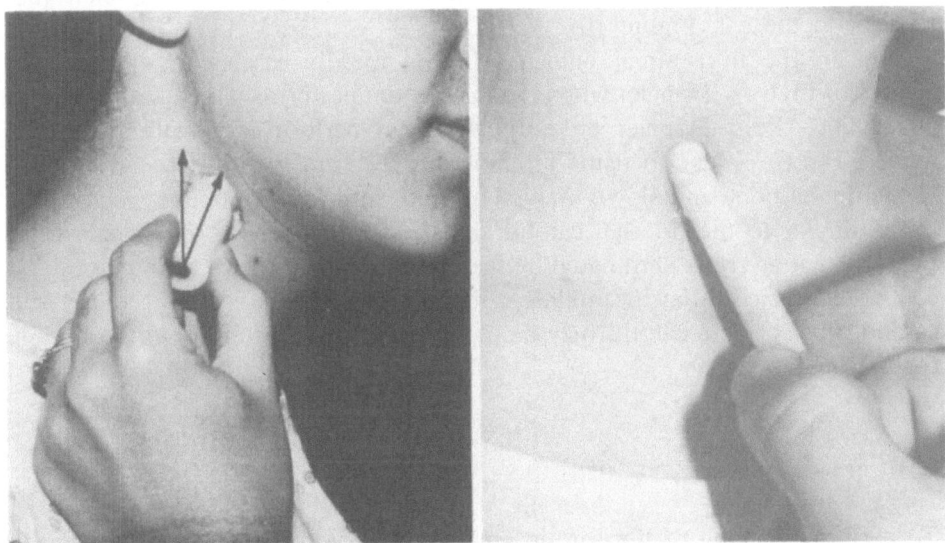

Figure 9a and b. Demonstration of hand-held technique for examining the external, internal, and common carotid arteries when technical difficulties arise in the development of the Doppler images.

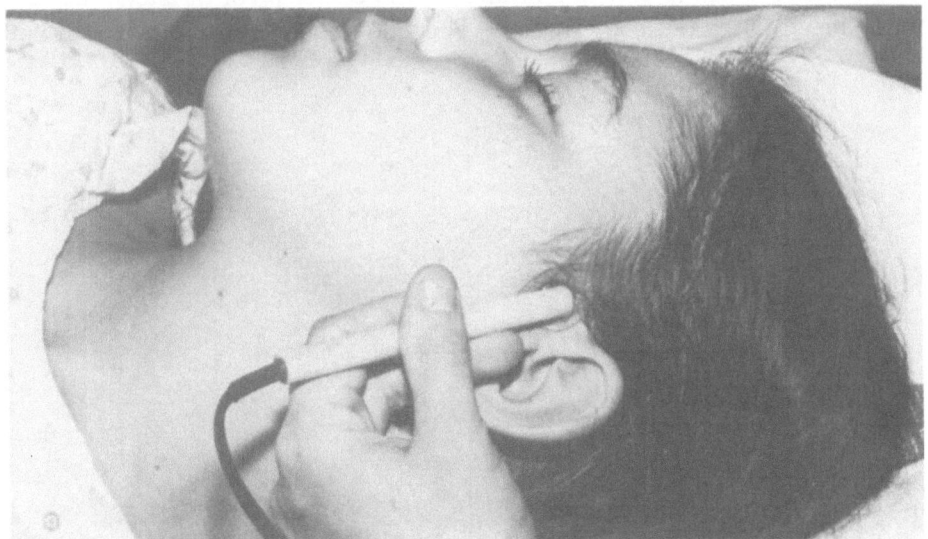

Figure 10. Doppler probing of the temporal artery with a 10 MHz probe.

The common carotid signal may also be obtained by hand holding the Doppler probe as shown in Figure 9b. Also of value in determining the hemodynamic state of the common carotid or the external carotid is Doppler probing of the temporal artery as it passes over the zygomatic arch just anterior to the ear (Figure 10).

Flow in the intracranial branches of the middle cerebral artery may be detected with C-W Doppler when the instrument performs with a high signal to noise ratio. (Pulse-Doppler presently does not perform well with this technique.) The C-W lens-focusing probe is pressed firmly against the scalp over the temporal bone and slowly moved around until a continuous type signal is heard similar to the internal carotid signal. Confusion with the signals from the temporal artery is eliminated by firm pressure on the face of the probe. To confirm suspicions that the middle cerebral artery source is from the opposite carotid, the opposite carotid may be compressed while listening to the middle cerebral artery signal.

2. DOPPLER IMAGING TECHNIQUES

To perform imaging of the carotid and vertebral vessels the patient is placed recumbent on a table with a firm bed (Figure 11). The chin is lifted and the cervical spine supported by comfortable padding behind the neck. In order for the body to relax into a stable position careful attention to the physical comfort and mental ease of the patient should be taken. The mechanical arm is suspended over the patient's head with the center pivot or lateral displacement directly over the body midline. This allows a 10° angle of the arm with

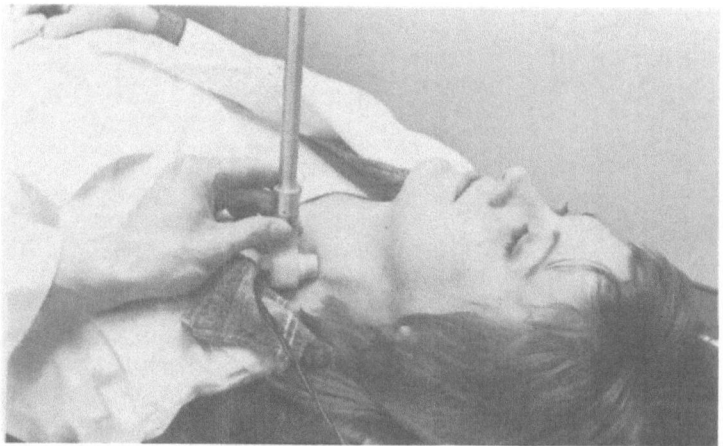

Figure 11. Position of the scanning arm for development of the Doppler image.

the surface of the table and the cornal planes of the body. The patient's chin is directed by 10° towards the opposite side. This arrangement usually gives maximum separation between the external and internal carotid arteries. The probe is mounted on the lower end of the arm with the sound beam directed at a 60° angle from the body axis or 30° from a perpendicular point to the arteries providing a cosine function of 0.5 when computing blood velocities from the Doppler equation. This arrangement approximates a lateral projection of the carotid bifurcation.

The carotid bifurcation is centered on the imaging screen by moving the probe mount controls so that the area between the clavical and the mandible are represented by the inferior-superior swing of the arm and the common carotid signal is represented in the middle of the anterior-posterior range of the image. Sound coupling jelly should be applied to the skin. Only sufficient pressure against the skin should be applied with the probe to ensure the elimination of air space. The carotid in the neck usually lie at a depth of 2 to 3 cm and run parallel to the skin surface. Because the probe positioning sensors represent only the anterior-posterior and the inferior-superior displacement and do not represent the lateral displacements, variations in skin pressure will not affect the image.

Imaging is begun using the common carotid which provides the strongest signal. Slight threshold control on the signal eliminates artifacts most of which are already reduced by the mixer in the electronic circuitry. By synchronization of probe movements with the pulse beat a cross-diameter stroke of the probe can be made with each beat while mapping slowly up the carotid channels. The internal signal as well as the differences in their audio qualities constantly monitored during the scannihg procedure. The external signal displays high pulsatility with little diastolic runoff, while the internal signal has a lower pulsatility with a high diastolic component.

Occasionally, it is difficult to determine the exact position of the bifurcation. In these instances, turn the beam switch off and reposition probe in the area of the distal internal, around the angle of the jaw. Once a strong internal signal is located, turn the beam back to the 'image' position, and proceed to image backward (posteriorly) toward the bifurcation. To locate the external, move superiorly from the distal internal signal until the more systolic external signal is intercepted. Trace this signal back to its source at the bifurcation. Where abnormal signals are detected, turn the beam switch to 'on' and draw a line on the image to show their precise location. With the beam in the on position, draw in the jawline to denote the relative location of the bifurcation. Before erasing the image, an instant picture is taken which becomes a part of the permanent record.

3. SELECTED AUDIO RECORDING

Once a Doppler image of the common carotid system is developed, make spot recordings of representative audio signals. Voice made notations on the 2nd audio channel are useful to designate the position of the probe. Finally a continuous sweep of the probe up the common-internal and common-external channels is helpful to confirm the selected recordings.

4. DOWN IMAGING

'Down imaging' is recommended for the low common carotid when: A) a bruit is heard low in the neck, and cannot be definitely attributed to the subclavian artery, and B) abnormal signals are detected low in the common carotid while 'up' imaging.

To 'down image' the low common carotid and vertebral artery as well, rotate the probe holder so the probe is directed in the inferior direction and

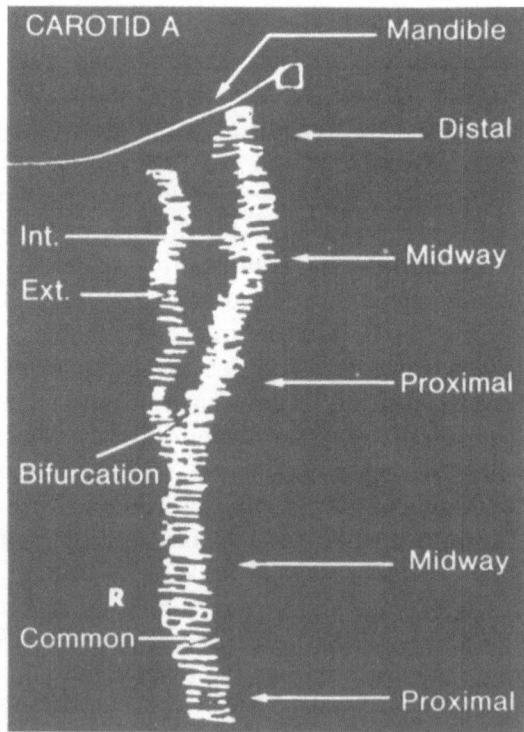

Figure 12. C-W Doppler image of the carotid bifurcation illustrating routine points for selected audio recordings.

compensate for the reversed direction by changing the signal polarity. Proceed to scan by moving in a posterior direction toward the clavicle, as far as the patient anatomy will permit. To locate the proximal vertebral, move slightly posterior, and find the vertebral 1–2 cm behind the carotids. It is often possible to image a short segment of the subclavian artery where it gives rise to the vertebral. When all signals have been identified and imaged, record the audio signals on tape and make a photograph (Figure 12).

5. PROBLEMS ASSOCIATED WITH THE DEVELOPMENT OF THE CAROTID IMAGE

Sometimes strong venous interference arises when imaging the carotid system. One method of alleviating this problem is by applying more pressure with the probe, thus obliterating the venous signal and allowing the stronger arterial signals to predominate, or by gently compressing the jugular vein distal to the probe. This problem has been alleviated by recent addition of bidirectional capability to the analogue signal. Only arterial headward flow is now imaged eliminating confusion of venous signals. Another problem associated with imaging is occasional inability to separate the internal and external arteries. A single vessel with discernible signals may be imaged to the angle of the jaw. To separate the external from the internal change the angle of the probe arm with respect to the midline plane and direct the patients chin slightly (10°) toward the opposite side.

REFERENCES

1. Von Reutern, Personal Communication, 1980.
2. Von Reutern, Pourcelot: Cardiac cycle dependent alternating flow in vertebral arteries with subclavian artery stenosis. Stroke 9(3):229-236, May-June 1976.

7. VASCULAR MURMURS

MERRILL P. SPENCER, M.D.

1. DEFINITION

Vascular murmurs, also called bruits, are audible sound, other than the normal pulse transients, generated in the arteries or veins. They usually have a random, blowing quality but may, in addition, contain a superimposed resonance.

Vascular bruits arise from vibrations of the walls of the larger vessels driven by turbulence in the blood flow streams and transmitted to the body surface where they can be detected with a stethoscope.

Stethoscopes possess two types of skin-contacting heads: the bell-type and the diaphragm-type. Both types utilize pneumatic tubes to transmit the skin vibrations to the ears. The bell-type contacts a small area of skin surface which acts as the sound transmitting 'diaphragm'. The diaphragm-type covers a broader area with a stiff membrane. The large, stiff membrane transmits a louder sound but filters out the lower bruit frequencies. The frequencies transmitted by the bell-type may be modified by pressure against the skin. A

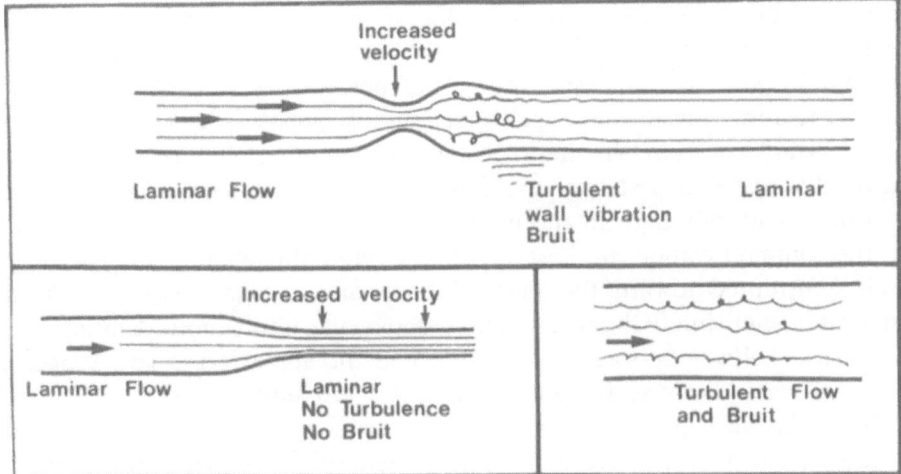

Figure 1. Three important arterial abnormalities which may or may not produce a bruit depending on the downstream channel widening.

lightly-applied bell is more sensitive to lower frequencies than is the diaphragm-type, but higher pressure will tense the skin and better transmit higher frequencies. The bell is preferred for better localization of bruits.

The most common cause of arterial bruits is a discreet narrowing (stenosis) of the blood flow channels with widening of the channel beyond the stenosis. Bruits may not be produced by narrowing of the blood channel if a downstream widening is not present. Bruits, however, may be produced in a large blood vessel by high velocity without stenosis (Figure 1).

2. MURMUR CHARACTERISTICS

The observer should evaluate and describe the following four major characteristics of all bruits:

Location and transmission
Intensity and loudness variations
Frequency and timbre
Duration and timing

3. LOCATION

The location of loudest intensity should be identified. The surrounding area of transmission of the bruit representing its spread to secondary intensities should be determined. Vascular bruits tend to spread in the direction of blood flow particularly in an arterial channel, and also are preferentially transmitted along the bones. For record-keeping, we recommend the following diagram (Figure 2) with an 'x' representing the position of loudest intensity and arrows representing the principal directions of spread over the skin surface.

Bruits arising from the internal carotid siphon at the base of the skull generally are heard best over the closed eyelid. The bruit the patient herself can hear is usually high in the internal or vertebral. Bruits at the bifurcation of the common carotid are best heard just below the angle of the jaw. If it is well transmitted toward the mastoid bone or the lobe of the ear, it may indicate a high internal carotid source above the bifurcation. A bruit in the mid-neck, halfway between the clavicle and the angle of the jaw, suggests a common carotid course but may represent a low bifurcation.

Bruits in the supraclavicular region at the medial end of the clavicle may represent subclavian or vertebral artery stenosis. Subclavian bruits may be transmitted along the axillary artery below the lateral end of the clavicle. Vertebral artery bruits tend to spread in a superior and posterior direction. Bruits in the innominate artery, at the origin of the left subclavian or in the

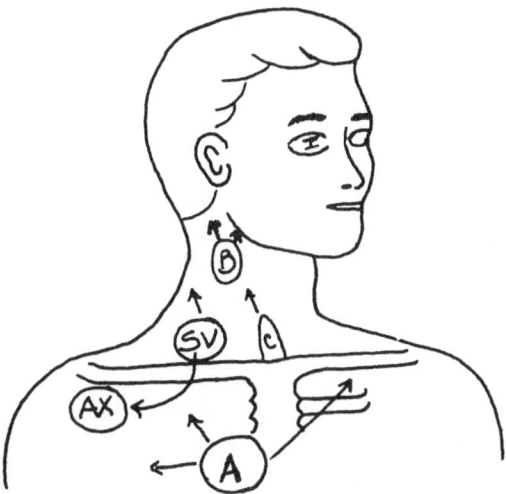

Figure 2 shows locations where bruits are heard and, illustrates their transmission mode over bone and arterial channels. B = bifurcation; C = common carotid; V = vertebral; S = subclavian; AX = axillary; A = Aorta; I = internal 'siphon'.

aortic arch, tend to be heard in the upper chest with wide rumbling quality transmission up both sides of the neck. Common carotid lesions in the neck near their origin have similar transmission modes.

4. INTENSITY

The loudness of a bruit may be clinically graded between Grade I and VI with Grade I being the barely audible bruit and Grade VI being one that can be heard with a stethoscope close to but not touching the skin. In addition, Grade VI vibrations may be felt with the fingertips in a sensation called a 'thrill.' Most bruits detected clinically of moderate loudness are designated Grade III or Grade IV, whereas Grade II or Grade V represent estimates between the two outside loudness grades and the average grade. See Figure 3.

As stenosis of an artery progresses, the loudness of the bruit tends to increase up to approximately 50% reduction in the lumen at which condition a maximum energy is released through turbulence and vessel wall vibration. This is because the volumetric flow through the stenosis is generally not compromised by this degree of obstruction, but the momentum and dissipating energy in downstream turbulence has greatly increased. With further stenosis, volumetric blood flow is reduced and the bruit becomes softer until, when the stenotic lumen is less than $\frac{1}{2}$ mm in diameter, it is difficult to detect

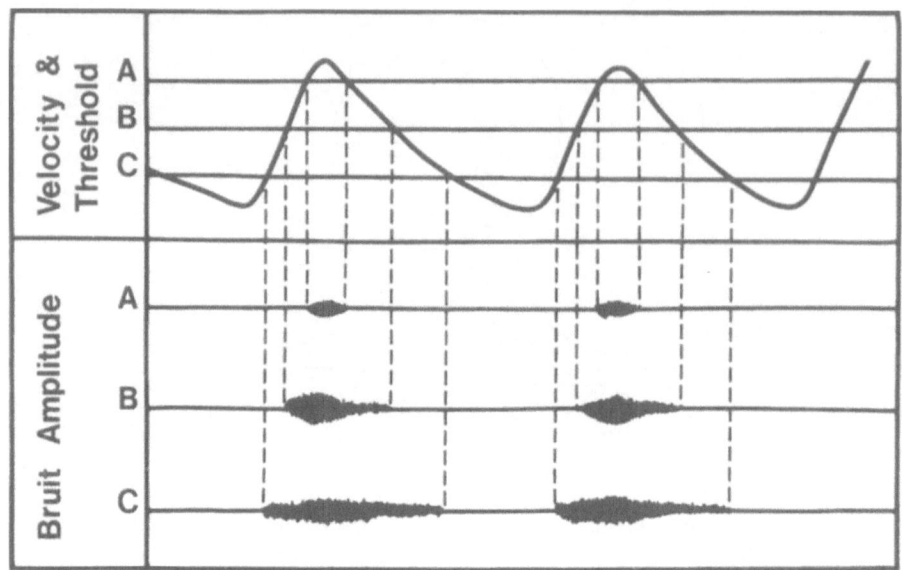

Figure 3. Diagramatic representation of how the blood turbulence threshold working on the arterial flow waveform changes the amplitude and duration of carotid bruits. 'A', 'B', and 'C' in the upper panel represent three stages of increasing stenosis with corresponding decrease in the turbulence threshold. 'A', 'B', and 'C' in the lower panel represent three bruits representing the three stages of stenosis selected in the upper panel. Note: the flow tracings are normalized to the same scale though 'A', 'B' and 'C' represent progressive increases in blood velocity.

with a stethoscope. If there are collateral channels available through which the blood flow is shunted to the normal vascular bed of the stenotic vessel, the bruit amplitude will decrease sooner and more rapidly. If there are no collateral channels, normal volumes of blood flow can pass through 1 mm lumen because of high velocity generated by a large pressure gradient.

5. FREQUENCY (TIMBRE)

All arterial bruits possess a blowing quality which means that there is a random noise-type audio spectrum. A superimposed humming or whining quality indicates periodic vibration of a flexible downstream arterial wall.

The upper frequencies of a bruit to increase as the stenosis approaches the most severe degrees. The upper frequency content of the bruit spectrum is related to the blood velocity (Figure 4). The upper frequency generally does not exceed 600 Hz and, therefore, moderate hearing losses of the observer do not affect his ability to recognize them. If a very faint, high frequency bruit of

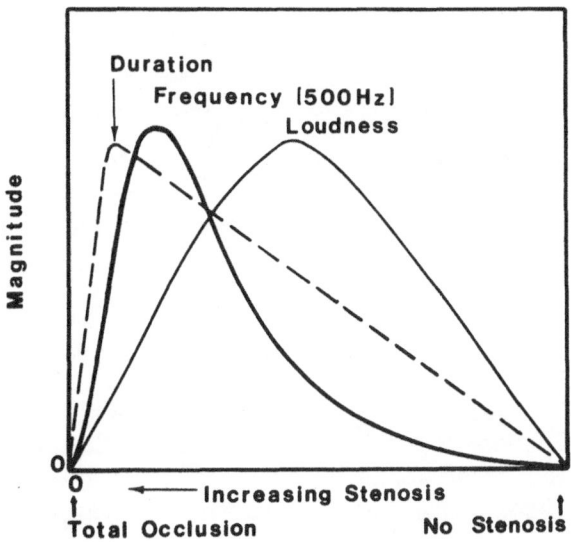

Figure 4. As stenosis increases, the magnitude of the bruit with respect to loudness, frequency, and duration also increases proportionally; however, seldom exceeds 500 Hz at which time it reverses until no bruit can be heard, even though the stenosis continues to increase.

a tight stenosis is heard or suspected, the diaphragm stethoscope should be used to collect the maximum vibratory information.

The higher frequency components provide a sense of 'presence' to the sound usually at the point of maximum intensity and immediately over the bruit source. The high frequencies are lost as the bruit spreads because the tissues tend to damp out the higher frequency components more than the low frequency components. The highest frequency qualities tend to be associated with bruits of longer duration within the cardiac cycle.

6. DURATION AND TIMING

With minor degrees of stenosis or irregularity in the arterial channel, the bruit will be of short duration in mid-systole. As the stenosis increases, the duration of the bruit tends to expand to become pan-systolic. With the tightest degrees of stenosis or with greater hemodynamic significance, the duration spreads into diastole and may become continuous throughout the cardiac cycle (Figure 5). Long duration, high frequency bruits are hemodynamically significant because there is a large pressure gradient throughout the cardiac cycle and indicates poor arterial collateral to the distal vascular bed.

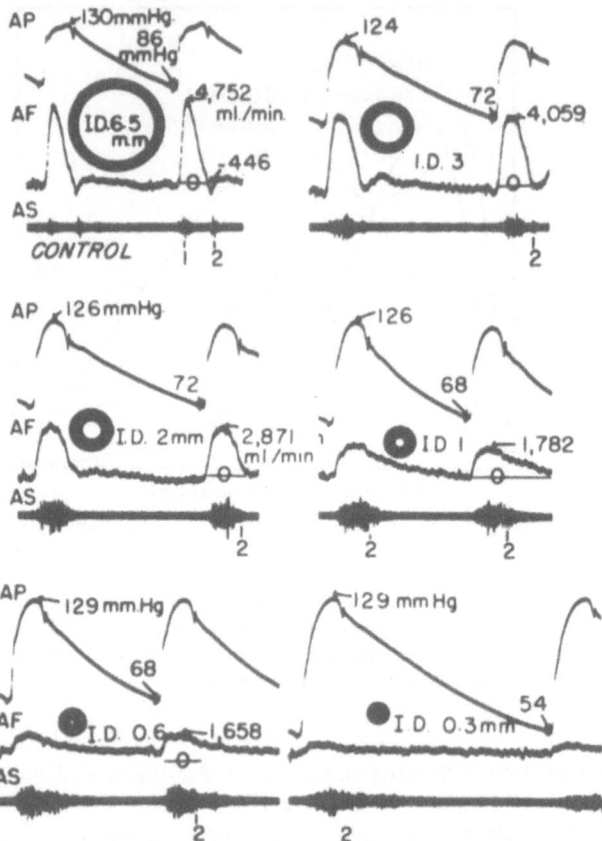

Figure 5. The sequence of events which takes place as a result of lumen reduction in experimental coarctation. The upper left-hand panel is the control, subsequent panels indicate the physiological changes which occur.

7. SUMMARY

Through careful evaluation of the location, intensity, frequency and duration of vascular bruits, a good estimate can often be made concerning the severity and hemodynamic significance of stenosis (Figure 4).

Bruits caused by arterial-venous fistulae tend to be of long duration, very loud and transmit widely. Because of their loudness throughout the cardiac cycle, 'designated machinery bruit,' they are generally not confused with a tight stenosis bruit.

REFERENCES

1. Spencer MP, Johnston FR, Meredith JH: The origin and interpretation of murmurs in coarctation of the aorta. Am Heart J 56:722, 1958.
2. Spencer MP, Fourney ME: Spectral analysis of murmurs produced in stenosis of large arteries. Physiologist 8 (3), 1965.

8. BLOOD FLOW IN THE ARTERIES

MERRILL P. SPENCER, M.D.

The arterial system is a many-branched elastic conduit for distribution of blood from the heart to all body tissues. Its calibre ranges from 4 cm for the human aorta to 4 µm for the capillaries. Over this wide range, the dynamics of each vascular segment may be described by various combination of 3 fundamental physical properties. Resistance, Inertance and Compliance, collectively referred to as Impedance.

1. DISCRETE ARTERIAL ELEMENTS

Resistance (R) arises from viscous losses in the blood flowing through the vessel segment. Hemodynamic resistance is analogous to electrical resistance which we symbolize as —⋀⋀—. Just as electricity is impelled by a voltage difference, blood always flows in the direction of the pressure gradient or pressure difference (ΔP). Resistance is found mainly in the small arterials or in larger arteries when disease process causes narrowing.*

Resistance is equal to:

$$R = \frac{\Delta P}{F}$$

where 'F' is flow in ml s^{-1} and ΔP is in mmHg. Also,

$$R = \frac{\Delta P}{v \cdot A}$$

where v = velocity of blood and A = cross-sectional area of the blood vessel. The large arteries such as the aorta and its larger branches normally have very low resistance because they are so wide that very little pressure drop occurs as the blood flows through them. Only when abnormally narrowed do they develop a significant pressure gradient in the direction of the blood flow. Resistance is inversely proportional to the 4th power of the radius of the artery lumen and proportional to its length. As a large artery gradually narrows due to the atherosclerotic plaque buildup, no significant increase in

---

* For short stenotic segments in large arteries: $\Delta P = \frac{1}{2}\rho\,(v^2_{\text{stenosis}} - v^2_{\text{proximal}})$.

resistance occurs until the lumen is reduced to less than 50% of its original diameter. If collateral circulation is poor, the increasing pressure difference may maintain normal flow until the lumen diameter is less than 2 mm i.d. At this point, however, the patient is in a critical situation and further reduction in lumen may produce a clinically significant effect.

If there is good collateral circulation for a stenotic artery, the flow will decrease faster than when there is poor collateral. This is because in the case of good collateral, the pressure gradient does not increase over a certain pressure level because it is supported by the collateral channels. If this pressure level is high enough for normal perfusion, total occlusion may take place without symptoms of cerebral ischemia.

During pulsating flow through a hemodynamic resistance, the waveform of the flow pulse rises and falls in phase with the pressure waveform (Figure 1A).

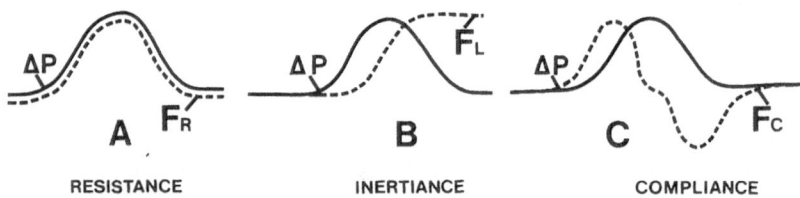

| RESISTANCE | INERTIANCE | COMPLIANCE |

Figure 1. Phase relationships between pressure gradient and flow form of the three types of impedances.

Inertance and Compliance, which together are called reactances, are two other flow impedance properties which greatly affect the pulsatile flow waveforms in the arteries.

Inertance (L) is the most apparent impedance in normal large arteries and exists primarily in the mass of the blood. It is analogous to electrical inductance symbolized as ⌒⌒⌒. Any change in electrical current through a coil of wire or an electrical inductance requires a peak of voltage difference in the direction of current flow to overcome the inductance of the coil. When the voltage is to a constant, it diminishes voltage difference to maintain current flow through the resistance of the coil which usually is low. Similarly, any change of blood flow in the large blood vessels is attended with an acceleration transient in the blood pressure gradient to overcome the inertance of the blood mass (Figure 1B). A more familiar example of the inertance property is that of pushing a person on an ice sled. One must push hard against the sled to accelerate it in order to get it going and pull to stop it, but after that, only enough push must be applied to overcome the small friction (resistance) of the runners.

Inertance in hemodynamics is equivalent to:

$$L = \frac{\Delta P}{dF/dt}$$

where dF is the rate of change of flow in $cm^3 s^{-2}$. Also, we define

$$L = \frac{\Delta P}{a \cdot A}$$

where a = the acceleration of the blood in $cm\,s^{-2}$ and A = cross-sectional area of the vessel in cm^2. Because inertance is defined in terms of volumetric acceleration, the larger the lumen cross-section, the smaller will be the inertance per unit length of vessel. 'L' increases directly with the increase in length of the vessel. Because resistance is low in the larger vessels, inertance together with the compliance produces high pulsatility of flow in the large arteries.

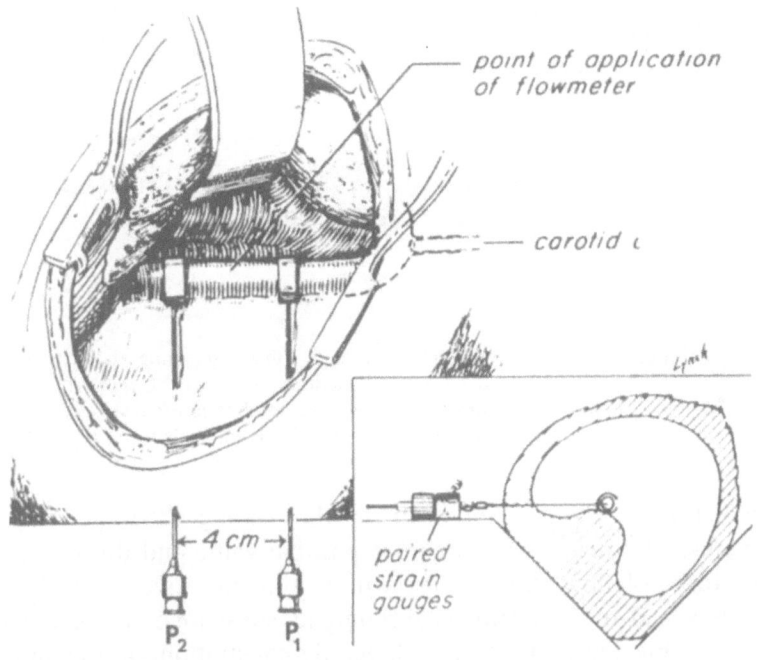

Figure 2. How two pressure measurements are made simultaneously along the aorta in order to record ΔP for Figure 3.

The property of inertance in the aorta was first demonstrated in 1966 by direct measurement of the pressure difference along a 4 cm segment through which volumetric flow was simultaneously measured. Figure 2 illustrates the experimental arrangement for measurement of two pressures simultaneously along the aorta.

By subtracting the downstream pressure (P_2) from the upstream pressure (P_1), the instantaneous pressure difference (ΔP) across the segment was recorded. The instantaneous blood flow was recorded with the square wave electromagnetic flowmeter applied between the pressure points.

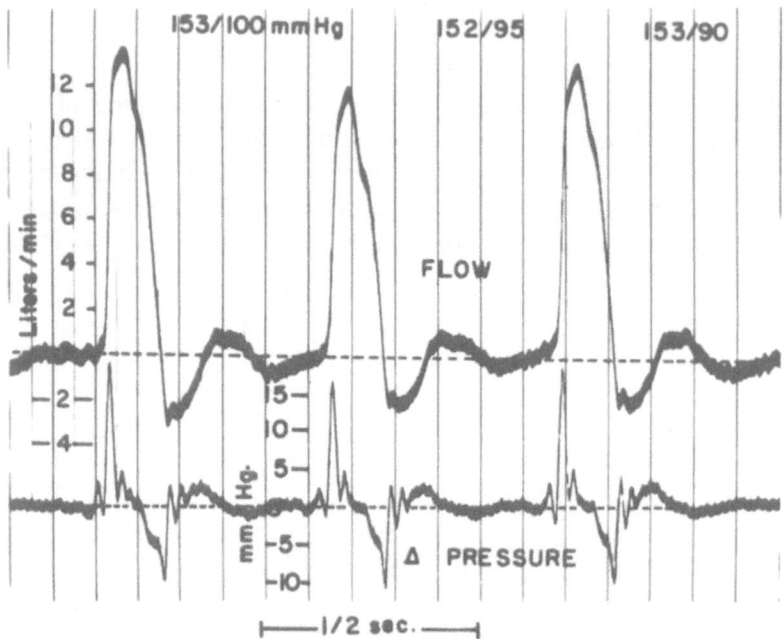

Figure 3. Relationship between flow and ΔP in the descending thoracic aorta. Each rise in flow is produced by a + acceleration seen on the ΔP tracing and each decrease in flow is produced by a negative acceleration (deceleration) transient in ΔP. Two backflow phases are seen on the F tracing during diastole.

By inspection of Figure 3, one can see that during the systolic upslope of the flow pulse, ΔP reaches a maximum positive value and during the following downstroke of flow, ΔP reaches a maximum negative value. This phase lead of ΔP ahead of F continues throughout subsequent oscillations in the heart cycle. This phase lead is a direct demonstration of the property of inertiance in the large arteries. The flow pulse in Figure 3 also demonstrates a marked backflow occurring at the end of systole. This oscillation is a prominent feature of the arterial 'resonant wave' which will be discussed later.

Figure 4 illustrates the property of inertiance in the cardiac ejection of the stroke volume into the ascending aorta. The flow tracing represents the time course of normal cardiac ejection as measured with the square-wave electromagnetic flowmeter. Ejection begins with a positive (+) ΔP representing an acceleration transient to open the valve and produce a steep systolic upslope

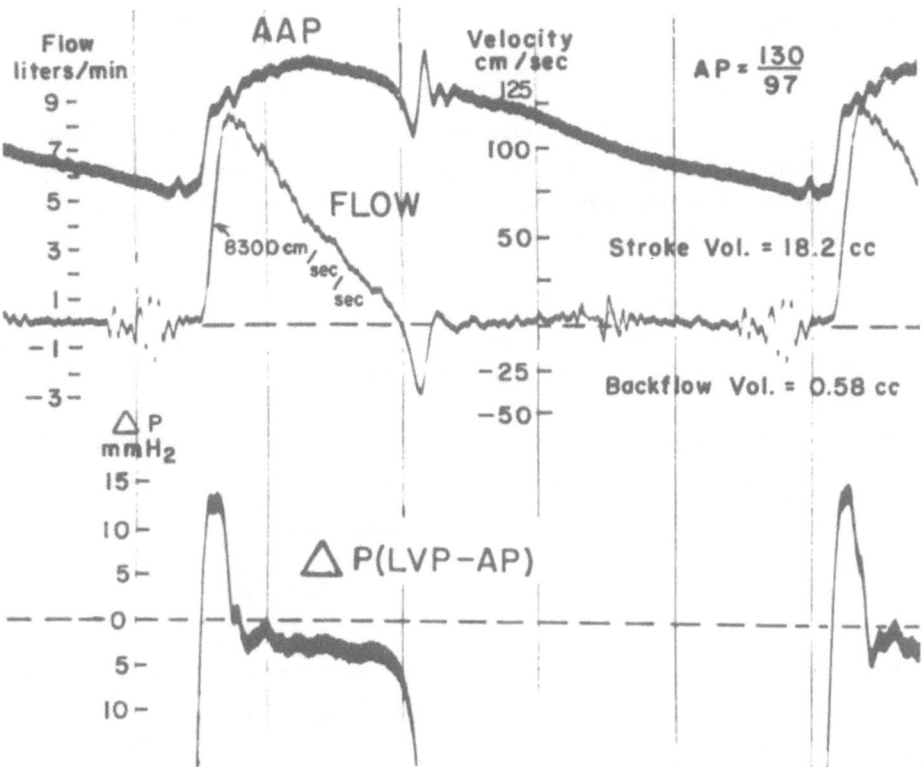

Figure 4. The effect of inertia of the blood during cardiac ejection into the ascending aorta produces a large but brief positive acceleration transient in early systole followed by a small but prolonged deceleration phase.

in the blood flow tracing. The flow reaches a peak at the end of the ΔP acceleration transient where ΔP reverses direction. Through the remainder of systole the blood is decelerated by a decrease of ventricular pressure slightly less than aortic pressure until cardiac ejection is complete and ventricular contraction falls off. The valve then closes with a brief backflow transient whose reflection on the aortic pressure is called the 'incisura." This ejection flow pulse is modified by the inertiance and compliance of the large arteries as it is transmitted to the periphery.

Inertance represents a non-stationary phenomenon due to time-varying changes in kinetic energy. Another stationary change in kinetic energy occurs where there is a stenosis or narrowing along a large vessel segment. At the entrance there is a spatial acceleration which is stationary in time. After Bernoulli, we defined the pressure drop (ΔP_B) as dependent on the blood density (ρ) and the velocity of the blood before the stenosis (v_1) and the velocity within the stenotic segment (v_2):

$$P_B = \tfrac{1}{2}\rho(v_2^2 - v_1^2)$$

If the vessel returns to a larger diameter, such as in a short stenotic segment in a smooth gradual way, the ΔP_B may be regained with no net loss in ΔP except for the viscous term. Note: please see Chapter 9 for discussion of Bernoulli's term when downstream turbulence exists.

Compliance (C) is a property of the arterial wall arising from its distensability and chiefly resides in the elastic fibers but also is contributed to by smooth muscle and fibrous tissue. Vascular wall compliance is analogous to electrical

Table 1. Three types of blood flow in the arteries.

	RESISTIVE	INERTIAL	COMPLIANCE
ELECTRICAL ANALOGY	—⋀⋀⋀—	—⋂⋂⋂—	—┤├—
FUNCTIONAL DEFINITION	$R = \dfrac{\Delta P}{V \cdot A}$	$L = \dfrac{\Delta P}{a \cdot A}$	$C = \dfrac{V}{\Delta P}$
PRESSURE, FLOW DEFINITION	$R = \dfrac{\Delta P}{F}$ F & ΔP IN PHASE	$L = \dfrac{\Delta P}{dF/dt}$ F LAGS BEHIND ΔP	$C = \dfrac{\int F \cdot dt}{\Delta P}$ F LEADS ΔP
MATHEMATICAL DEFINITION	$R = \dfrac{8\eta 1}{\pi\, r^4}$	$L = \dfrac{\rho 1}{\pi\, r^2}$	$C = \dfrac{2\pi\, r^3}{E}$
ANATOMICAL EXAMPLE	P_1 R P_2	P1 L P2	P1 ⋯ P2

P = BLOOD PRESSURE IN DYNES/CM^2.
ΔP = PRESSURE DIFFERENCE BETWEEN 2 POINTS.
F = BLOOD FLOW IN CM^3/SEC.
V = BLOOD VELOCITY IN CM/SEC.
a = ACCELERATION OF BLOOD IN CM/SEC^2.
V = VOLUME OF BLOOD IN VESSEL SEGMENT IN CM^3.

A = VESSEL CROSS-SECTION IN CM^2.
1 = LENGTH OF VESSEL SEGMENT IN CM.
r = RADIUS OF VESSEL IN CM.
η = BLOOD VISCOSITY IN DYNE SECONDS/CM^2.
E = MODULUS OF ELASTICITY.
ρ = BLOOD DENSITY IN GMS/CM^3.

capacitance which is symbolized as —| |—. Just as an electrical capacitance represents the ability to accumulate a charge of electricity and discharge it back into the same circuit, so compliance is the ability of the arteries to expand and take up a volume of blood during systole, then discharge it along the arteries during diastole.

Compliance has been defined as:

$$C = \frac{\Delta V}{\Delta P}$$

where ΔV is the change in volume of blood (in cm^3) for any vessel segment and ΔP is the pressure difference between the inside of the vessel and the outside of the vessel produced by ΔV.

The property of compliance was expressed in the early 'windkessel' concept of the aorta which considered it to rapidly take up the cardiac stroke volume during systole and slowly discharge it during diastole through the peripheral resistance. Compliance of an artery varies directly with the 2nd power of the radius and directly with its length. Table 1 summarizes the 3 discrete arterial parameters.

2. COMBINED ARTERIAL MODELS

Figure 5 illustrates the windkessel concept as a simple electrical analogy. The heart is represented as a flow generator with an ejected flow pulse 'F.' The fraction of F flowing in and out of the compliance (capacitator) C is designated f_1 and that fraction flowing through the peripheral resistor R is designated f_2. The changes in V do not follow P closely because the inertial element is not represented in the model.

This model of the arterial tree explains the gross rise and fall characteristic of the arterial pressure and shows how flow runs off through the peripheral resistance during systole as well as diastole. This model is insufficient to explain other diagnostic characteristics of the peripheral arterial pressure and flow pulses. The windkessel model does not explain how there is a higher systolic pressure in the legs than in the arm. It does not explain backflow phases in the flow pulse and does not explain the dichrotic notch in the pressure pulse.

A more complete and clinically useful model of the hemodynamics of the aorta and its major branches is illustrated in Figure 6.

Here the model of the arterial tree is expanded to 2 windkessels represented by 2 R–C circuits and connected by an inertial element, L. L represents the mass of blood in the aorta connecting the upper aorta and its branches with the abdominal aorta and its branches. The heart pumps directly into C_1, representing the compliance of the aortic arch and its immediate branches.

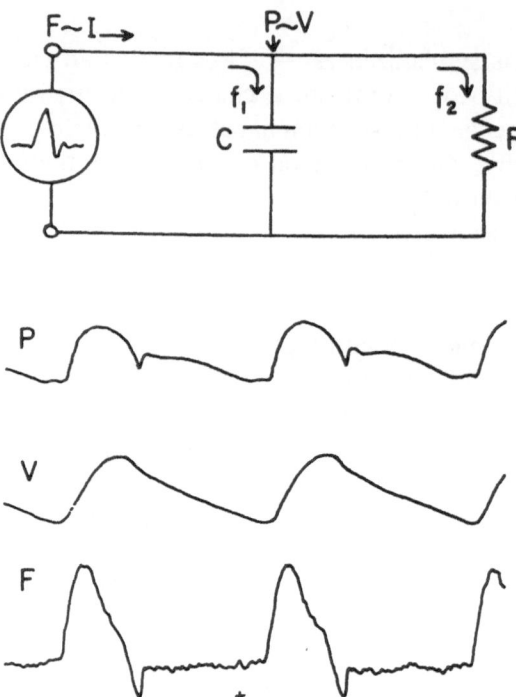

Figure 5. The 'windkessel' model of the arteries demonstrated as a simple R-C electrical circuit. It is not sufficient to explain the incisura and other details of the actually measured pressure. F and P are measured, V is computed in the analogue model.

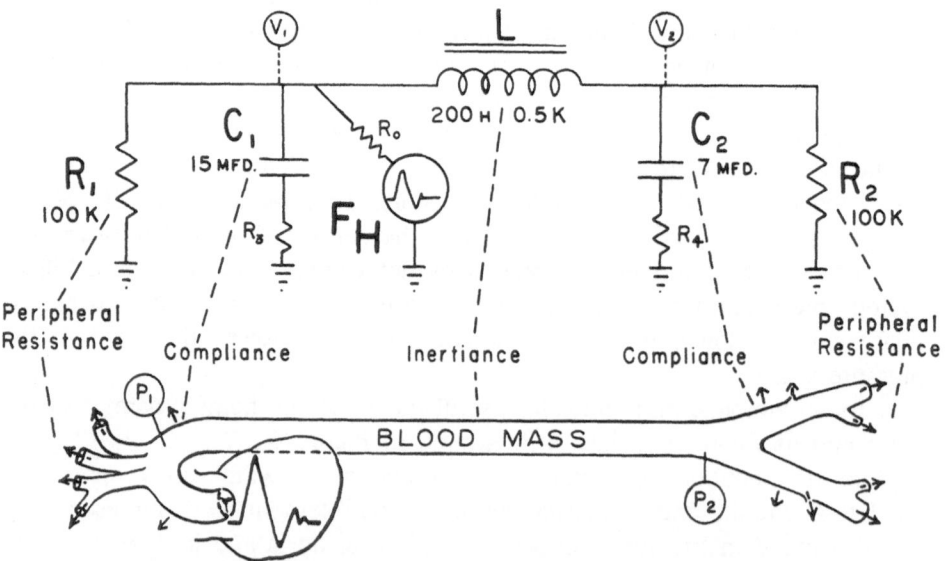

Figure 6. A model of the hemodynamics of the aorta and its major branches which explains many clinically important features of flow and pressure pulses.

The upper windkessel initially absorbs the left ventricular stroke ejection 'bolus'. In early systole while the inertiance of blood in the descending aorta impedes flow into C_2 but after the acceleration transient passes, the flow pulse moves down the aorta to be absorbed by the C_2 windkessel. As the pressure in the lower windkessel then peaks out, the flow and pressure waves are reflected back up the aorta producing a backflow throughout the descending aorta.

According to this model, the arterial tree is a liquid filled elastic tube which is set into oscillation by each beat of the heart. The combination of the 2 capacities with the blood mass lumped as a middle element produces resonant flow waves. The resonant and the 'standing' pressure wave of Hamilton are part and parcel of the same interaction of inertiance and compliance. The dichrotic notch so prominent in the peripheral pressure and volume pulses is a representation of the standing wave.

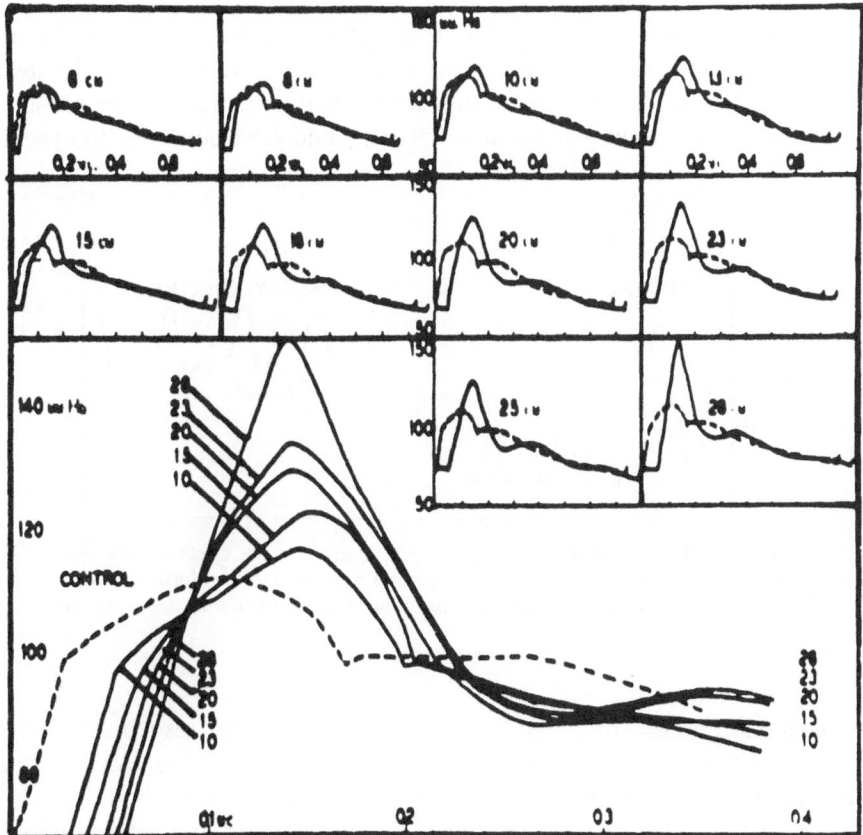

Figure 7. Development of the standing wave in the pulse as it is transmitted to the lower aorta and femoral artery (according to Hamilton).

Figure 7 illustrates how the standing wave builds up in the peripheral arteries. The peak systolic pressure in the femoral artery is normally greater than that of the arms because C_2, of which the femoral artery is a part, is approximately 1/5 the size of C_1, of which the brachial artery is a component. When the flow pulse enters the smaller C_2, the pressure builds higher during systole than it did when the flow pulse first entered C_1. The mean pressure in the arms and legs averaged over the heart cycle is very nearly equal because, as stated earlier, the large artery resistance does not produce a large pressure drop. The excess pressure in the femoral artery during systole is made up during diastole by the dichrotic notch pressure which is, at the time of its occurrence, lower than the upper aorta pressure.

3. PERIPHERAL FLOW PULSES

As the resonant flow wave is transmitted to the periphery, the backflow phase persists when the downstream resistance is high, such as in the resting extremities (Figure 8). Two conditons diminish the resonant wave amplitude: vasodilation of the downstream small arteries and obstruction of the proximal artery.

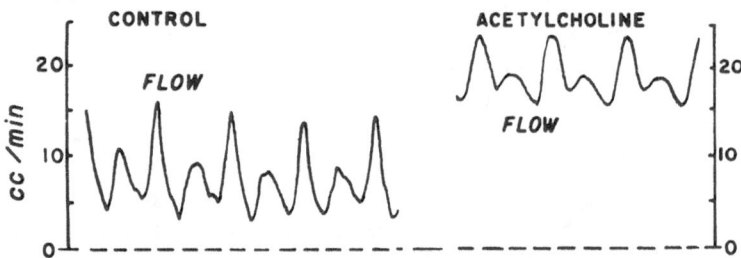

Figure 8. Blood flow in a small peripheral artery and the effect of vasodilation. The control flow may be considered a resonant flow form which is converted to resistant flow by the injection of acetylcholine into the arterial channel.

Vasodilation raises the diastolic flow and dampens the resonant wave. This can be demonstrated on a normal subject by listening to the Doppler sounds from the brachial artery while making a tight fist and releasing. While the fist is clenched the resonant wave produces systolic forward and reverse flow only because of the high resistance produced by muscular compression of the downstream small arteries. Upon release of the clenched fist, reactive hype-

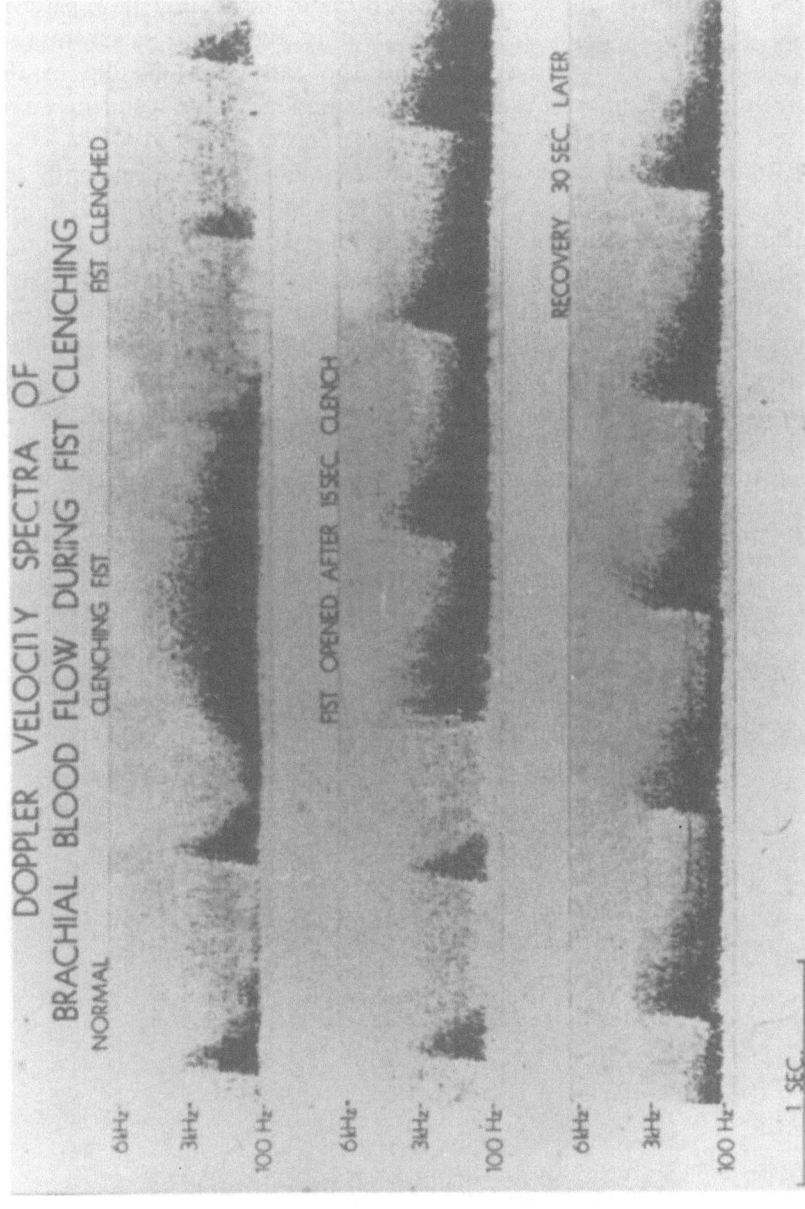

Figure 9. Vasodilation produced in a normal subject demonstrating increased diastolic flow and reduced pulsatility (upper panel). Middle panel illustrates elevation and diminution of the resonant wave. The lower panel shows the resting flow pattern 30 seconds after release of clenched fist.

108

emia in the distal bed produces increased flow and increased flow velocity in the brachial artery. Two features are particularly noticeable: 1) high diastolic flow with a decrease in the pulsatility and 2) elevation and diminution of the resonant wave. By observing the gradual return to the resting flow pattern, one can see on the analogue tracing and hear in the audio spectrum that diastolic backflow in the resting limb and the early diastolic dip in the vasocilation limb represents the same basic phenomenon, the resonant wave, superimposed on various levels of steady flow (Figure 9).

Figure 10 illustrate that resistive flow and resonant flow independently act to produce a variety of peripheral flow pulses. Tracings of Figure 10 a, b, and c represent resistive blood flow from increasing peripheral runoff through vasodilation. While 1, 2, and 3 represent reactive flow (resonant flow) with increasing stiffness of artery wall producing various resonant frequencies. An infinite number of combinations produces a wide variety of analogue flow pulses seen in the extremities. Six varieties are shown in Figure 10. The normal arterial flow waveforms are distorted by proximal obstruction in recognizable ways. These distortions and their use in diagnosing subclavian and innominate artery stenosis are discussed in Chapters 1 and 13.

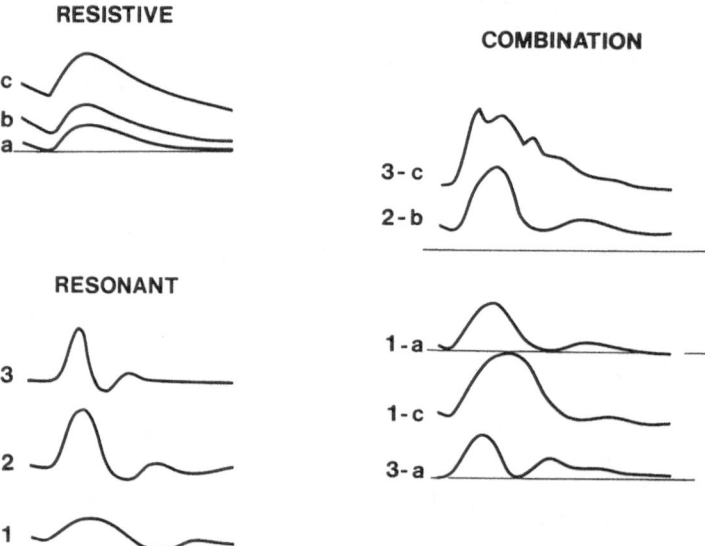

Figure 10. Resistive and resonant flow waveforms combine to produce a variety of individual flow pulses. Resistive forms a, b, and c represent increasing runoff from decreasing peripheral resistance. Resonant forms 1, 2, and 3 represent increasing frequency usually due to increasing stiffness of the arterial tree. Five combinations are shown as examples of types of blood flow and velocity pulses.

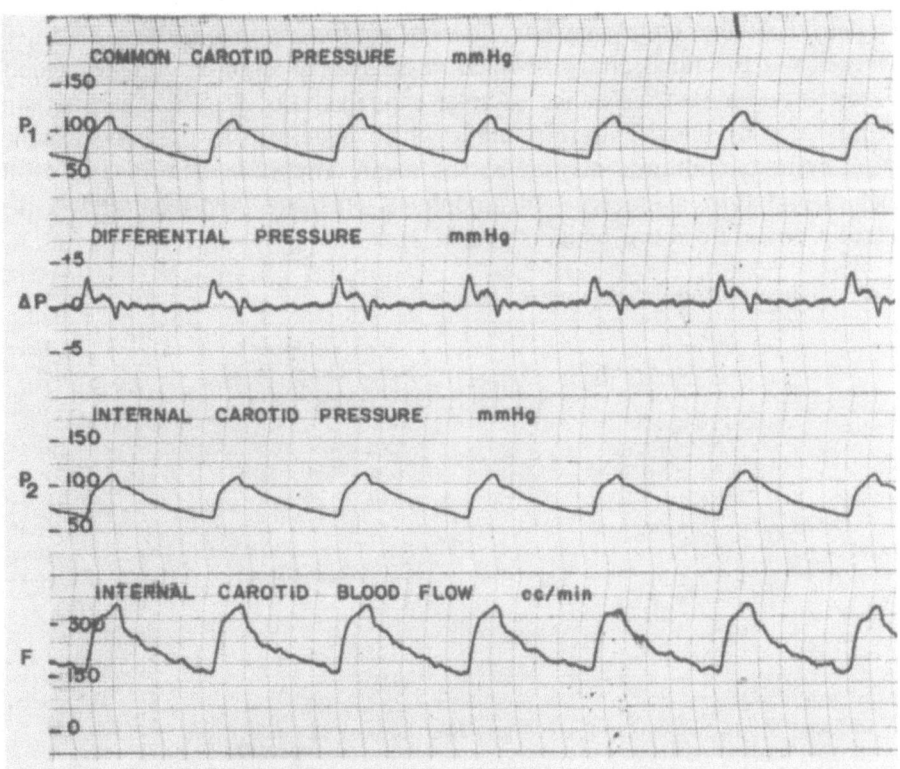

Figure 11. Normal hemodynamics of the internal carotid artery. The blood flow wave form closely tracks the pressure pulse.

4. CHARACTERISTICS OF NORMAL CAROTID BLOOD FLOW

Figure 11 illustrates the normal pulsatile wave form of human internal carotid blood flow signals measured with the electromagnetic flow meter simultaneously with P_1, P_2, and ΔP. It is seen that the inertial flow pulse wave form closely tracks the internal arterial pressure pulse, both of which are superimposed on a large static 'DC' component which produces considerable displacement of the pulsations from the zero references. Inspection of the differential pressure, ΔP, discloses minor features of both inertial and resistive flow. The first peak of ΔP and early systole corresponds to a 'hump' on the upstroke of F and represents the acceleration transient. Immediately following this transient, in mid-systole, is a more rounded wave which corresponds to the maximum systolic flow. This is followed immediately by a deceleration transient. During diastole, an almost imperceptible pressure gradient exists. The normal resistance of the internal carotid channel, R_1, of human subjects is 0.001 PRU's/cm where one PRU represents . mmHg ml^{-1} min.

The relatively large diastolic flow is characteristic of both the internal carotid and the renal arteries, which vessels carry large amounts of blood to feed the two lowest resistance vascular beds in the body. This characteristic is represented by a low pulsatility index which is defined as the end diastolic to peak systolic amplitude divided by the mean amplitude. The index for internal carotid flow averaged 1.10 among 48 pre- and post-repair flows in 35 carotid endarterectomy patients (Table 2).

Table 2. Human internal carotid pulsatility index.

	Stenosis pre-endarterectomy	Normal diameters post-endarterectomy	Combined overall
F_{EMF}	# = 13	13	48*
	$\overline{X}$ = 1.12	1.01	1.10
	Sx = 0.39	0.18	0.30
	S$\overline{x}$ = 0.11	0.05	0.04
	f_1	f_2	Combined
$V_{Doppler}$	x = 31	32	63
	$\overline{X}$ = 1.22	1.11	1.16
	Sx = 0.36	0.28	0.32
	S$\overline{x}$ = 0.06	0.05	0.04

* Includes 22 measurements in which pre-repair flows were not determined.

The time mean internal carotid blood flow ($\overline{F}$) measured in 31 carotid arteries immediately after endarterectomy was 194 ± 78.3 ml/min. when the mean blood pressure was 107 ± 18.4 mmHg. The mean hemodynamic resistance of the unilateral carotid-brain vasculature (P_1/F_1) averaged 0.59 ± 0.25 mmHg ml^{-1} min.

5. DOPPLER FREQUENCIES, BLOOD VELOCITIES AND FLOW

The spectral distribution of frequencies representing blood velocities in the internal carotid artery of a healthy young subject are seen in Figure 12. The concentration of energy near the maximum frequency edge of the spectrum gives a normal 'smooth' audio quality to the signal. The figure also illustrates the definitions of temporal mean and spatial mean velocities and relates these to blood flow.

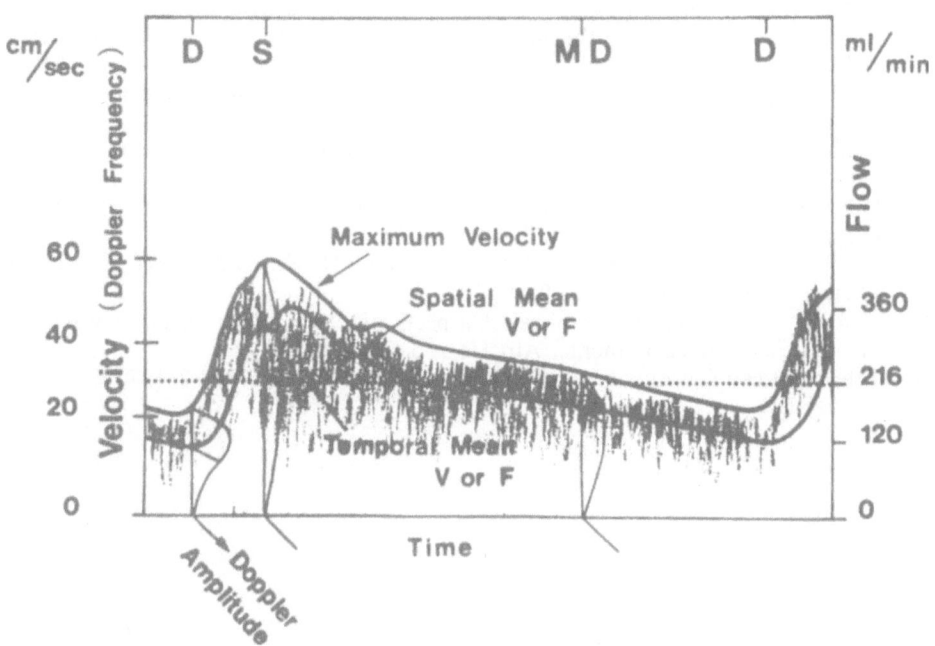

Figure 12. Normal Doppler spectrum of frequencies (velocities) in the internal carotid.

REFERENCES

1. Spencer MP, Denison AB Jr: Aortic flow pulse as related to the differential pressure. Circ Res 4:476, 1956.
2. Spencer MP, Johnston FR, Denison AB: Dynamics of the normal aorta: 'inertiance' and 'compliance' of the arterial system which transforms the cardiac ejection pulse. Circ Res 6:491, 1958.
3. Spencer MP, Denison AB Jr: Square-wave electromagnetic flowmeter for surgical and experimental applications. Methods in med research, vol. III, ed Bruner. Year Book Publishers, 1960, p 321.
4. Spencer MP: Differential pressure measurements: paired transducer system. Methods in med research, vol. VIII, ed Bruner. Year Bood Publishers, p 341.
5. Spencer MP, Denison AB Jr: 1960, An explanation of the major features of the arterial pulse by means of a simple electronic analogy. Fed Proc 19:87, 1960.
6. Spencer MP, Okino H, Denison AB Jr, Berry RL: Electronic and mathematical models of the circulatory system. Digest of the 1961 (4th) International Conference on Medical Electronics, New York, 1961, p 144.
7. Spencer MP, Greiss FC: Dynamics of ventricular ejection. Circ Res 10:274, 1962.

112

8. Spencer MP, Denison AB Jr: Pulsatile blood flow in the vascular system. Handbook of physiol, section 2, Circulation, vol. II, chapter 25, sec ed Hamilton. Am Physiol Soc, 1963.
9. Warner HR: A study of the mechanism of pressure wave distortion by arterial walls using an electrical analogue. Circ Res 5:79, 1957.
10. Hamilton WF, Dow P: An experimental study of standing waves in the pulse propogated through the aorta. Am J Physiol 125:48, 1939.
11. McDonald DA: Blood flow in the arteries. Baltimore: William and Wilkins, 1960.
12. Green HD: Circulatory system: physical principals. Medical physics, ed: Glasser. Chicago: Year Book Publ, vol. 2, 1950, p 228-251.
13. Okino H, Fujisaku K, Sakaguchi D, Sasamoto H: Pulsatile blood flow in the arterial system. Respir & Circ 8:49, 1960.
14. Van der Tweel LH: Some physical aspects of blood pressure, pulse wave and blood pressure measurements. Am Heart J 53:4, 1957.
15. Peterson LH: The dynamics of pulsatile blood flow. Circ Res 2:127, 1954.

9. HEMODYNAMICS OF CAROTID ARTERY STENOSIS

MERRILL P. SPENCER, M.D.

It is generally agreed that at least one-third of Strokes arise from atheroscle-rotic lesions developing on the extracranial arterial channels. The bifurcation of the common carotid artery in the neck is a site particularly prone to develop plaques. The adverse effects of carotid atherosclerotic plaques are manifest through two effects on brain perfusion: 1), embolism to the brain and eye from intimal ulcerations, and 2), a reduction in hemispheric flow. The purpose of this chapter is to understand the local Doppler velocity signals and the local pressure-flow relationships associated with stenosis of the caro-tid arteries in order to quantitate the degree of carotid narrowing and its effect on brain perfusion.

1. LOCAL DOPPLER CHARACTERISTICS

Figure 1 illustrates the local Doppler audio qualities associated with carotid artery stenosis. The diagram in 1a is the flow situation present in normal arterial channel. The normal smooth quality of the Doppler audio spectrum, representing laminar blood flow, is illustrated in Figure 2 and Figure 3. The concentration of energy near the maximum frequency at the upper edge of the spectrum indicated that most of the blood flow is moving near the maximum velocity and that a relatively small amount of blood is moving at a lower velocity. Young elastic arteries, with good extensibility, often produce a low frequency thumping at the beginning and end of systole which may be represented on the spectrum by a concentration of low frequencies and artifactual blanking of the spectrum during those phases. The low frequency thumping quality arises from the Doppler detection of the motion of the arterial wall.

Figure 1b illustrates a narrowing of the channel, with tapering of the entrance and exit producing an increased blood velocity and Doppler frequen-cy but with laminar flow maintained. When the exit from the distorted channel is sufficiently abrupt, the normal laminar flow streams are broken into turbulence which produces a Doppler signal which may be described as fluttering in quality and illustrated in Figure 1c. These fluttering signals are

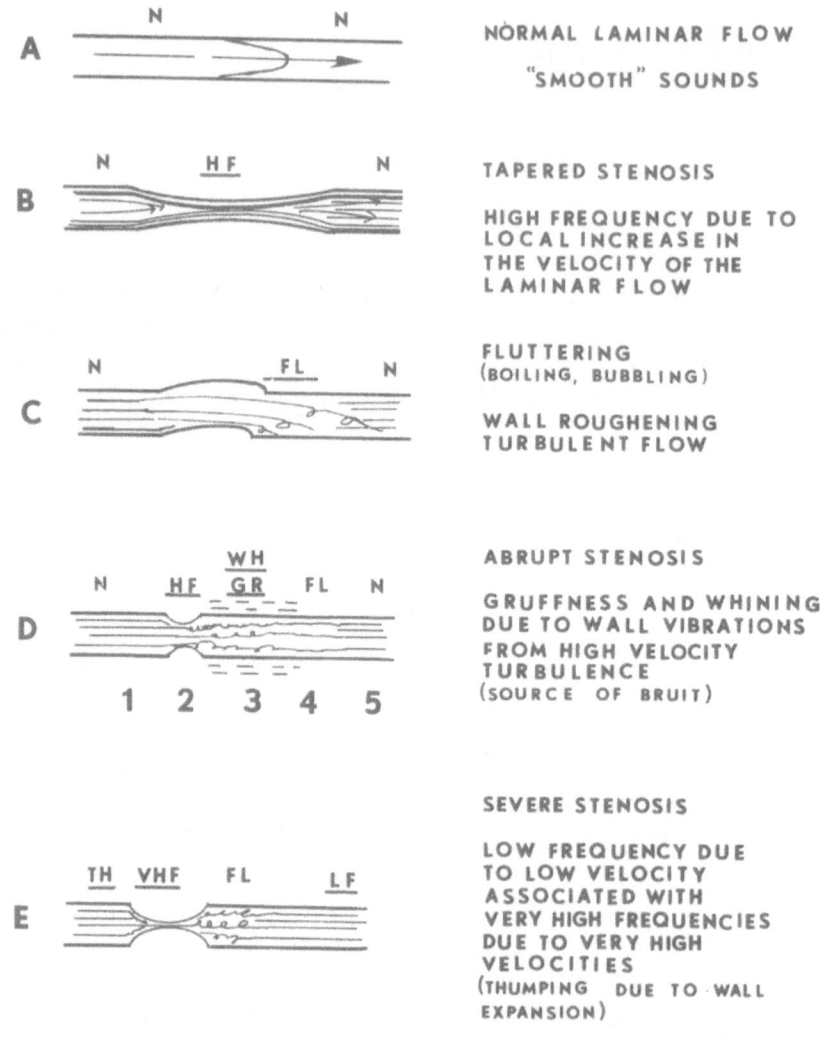

Figure 1. Local Doppler audio qualities in carotid artery stenosis.

represented on the spectrum by random irregularities in the upper maximum frequency and by spectral broadening. There may be no effect on mean flow through the channel, and the presence of fluttering-only signals diagnose a non-obstructing plaque.

Carotid artery stenosis is usually associated with a fully developed group of characteristic signals which may be divided into five zones (Figure 1d). Zone 1 is immediately upstream to the stenosis and may be of normal quality. Zone 2 is represented by high frequency signals directly within the narrowed segment and also immediately downstream in the exit channel. Zone 3,

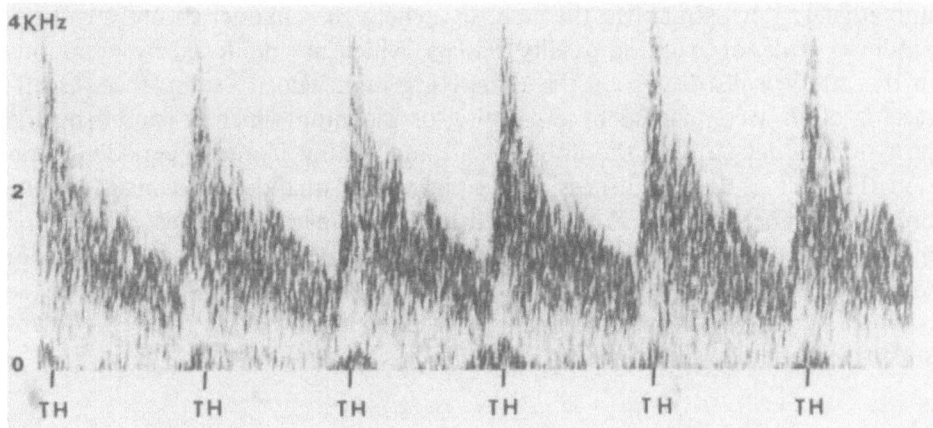

Figure 2. Normal smooth Doppler audio spectrum from internal carotid of a 23-year-old female. Note concentration of velocity frequencies near maximum frequency throughout pulse cycle. Expansion of flexible artery wall produces low frequency thumping (TH) in early systole. The maximum systolic frequency is 4 KHz.

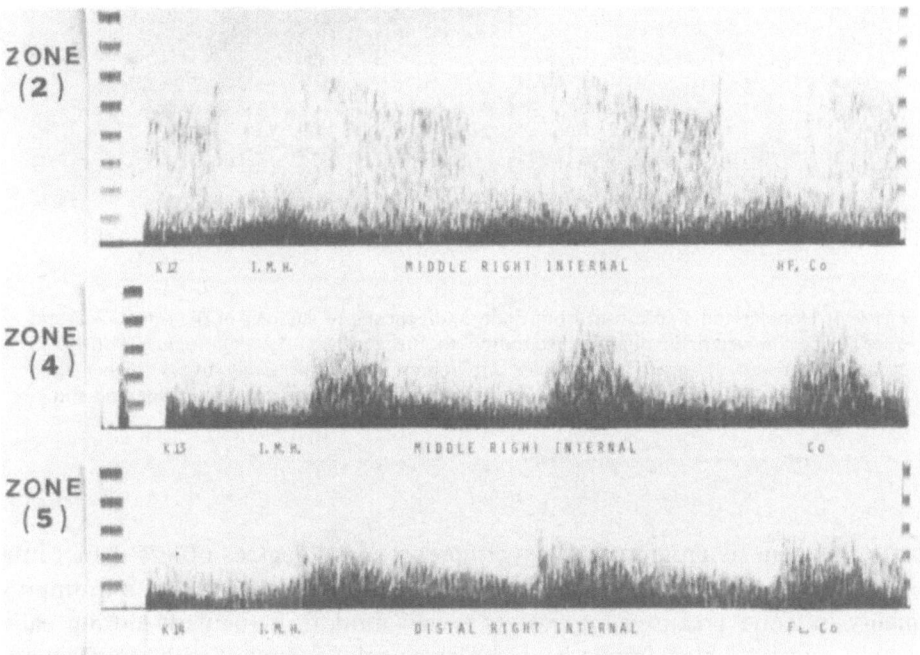

Figure 3. Doppler audio spectra from Zones 2, 4 and 5 demonstrate high frequency, coarse and fluttering signals.

116

immediately downstream to the stenosis, where the channel abruptly widens, produces gruff, or grunting quality signals, which are produced by vibrations of the artery walls driven by the underlying high velocity turbulence. Gruffness is often accompanied by a whining or moaning which is caused by the post-stenotic jet striking the arterial wall and setting it into a periodic vibration (Figure 4). Both gruffness and whining are qualities also heard in the bruit upon auscultation. Zone 4, further downstream, produces a fluttering quality signal as the vortex velocity of the turbulence diminishes. If sufficient length of artery is available for examination, Zone 5 may be identified as normal signals when the laminar flow resumes three to five cm downstream (Renneman and Spencer 1979).

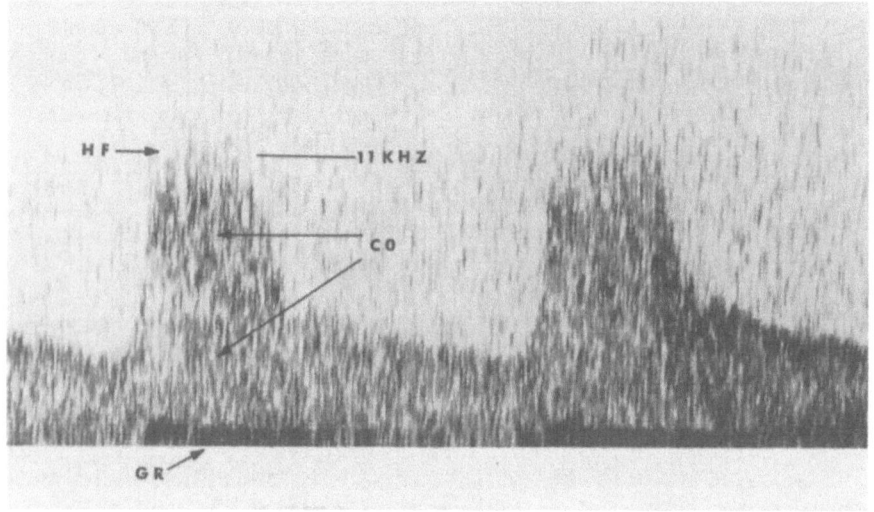

Figure 4. Doppler audio spectrum from Zone 3, diagnostic of stenosis of the internal carotid artery. The characteristic qualities (sounding to the ear) are: 1) high frequency (HF), 2) 'coarse' (CO) and 3) 'gruff' (Gr). These are represented respectively by: a. higher than normal maximum frequency envelope, b. the even distribution of spectral broadening and c. systolic high amplitude, low frequency (darkening) in the 0–500 KHz range.

As the stenosis progresses to severe preocclusive degrees of less than 1 mm in diameter, a special set of signals can be identified consisting of a thumping quality in Zone 1 caused by excessive wall motion, particularly during early systole, and very high frequency Doppler signals in Zone 2 with low frequency systolic-only signals in the downstream zones. Zone 3 generally does not produce the gruff quality but fluttering may be detected in Zones 4 and 5.

2. PRESSURE, FLOW, VELOCITY AND DIAMETER RELATIONSHIPS

Prior to the availability of the non-invasive transcutaneous Doppler ultrasonic velocity detector, the hemodynamics of arterial stenosis was investigated with measurements of blood flow with the electromagnetic flow meter and the pressure gradient across the narrowed arterial segment. Such measurements require surgical exposure for the application of the flow meter probes and the insertion of pressure measuring needles. The electromagnetic flow meter measures the instantaneous volumetric flow across the artery lumen integrating the velocities of all the flow streams. In this section we will present pressure-flow data in experimental carotid artery stenosis related to Doppler velocity recordings and utilize electrical/mathematical modeling and graphic analysis to further understand the hemodynamics of carotid artery stenosis.

The time of surgical application of the Selverstone clamp for treatment of intracranial aneurysm allowed the opportunity for study of the local hemodynamic effects of graded carotid stenosis. Figure 5 illustrates the positioning of the Selverstone clamp on the common carotid at the bifurcation, the electromagnetic flow meter probe on the internal carotid artery, and pressure recording of needles inserted below and above the clamp. The interposition of the external carotid branch between the clamp and the internal carotid flow probe does not significantly affect the interpretation of the data presented.

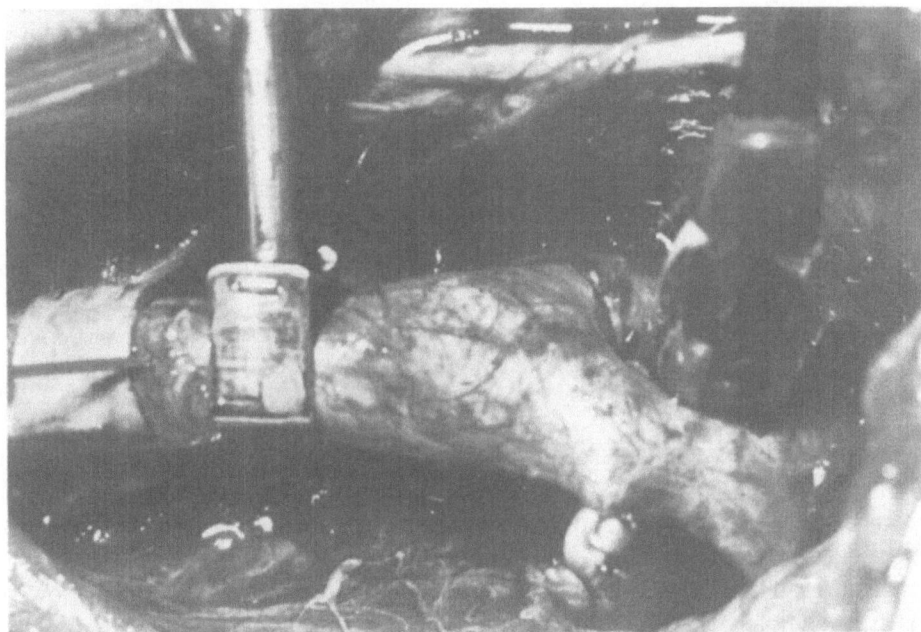

Figure 5. Surgical application of the Selverstone clamp for treatment of intracranial aneurysm.

Figure 6 illustrates typical progressive changes in the flow and pressure gradient in the artery during graded construction and release of the clamp. The inverse proportional relationship between flow and pressure difference is seen. It is further observed that when the carotid is completely obstructed, there is a residual pressure ('stump' pressure) in the distal carotid due to collaterals. Slight residual flow in the internal carotid is produced by minimal flow from the external carotid but most of the residual pressure arises from collaterals (Spencer et al. 1966).

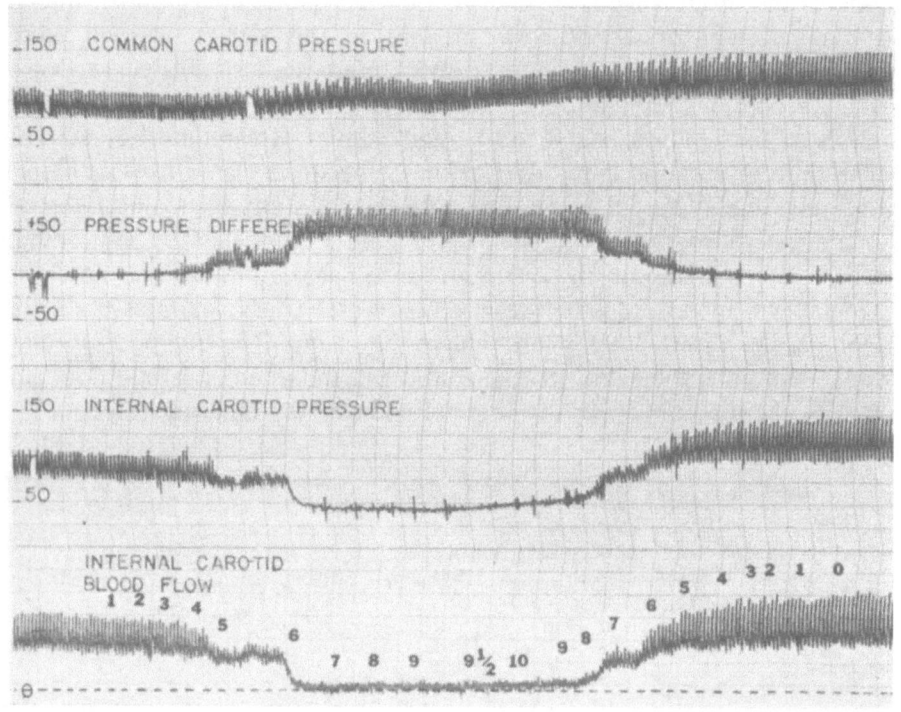

Figure 6. Progressive changes in flow and pressure as the selverstone clamp (shown in Figure 5) is constricted and released. The numbers 1–10 in the lower panel represent 'turns' of the clamp.

A more detailed analysis may be seen in Figure 7 which represents an impedance plot of instantaneous flow and pressure difference. It is seen that considerable reduction in the vessel lumen is necessary before flow was significantly affected. Five turns of the clamp represents approximately 50 percent reduction in the lumen and less than 10 percent reduction in flow. It is further noted that a critical stage occurs at this time when turns 6, 7, 8, and 9 produce a profound reduction in carotid flow.

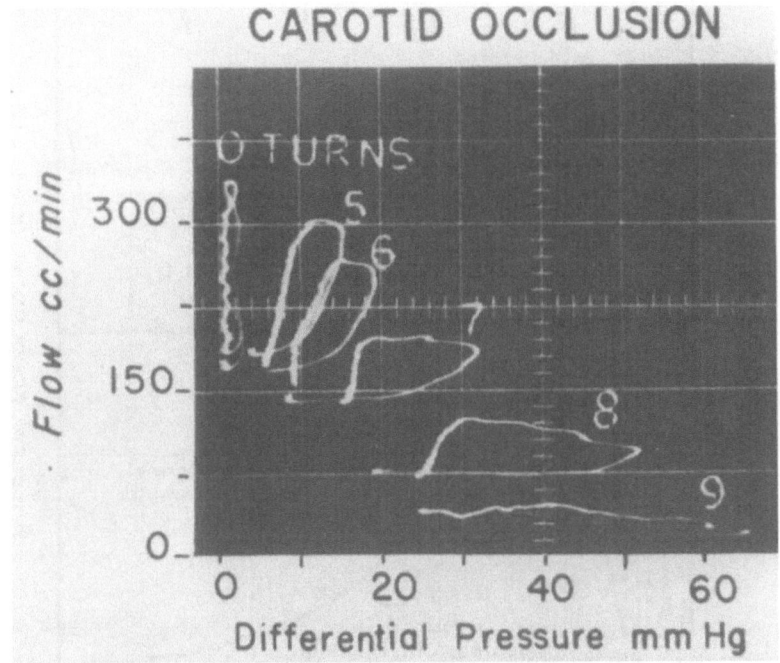

Figure 7. Represents impedance plot of instantaneous flow and pressure. Turns of the clamp 0, 5, 6, 7, 8, and 9 are represented. Impedance loops move counterclockwise.

In 8 carotid constriction patients, the pressure, flow relationship was uniformally found to be inversely proportional according to the following equation:

$$F = (B - \Delta P)/R$$

This equation represents the resistive flow so characteristic of the internal carotid artery where F, the flow in ml per minute, and ΔP, the pressure gradient in mm Hg, and resistance (R) is the ratio of flow to ΔP. B represents the maximum ΔP developing upon total occlusion of the carotid artery.

3. THEORETICAL VELOCITY DOPPLER RELATIONSHIPS

Since F is represented by the product of the cross sectional area (A) and the velocity (v), we may compute from these human experiments a mean lumen diameter to represent each value of R during the graded stenosis. We assume a nominal value for viscosity as 0.08 Poise and a stenosis length of 1 mm.

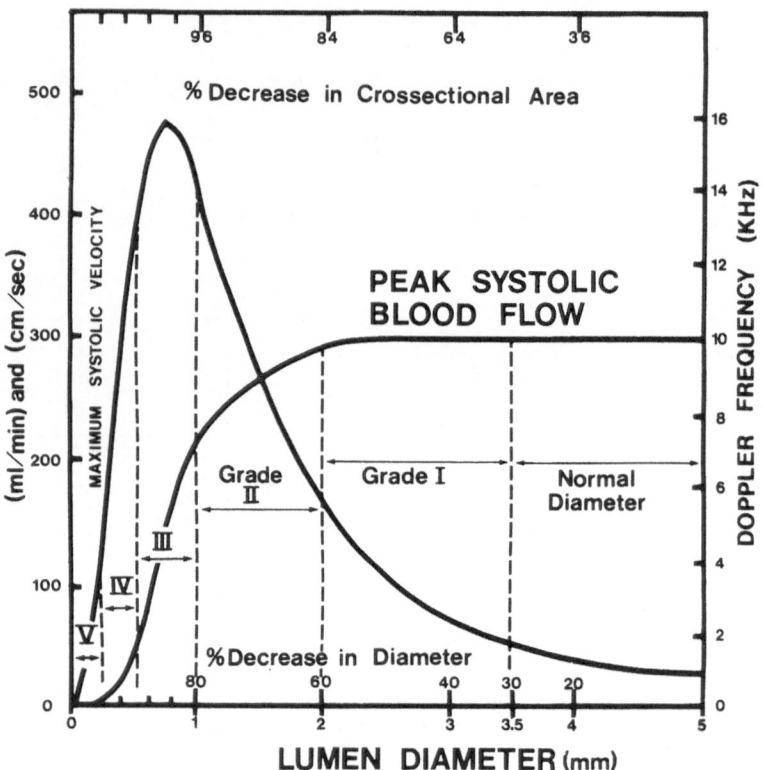

Figure 8. Theoretical relationships between blood velocity and flow in graded stenosis assumed to be smooth and axisymmetric. The effects of turbulent flow in abrupt stenosis is not considered. Settings for collateral and brain vascular resistance are in the normal range for humans. (Spencer and Reid 1979).

Figure 8 illustrates a resultant calculated relationship between instantaneous flow and instantaneous velocity for each computed lumen diameter. The data utilized from a patient with a maximum ΔP of 40 mm of mercury and whose initial internal carotid flow was 300 ml per minute. Also represented is the corresponding Doppler audio frequency using a 5 MHz probe angled at 30 degrees normal to the artery axis. Several important observations can be made:

1. Flow is not reduced below 10 percent of its initial value until the arterial diameter is less than 1.2 mm, regardless of the initial diameter. During this early phase of stenosis, the velocity increases with the inverse square of the diameter, i.e.:

v and $f \propto 1/D^{-2}$.

2. When the diameter (D) is reduced below 1 mm, a critical phase is reached where a small change in D produces a great change in F; v reaches a maximum when F reaches one half of its initial value ($\frac{1}{2}$F). In the case illustrated, v was calculated to reach 480 cm per second when $\frac{1}{2}$F was 150 ml per minute, and the diameter was only 0.75 mm.

3. As the stenosis proceeds towards occlusion, the decreasing velocity and consequent Doppler frequencies, pass back through the same range produced by the early and lesser degree of stenosis.

4. THE EFFECTS OF COLLATERALS ON F AND v

In the 5 patients studied with the Selverstone clamp, the 'stump' pressure when the common carotid is occluded, P ranged from 30/27 to 76/65 mm Hg (Table 1).

Table 1. Pressure studies in Selverstone clamp patients.

Patient	P_{sys}	ΔP_{max}	P_{stump}
FW	190	116	74/67
KP	142	66	76/65
EP	120	68	52/40
AK	104.5	69	36/33
JG	100	70	30/27.5
WW		65	
RH		63	
IT		95	

These figures demonstrate the wide range of collateral circulation available to support the pressure and flow in the Circle of Willis. These variations in collateral will alter the velocity and blood flow within the stenosis. To understand the influence of this collateral circulation, and in order to predict the effects of stenosis on brain perfusion, a model of the carotid blood supply to the Circle of Willis was conceived (Figure 9). In this model P_1 represents the

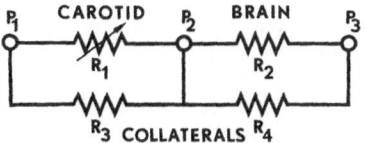

Figure 9. A model useful in understanding the influence of collateral circulation on brain perfusion.

common carotid arterial pressure; P_2 represents the pressure in the distal internal carotid and the Circle of Willis, and P_3 represents the jugular vein pressure. R_1 represents the varying resistance of the carotid stenosis, R_2 the resistance of the brain perfused by the internal carotid, and R_3 represents all channels potentially serving as collateral for the internal carotid. R_4 represents vascular resistance of the tissues normally supplied by the collateral arteries which drain into the jugular vein. In the normal, non-stenotic situation, R_1 is very small in comparison to R_3 and, therefore, the flow through R_1 is divided between R_2 and R_4.

The theoretical effect of extreme variations in collateral on carotid F and v is shown in Figure 10.

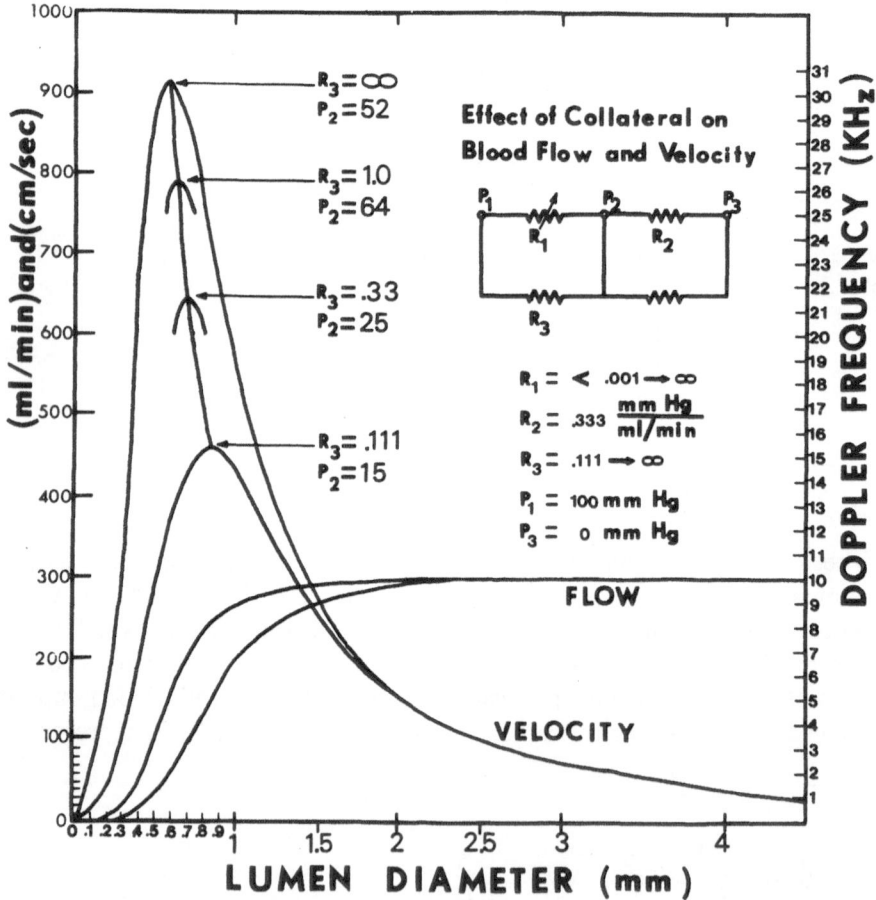

Figure 10. The effect of collateral circulation on blood flow and velocity in carotid stenosis. See text for definitions in the resistive model.

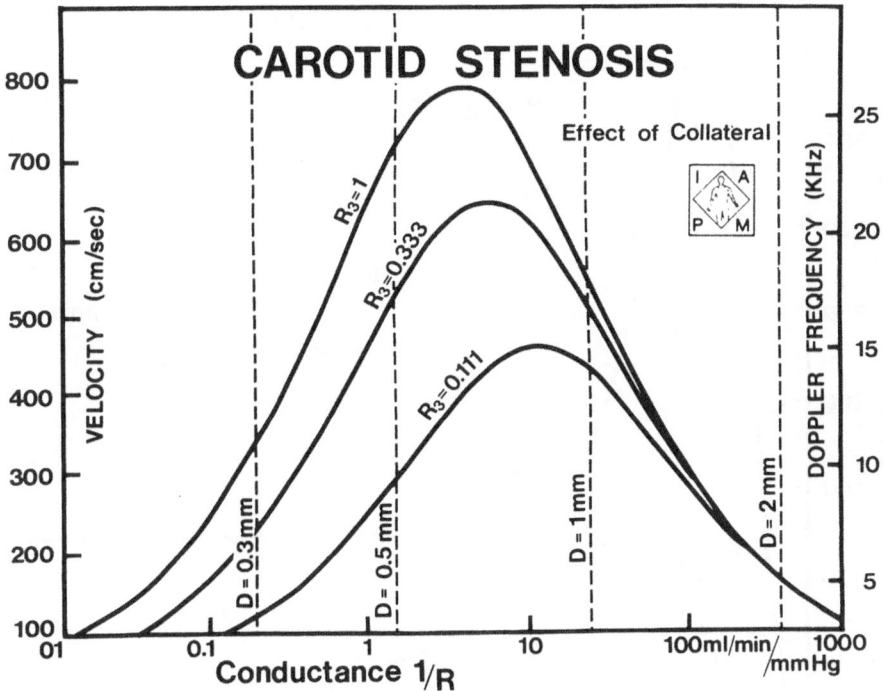

Figure 11. A Replot of the data in Figure 10. Plotting conductance on a log scale accentuates the great effect in the critical stages of collateral circulation.

The effect is seen only when the stenosis reaches the critical dimensions less than 2 mm of diameter. Figure 11 illustrates the same data in a way that expands the effects seen during the critical phases of stenosis. Here velocity is plotted against the conductance $(1/R)$ of the stenosis, against the corresponding velocity when R_3 varies between 1 and 0.111. Again it is seen that increasing velocities down to 2 mm diameter may be predictive of resistance of diameter regardless of collaterals, but at diameters of 1 mm and less the velocity will vary considerably with the collateral availability.

5. EFFECTS ON BRAIN PERFUSION

Figure 12 demonstrates that hemispheric perfusion cannot diminish more than 50% of its normal value when total occlusion of the internal carotid occurs if there is equal resistance (conductance) of the collateral channels and the brain vasculature. If collateral resistance is less than brain resistance, as often occurs, brain perfusion may not be affected.

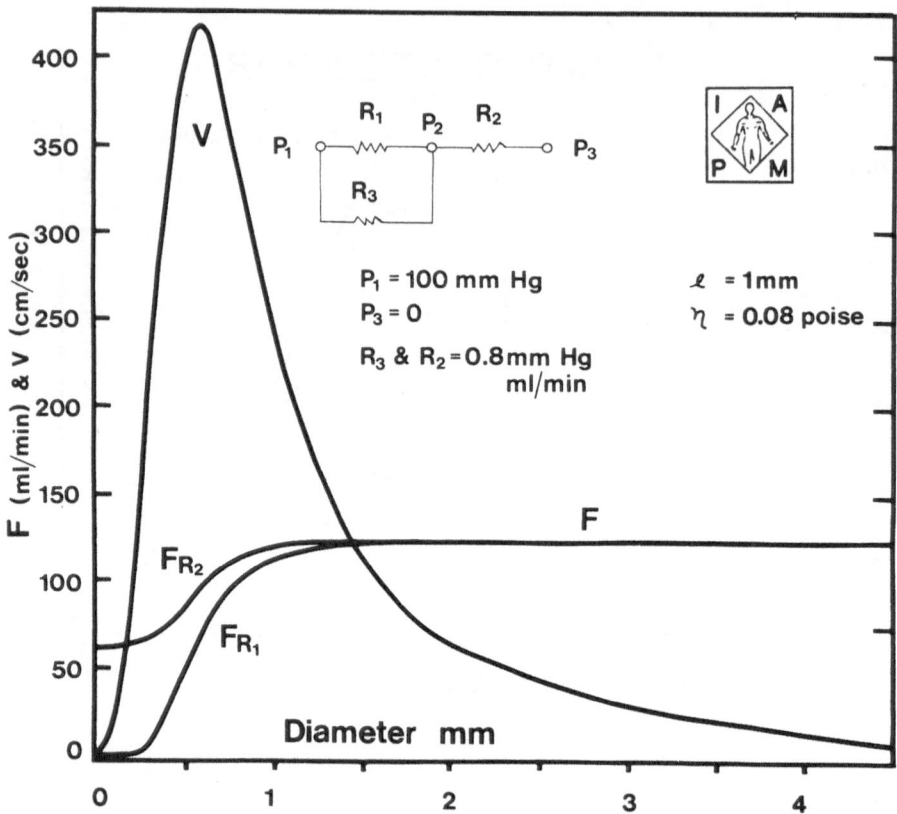

Figure 12. Effect of carotid stenosis on brain perfusion.

Brain resistance of vascular channels served by 23 internal carotids, calculated from pressure and flow measurements following endarterectomy, varied from 0.2 to 1 mm Hg/ml/min and averaged 0.6. The data to calculate collateral resistance was not available, but measurements of stump pressure and Doppler evaluations of collateral circulation and Circle of Willis pressure indicates that collateral resistance does not vary outside the limits of 0.1 and 1 mm Hg/ml/min and averages around 0.3.

Immediately following carotid occlusion, brain perfusion falls significantly, averaging 50% of control in 19 patients (Waltz et al. 1972) and falling to 35% in 45 patients of another study (Jenett et al. 1976).* However, in patients with longstanding complete occlusion of one or both carotids, cerebral blood flow (CBF) was reduced by an average of only 12% and the lowest CBF was 40 ml/min/100 gms, a reduction of 27% (Adams et al. 1963). No statistically

---

* Internal carotid obstructions caused a greater decrease than did common carotid obstructions.

significant improvement in CBF results from carotid endarterectomy of stenotic lesions (O'Brien et al. 1967, Adams et al. 1963). Combined carotid-vertebral lesions or aortic arch lesions do depress CBF.

It therefore appears certain that obstruction by stenosis or occlusion of the internal or common carotid artery, as it develops in atherosclerosis, does not produce clinically significant brain ischemia. Presumably, the gradual onset of the stenosis allows time for the development of collateral channels.

6. EXPERIMENTAL STENOSIS IN SHEEP CAROTIDS

To experimentally test the validity of the carotid flow predictions of the model, we produced graded stenosis of the common carotid in adult sheep while measuring flow and pressure difference. Since sheep have extremely rich collaterals for the common carotid artery, the contralateral carotid was ligated to produce conditions more similar to the human carotid. Graded stenosis was produced with a flexible wire snare. Blood velocity was recorded with the 5 MHz C-W Doppler probe angled at 60 degrees from the vessel axis and the volumetric blood flow was measured simultaneously with the square wave electromagnetic flow meter. Real time spectral analysis was performed on the Doppler audio signals using the Kay sonogram. From the spectrum and the probe angle, we determined the peak maximum systolic velocity present during each grade of constriction. The set of sheep stenosis considered to be most complete and most accurate is presented in Figure 13.

The maximum ΔP developed upon complete occlusion, even with the opposite carotid occluded, was 51 mmHg. The diameter on the abscissa of this plot is a computed one, utilizing instantaneous F and v max. As in Selverstone clamp patients and the theoretical model, the maximum frequency is reached at the time of 1/2 initial flow and 1/2 final ΔP, but this occurred at 1.4 mm diameter, somewhat greater than predicted. The maximum velocity reached (284 cm/sec) occurring when ΔP was 26 mmHg i.e. when 1/2 of the total pressure head was potentially available at the time of total occlusion (1/2 ΔP_{max}). In the experiment, R_2 and R_3 were both calculated to be 0.37 PRU's when the mean arterial pressure was 112 mmHg. R_3 was calculated at this stage (grade III stenosis) as:

$$R_3 = 1 / \left(\frac{1}{R_1} + \frac{1}{R_2} \right)$$

The experimental values for R_3 were close to the selected values for theoretical R_2 and R_3 of Figure 8, and are in the middle of the range chosen for the collateral study of Figure 10.

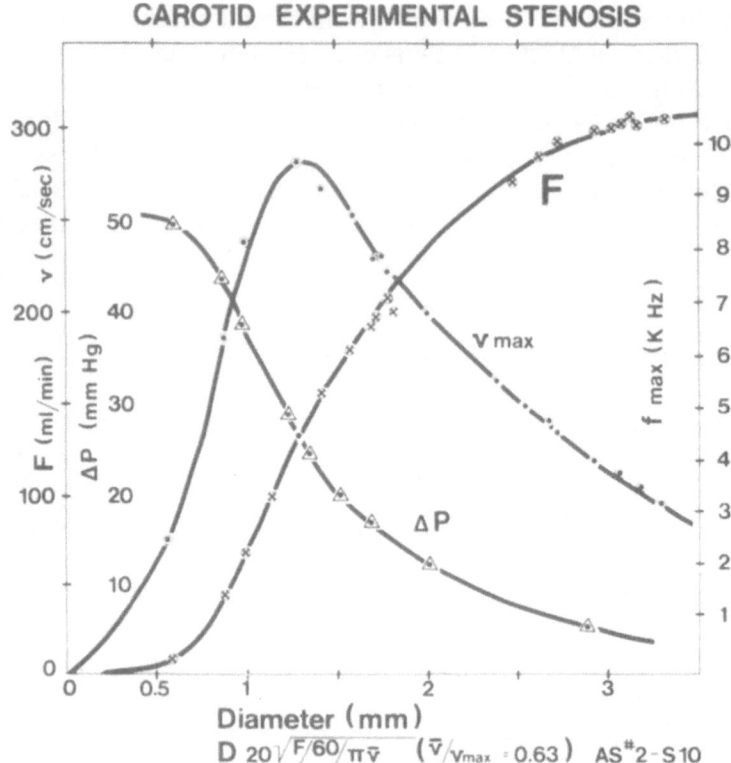

CAROTID EXPERIMENTAL STENOSIS

Diameter (mm)

$D\ 20\sqrt{F/60}/\pi\bar{v}$ $(\bar{v}/v_{max} = 0.63)$ $AS^{\#}2-S10$

Figure 13. Experimental effects of stenosis on blood velocity and flow in a sheep's carotid artery. Critical stenosis indicated by maximum velocity occurs at 1 mm effective diameter.

The principal discrepancy between theory and experiment appears to be the magnitude of the experimental velocity which is less than the theoretical one by a factor of 2.3. This deviation is shown in Figure 14 and may be explained by a pressure head loss caused by turbulence downstream from abrupt stenosis. This non-linear deviation is not entered into the model but is taken up in the discussion of Reynold's numbers.

The total pressure drop across a stenosis is $\varDelta P_s$, the sum of $\varDelta P_R$ of Poiseville (due to viscous loss) and $\varDelta P_B$ due to unregained kinetic loss of Bernoulli:

$$\varDelta P_s = \varDelta P_R + \varDelta P_B .$$

In terms of cross-sectional area:

$$\varDelta P_s = \frac{8\eta_s^!\pi}{A_s^2} \times F + \tfrac{1}{2}\rho(1/A_s^2 - 1/A_1^{l2})\,F^2$$

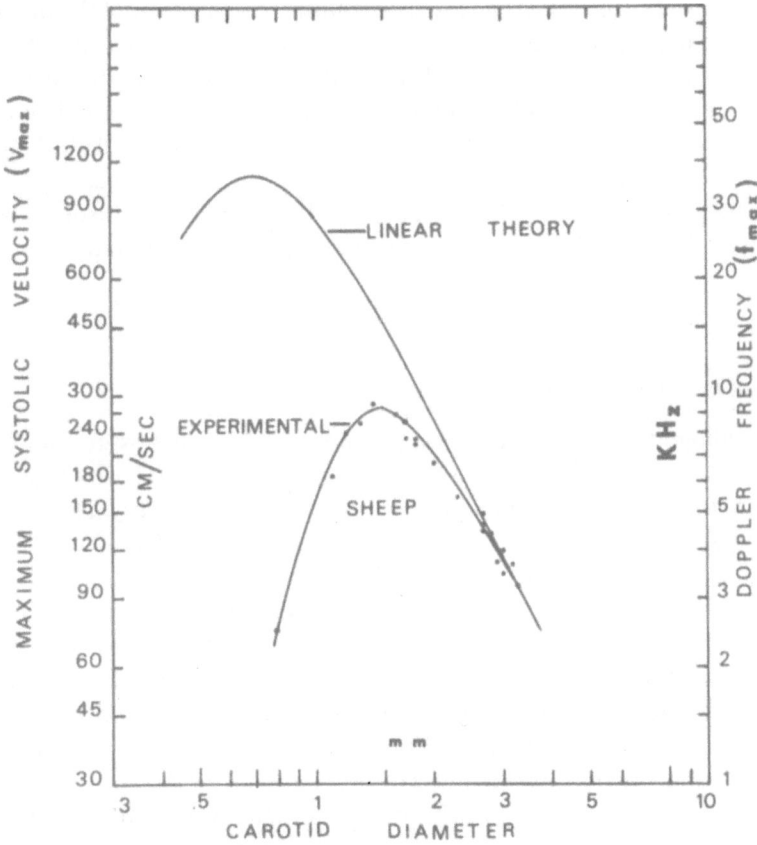

Figure 14. Deviation from linear theory of experimental stenosis velocities.

Where A_s = cross-sectional area in stenosis
  l_s = length of stenosis
  A_l = cross-sectional area proximal to stenosis.
In moderate and severe stenosis, A_s is less than half A_l, therefore $1/A_l^2$ can be neglected and ΔP_s is inversely proportional to A_s^2 in both the Poiseville and Bernoulli terms. At high volume flows of Grade I, II, and III carotid stenosis, ΔP_s is proportional to v_s^2 and the distal carotid intracranial pressure may be estimated from the Doppler frequency (f_{max}). In the sheep experimental data, ΔP_s was found to be calculable from:

$$\Delta P_s = f_{max}^2/3.3$$

so long as turbulence could be recognized in the Doppler signal.

We must conclude that stenosis velocities, as predicted by considering smooth stenosis only, are approximately twice those found in patients and experiments with abrupt stenosis. Maximum velocities of 500 cm/sec may, however, be expected in smooth stenosis and poor collaterals. It appears that the experimental sheep data provides a better description of the real relationship than does the theoretical prediction. The theoretical predictions were based on smooth-type of stenosis without turbulence, and turbulence is known to occur in most cases of stenosis of human subjects. It appears non-linearity introduced by turbulence in downstream stenosis is a likely explanation for the discrepancy between the theoretical and experimental data.

7. CLINICAL APPLICATIONS

The foregoing concepts of Doppler frequency relationships to stenosis and blood velocity were tested in two Seattle vascular clinics. The highest Doppler frequency found at the origin of the internal carotid artery at the time of imaging was compared with the minimal internal carotid diameter measured on x-ray arteriography films (Figure 15).

All patients during one calendar year were utilized if Doppler data and films were usable. If there was no stenosis present on the x-ray film the internal diameter was measured 0.5 cm from the origin where Doppler frequencies are routinely recorded on magnetic tape. Figure 15 illustrates the relationship found between the maximum systolic frequency and the smallest diameter found on the available x-ray films.

The ordinates used are logarithmic in order to spread out the points representing the smallest diameter and to compress the frequency range. On such ordinates the theoretical relationship represented between frequency (velocity) and effective diameter approaches a straight line since the square of the diameter is proportional to the Doppler frequency.

From Figure 15 it is apparent that Doppler frequencies found in carotid stenosis do generally follow the experimental relationship, but scattering around a trend less than the theoretical frequency. Much of the scatter in Figure 15 is due to problems of the x-ray in identifying the true luminal diameter. The great difference in the highest frequency obtained in patients and the highest theoretical frequency is undoubtedly due to downstream turbulence which develops in higher degrees of stenosis. Turbulence which reduced available head pressure to move blood was not accounted for in the theoretical relationship.

Clinically useful 'rules of thumb' arise from the quantitative exercise of Figure 15.

1. If the maximum systolic Doppler frequency at the origin of the internal exceeds 5 KHz a stenosis diameter of less than 3.5 mm is probably present.

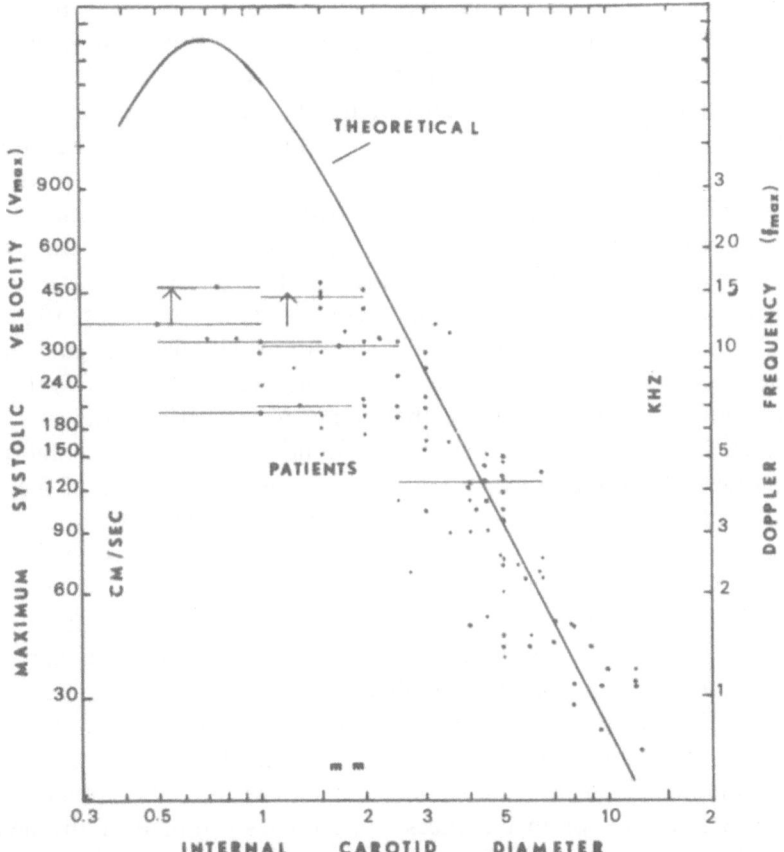

Figure 15. Maximum systolic frequencies found in patients and their corresponding carotid diameter, compared with theoretical relationship expected in smooth
(non-abrupt) stenosis. Deviation begins at 3 mm stenosis diameter, and increases
to limit greatest maximum velocity to 460 cm/sec: The horizontal lines represent
unusual uncertainty (greater than ±0.5 mm) in the diameter measurement. The
vertical arrows represent that we were not able to measure the maximum
frequency because of limitations of the magnetic tape from which spectral analysis was obtained.

2. If a frequency higher than 10 KHz is recorded, the narrowest x-ray
diameter likely to be found will be less than 2.5 mm.

In the clinic without spectral analysis available an excellent prediction of
what will be found at angiography can be performed by use of several
clues.

1. In a given patient an estimate of the ratio of the frequency found
downstream to the stenosis, at the angle of the jaw, and the frequencies
found within the stenosis provides an estimate of percent of stenosis present.

In the normal carotid, with a bulbous 'take off' of the internal, the frequencies increase as the artery lumen tapers to its usual 5 mm diameter at the jaw line. Subtle degrees of stenosis of the internal origin can be diagnosed if attention is paid to the downstream/origin frequency ratio.

2. When a very high frequency is heard from the origin of the internal, a highly important diagnosis of critical grades of stenosis can be made. If for example, the downstream frequencies are perceived by the hearing to be less than the normal carotid frequencies (i.e. less than 1 Kz) when the proximal 'stenosis frequency' is very high (i.e. greater than 5 KHz) one can conclude that the effective diameter of the artery within the stenosis is less than 1 mm. It should be noted that x-ray uncertainties of 'true' diameter and effective cross sectional area are greatest when lumen diameters are 1 mm or less. Doppler signals are more accurate than x-ray in critical stenosis.

3. When Doppler high frequencies are found to be weak and highly localized a critical stenosis is present. Often respiratory movements of the patient are sufficient to move the stenosis in and out of the Doppler beam. One of the great values of imaging is the assistance it provides in making a thorough and systematic search for high frequency signals at the origin of the internal. When critical threadlike 'preocclusive' stenosis is present, identification of the bifurcation and the location of the internal origin imaging narrows the field of search to enhance the possibility of finding the diagnostic signals. Hand-held Doppler probes of the bifurcation region and opthalmic artery or its branches often fail when imaging succeeds in detecting critical stenosis.

4. A combination of imaging signals and signals from the opthalmic artery in the posterior orbit often enhances the Doppler estimate of the degree of stenosis. For example, in the situation where high frequencies are found from the internal and opthalmic flow signals are normally directed, compression of the contralateral common carotid can establish whether the opthalmic flow is arising from the opposite carotid through collaterals or establish its source from the homolateral internal. In the former situation the diagnosis of the hemodynamically significant stenosis of the internal can be made. In the later situation the stenosis is non-hemodynamically significant (Grades I or II).

The information provided in this chapter is consistant with the concept that strokes developing from carotid stenosis arise from emboli at the stenotic site. Local brain perfusion defects producing the stroke are not detectable with flow measurement techniques applied to the extracranial blood vessels. The need for Doppler evaluations of the carotid bifurcation is based on; the stroke prevention assistance of finding operable lesions, evaluation of the collateral circulation, x-ray angiography evaluation of surgical hemodynamic results, following the progress of lesions, and assisting in the identification of embolic sources. Those and other examples of these, and other uses of the cerebrovascular evaluation are presented in subsequent chapters.

REFERENCES

1. Adams JE, Smith MC, Wylie EJ, Leake TB, Halliday B: Cerebral blood flow and hemodynamics in extracranial vascular disease: effect of endarterectomy. Surgery 53(4):449-55, April 1963.
2. O'Brien MD, Veall N, Luck RJ, Irvine WT: Cerebral-cortex perfusion-rates in extracranial cerebrovascular disease and the effects of operation. The Lancet, August 19, 1967: 392-395.
3. Reneman RS, Spencer MP: Local Doppler audio spectra in normal and stenosed carotid arteries in man. Ultrasound in Medicine and Biology 5(1):1-11, Pergamon Press, 1979.
4. Spencer MP, Johnson DL, Lawrence GG, Tytus JS, Hill LD: Evaluation of cardio-vascular lesions by means of an impedance plot at the time of surgical correction. Bulletin 20(1):1-12, The Mason Clinic, March 1966.
5. Spencer MP, Reid JM: Quantification of carotid stenosis with continuous-wave (c-w) Doppler ultrasound. Stroke 10(3):326-330, May-June 1979.
6. Waltz AG, Sundt TM, Michenfelder JD: Cerebral blood flow during carotid endar-terectomy. Circulation 45(5):1091-1096, May 1972.

10. AUDIO SPECTRAL ANALYSIS

Robert S. Reneman, M.D.

In continous-wave (c-w) Doppler flowmeters the received spectrum of frequencies is often processed to an analog tracing, representing the average velocity as an instantaneous function of time (Figure 1). In this technique

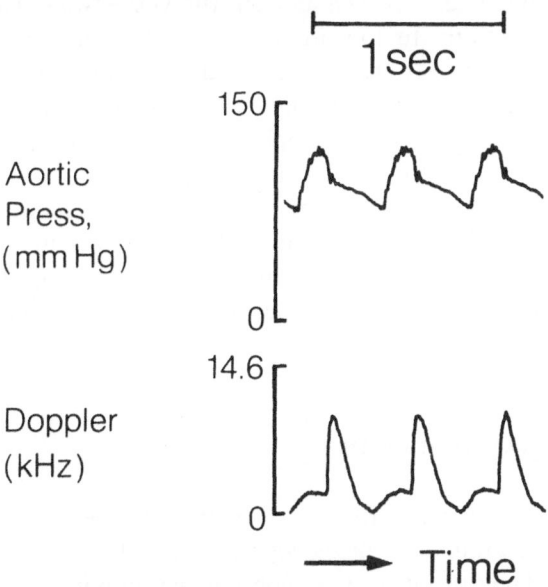

Figure 1. Aortic pressure curve and instantaneous flow tracing as recorded in the femoral artery of the dog with a 10 MHz c-w Doppler flowmeter, using a zero-crossing technique. The analog flow tracing represents the average velocity as an instantaneous function of time.

valuable information present in the Doppler signal is ignored [1]. Besides, the processing of analog tracings is subject to errors, especially when zero-crossing meters are used [2, 3]. Despite these disadvantages, analog tracings are most commonly used because investigators are acquainted with these types of tracings, resembling the instantaneous blood pressure wave form. In this chapter the limitations of analog tracings are summarized and audio spectrum analysis is discussed as an alternative way of analyzing received Doppler information.

134

1. THE DOPPLER SIGNAL

In Doppler flowmeters a beam of ultrasonic waves (at MHz level) is transmitted from a vibrating crystal diagonally through the vessel wall into the bloodstream. Ultrasound backscattered from particles in the flowing blood, mainly the red cells, is shifted in frequency by an amount proportional to the velocity of these particles. This frequency shift, which is retrieved by mixing the transmitted and received signals, is in the audio range and is called the Doppler signal. Information about the direction of blood flow can be derived when special demodulation techniques are used [4, 5].

In C-W Doppler flowmeters, the Doppler signal contains power backscattered from red blood cells as well as from the vessel wall. The signals induced by lateral wall motion are low in frequency, but high in amplitude. Their amplitude is approximately thirty times higher than that of signals induced by moving red blood cells. To diminish the influence of vessel wall motion signals and noise beyond the Doppler frequency band, the output of the demodulator is passed through a bandpass filter.

The Doppler signal does not contain one single frequency, but a spectrum of frequencies (the Doppler spectrum). The variations in frequency distribution depend on such factors as unequal distribution of the red blood cell velocity over the cross-sectional area of the vessel, variations in the blood cell interspaces and divergence and non-uniformity of the sound beams [6].

2. ANALOG SIGNAL PROCESSING

Determination of the mean frequency of the Doppler spectrum and conversion of the signal into an analog signal is usually performed with a zero-crossing meter. The output is an analog voltage proportional to the number of zero-crossings per unit of time. To diminish the counting of zero-crossing not related to blood flow velocity, the comparator voltage of the Schmitt-trigger is set at a relatively high level. In this mode the zero-crossing meter will not be activated by low level signals (e.g. noise).

Difficulties encountered in this signal processing technique were examined previously [2, 3]. The zero-crossing meter does not exactly measure the mean frequency of the Doppler spectrum, corresponding to the average velocity, but a value higher than the mean Doppler frequency [6, 7]. This systematic error depends on the shape and the width of the Doppler spectrum, the broader the spectrum the larger the error.

The zero-crossing meter appears to be accurate only for a single frequency or a relatively narrow frequency spectrum [6]. This limits the applicability of zero-crossing meters in combination with C-W Doppler system, where a wide spectrum is fed into the meter. In pulsed Doppler devices, small sample volumes are taken over the cross-sectional area of the blood vessel so that a narrow frequency spectrum is offered to the zero-crossing meter. Hence the error made in determining the mean frequency of the Doppler spectrum is smaller in these devices. An additional disadvantage of zero-crossing meters is that the output is independent of the amplitude of the audio-signal only at higher input levels (Figure 2). Increasing the peak-to-peak voltage of the audio-signal, however, is associated with amplification of noise, resulting in a shift of the instantaneous flow velocity tracing from the zero line.

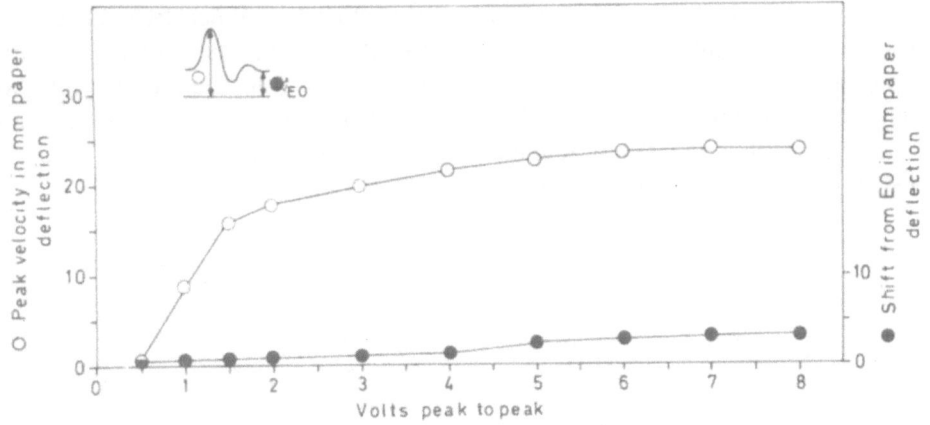

Figure 2. The peak velocity reading in the femoral artery and the shift of the instantaneous tracing from the electrical zero (EO) line as a function of peak-to-peak voltage of the audio signal during systole. From Reneman and Spencer [3].

This is especially a problem when the signal to noise ratio is poor (less than 10). Higher cut-offs at the lower end of the bandpass filter can largely prevent this shift [3], however, at a cost of lower flow velocity information. Artificial shifting from the zero line should be anticipated because in cerebral vascular disease valuable information can be derived from the systolic and diastolic amplitudes of the analog velocity tracings of the common carotid artery [8].

Recently and alternative method has been described to determine the mean velocity from the Doppler spectrum [9, 10]. This method looks promising because it properly takes into account the spectral distribution of frequencies and avoids the problems encountered in zero-crossing meters. This processing method, however, has been tested only under stable flow conditions. Information about its accuracy, when pulsatile flow is present, is required to appreciate the advantages of the method.

In spite of this possible improvement in the processing of analog tracings in c-w Doppler flowmeters, the use of these tracings has limitations. Although shape analysis and the systolic and diastolic amplitudes of the analog velocity tracing do give important information about the site and severness of arterial stenosis (see 11 for review) valuable information, present in the Doppler signal, is eliminated in this technique. More detailed information can be obtained from the Doppler signal when audio spectrum analysis is used [12].

3. AUDIO SPECTRUM ANALYSIS

In audio spectrum analysis, sonagrams are produced in which frequencies are given as an instantaneous function of time and the intensity of the pattern represents the amplitude of the frequencies, indicating the number of red blood cells moving at a given velocity (Figure 3). From sonagrams, information can be obtained about maximum blood flow velocity and the velocity distribution of red blood cells, giving insight in the flow pattern [13].

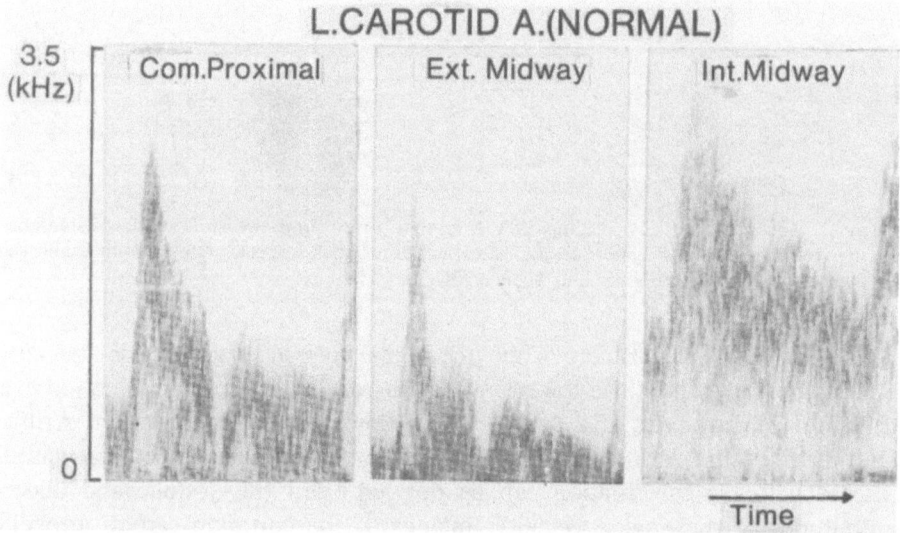

Figure 3. Sonagrams recorded in the common, external and internal carotid arteries in a volunteer without symptoms of cardiovascular disease. Proximal = just above the clavicle. Midway = halfway between the bifurcation and the mandible.

These are important variable in evaluating the peripheral arterial circulation. The maximum velocity can, for example, be used to diagnose lesions in arteries [1] or to estimate the degree of arterial stenosis [14]. Since changes in flow pattern along narrowed arteries occur at relatively slight degrees of stenosis [15, 16, 17], it is rather likely that the detection of these flow disturbances will contribute to the early diagnosis of arterial disease.

In laminar flow, the outline of the sonagram, defined as the line following the maximum frequencies during the cardiac cycle, is regular (Figure 3). In turbulent flow this outline becomes irregular due to the random changes in flow velocities occuring at any time during the cardiac cycle (Figures 4 and 5).

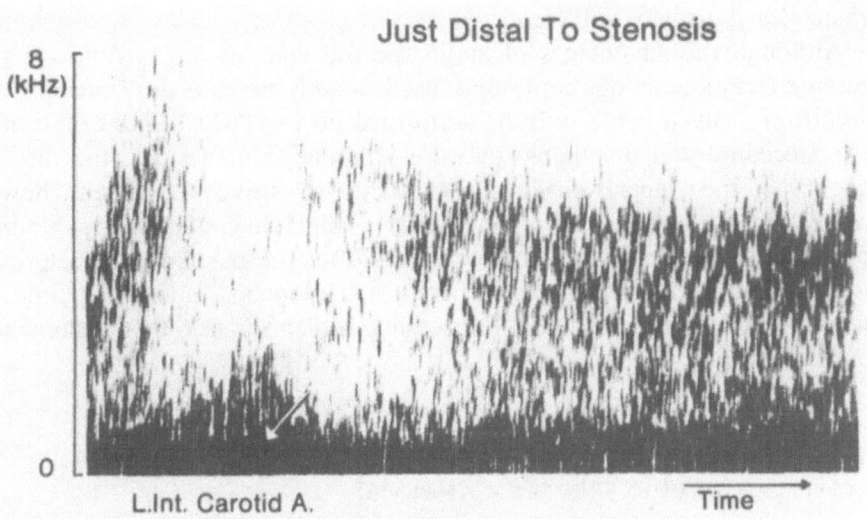

Figure 4. Sonagram as recorded in the internal carotid artery just distal to a relatively short stenosis of 67%. Note the high amplitude low frequency components during systole due to vessel wall vibration (see arrow). From Reneman and Spencer [13].

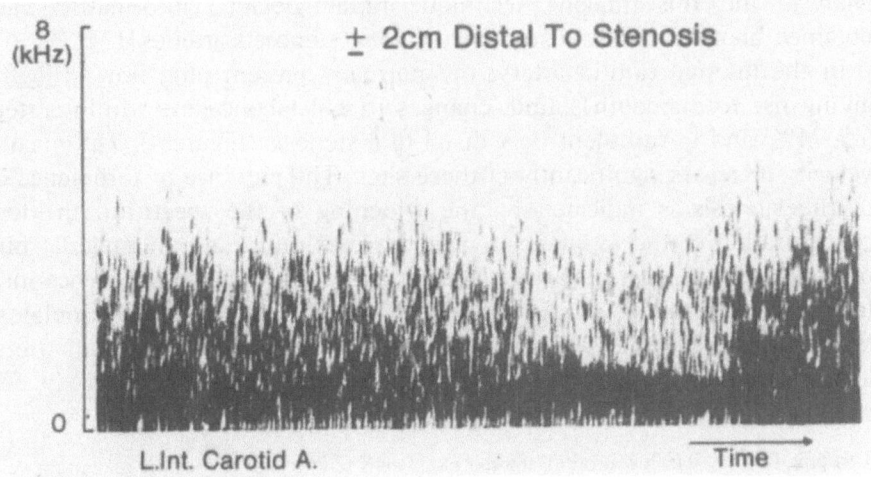

Figure 5. Sonagram as recorded in the internal carotid artery approximately 2 cm downstream to a stenosis. Same patient as in Figure 4. From Reneman and Spencer [13].

In the presence of high amplitude low frequencies due to lateral wall motion, high frequencies are often not presented on the sonagram. In this situation additional filtering at the lower end of the bandpass is required to attenuate these low frequencies in order to demonstrate the presence of high frequency information [13]. An increase in roll-off rate rather than increasing the cut-off frequency is usually sufficient.

Although the advantages of audio spectral analysis are obvious, this processing technique is not commonly used, mainly because until recently audio spectrum analysis could only be performed off-line, which is a time-consuming procedure and unsuitable for clinical application. Besides, the mean frequency of the Doppler spectrum is difficult to derive. At present, however, several on-line systems are commercially available [e.g. 18]. Beside the on-line presentation of sonagrams, these systems offer the possibility of determining the maximum and mean velocity as an instantaneous function of time. This requires, however, additional processing which makes the system rather expensive.

4. THE COMBINATION OF C–W DOPPLER FLOWMETER WITH IMAGING SYSTEM AND AUDIO SPECTRUM ANALYSIS

Beside the assessment of blood flow velocity, c-w Doppler flowmeters are used to imaging the circulation (see Chapters 3 and 4), allowing determination of the site of local blood velocities. The site of carotid artery stenosis can be determined with this technique [19, 20, 21]. By combining audio spectrum analysis and this imaging technique rather detailed information can be obtained about the flow disturbances along stenosed arteries [13].

In the internal carotid artery, the normally present plug flow* (Figure 3), giving rise to a smooth sound, changes to a parabolic flow within a stenosis (65–74%) and to turbulent flow distal to a stenosis (Figure 4). The maximum velocity increases significantly at these sites. The presence of turbulence distal to the stenosis is indicated by the widening of the spectrum, the loss of concentration of the frequencies near the maximum and an irregular outline of the sonagram. Just distal to a stenosis the high velocity turbulence induces lateral wall vibration, producing a gruff quality sound which simulates the bruit heard with the stethoscope. In the sonagram, lateral wall vibration appears as high amplitude low frequencies, less than 675 Hz for a 5 MHz

---

* In plug flow (= flat flow profile), the red blood cells tend to travel near the maximum velocity, giving rise to a concentration of frequencies near the maximum frequency. In parabolic flow, the red blood cells are travelling at various velocities, resulting in widening of the spectrum and a more or less even distribution of frequencies over the spectrum. Plug flow and parabolic flow are laminar flow patterns.

Doppler instrument, usually throughout systole (Figure 4). High-amplitude low-frequency components are occasionally seen in sonagrams of normal carotid arteries. In normal arteries, however, these low frequencies are present in systole only during acceleration and deceleration of blood flow. The gruff quality sound and the high amplitude low frequencies disappear approximately 2 cm downstream to the stenosis. At this site, the maximum frequencies of the sonagram decreases significantly, as compared with just distal to the stenosis but all signs of turbulence persist (Figure 5). The low velocity turbulence produces at this site a boiling or fluttering quality sound. Three to 4 cm downstream to a stenosis flow has become laminar again as indicated by the generally regular outline of the sonagram and the tendency of the frequencies to concentrate near the maximum frequency (Figure 6).

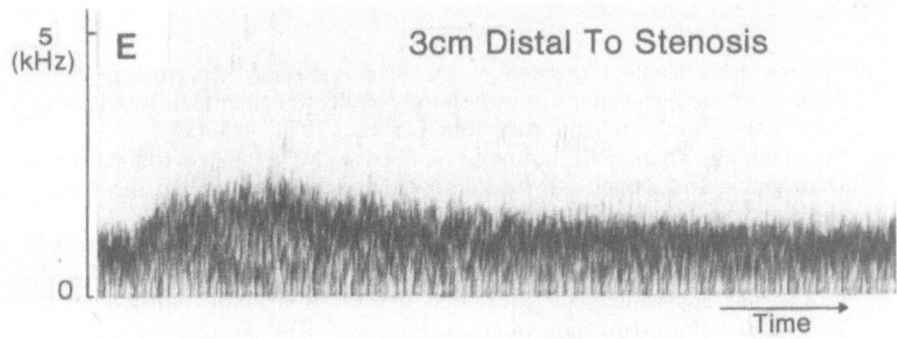

Figure 6. Sonagram as recorded in the internal carotid artery approximately 3 cm downstream to a stenosis. Same patient as in Figure 4. From Reneman and Spencer[13].

5. CONCLUSIONS

Although Doppler analog velocity tracings do give valuable information about the site and severness of arterial stenosis, the use of these tracings has its limitation. Beside the difficulties encountered in the processing of analog tracings, valuable information, present in the Doppler signal, is eliminated in the technique.

More detailed information can be derived from the Doppler signal when audio spectrum analysis is used. This method gives information about the maximum blood flow velocity, the velocity distribution of the red blood cells — giving insight in the flow pattern — and the degree of lateral wall motion.

By combining a c-w Doppler flowmeter with imaging system and audio spectrum analysis rather detailed information can be obtained about the flow disturbances along narrowed arteries. Since these disturbances occur at relatively slight degrees of stenosis, their detection may contribute to the early diagnosis of arterial disease.

Whether audio spectrum analysis can be considered as an alternative or a complement to analog velocity tracings in evaluating the peripheral arterial circulation in man, remains subject to further clinical investigation.

ACKNOWLEDGEMENT

The author of this chapter is indebted to Mrs Mariet de Groot for her help in preparing the manuscript and to Dr. Arnold Hoeks for his stimulating discussion.

REFERENCES

1. Gosling RG: General discussion: the usefulness of zero-crossing meters. In: Cardiovascular applications of ultrasound (ed RS Reneman). Amsterdam/London/New York: North-Holland/American Elsevier, 1974, 455-456.
2. Reneman RS, Clark HF, Simmons N, Spencer MP: In vivo comparison of electromagnetic and Doppler flowmeters: with special attention to the processing of the analogue Doppler flow signal. Cardiovasc Res 7:557-566, 1973.
3. Reneman RS, Spencer MP: Difficulties in processing of analogue Doppler flow signal; with special reference to zero-crossing meters and quantification. In: Cardiovascular applications of ultrasound (ed RS Reneman). Amsterdam/London/New York: North-Holland/American Elsevier, 1974, 32-42.
4. McLeod FD: A directional Doppler flowmeter. Digest of Seventh International Conference on Medical and Biological Engineering, Stockholm, 1967, 213.
5. Strandess DE, Kennedy JW, Judge TP, McLeod FD: Transcutaneous directional flow detection: a preliminary report. Am Heart J 78:65-74, 1969.
6. Peronneau P, Hinglais J, Pellet M, Leger F: Vélocimètre sanguin par effet Doppler à émission ultra-sonore pulsée. L'Onde électrique 50:369-384, 1970.
7. Rice SO: Mathematical analysis of random noise. Bell System Tech J 23:1-162, 1944.
8. Mol JMF, Rijcken WJ: Doppler haematotachographic investigation in cerebral circulation disturbances. In: Cardiovascular applications of ultrasound (ed RS Reneman). Amsterdam/London/New York: North-Holland/American Elsevier, 1974, 305-314.
9. Arts MGJ, Roevros JMJG: On the instantaneous measurement of blood flow by ultrasonic means. Med Biol Engng 10:23-34, 1972.
10. Reid JM, Davis DL, Ricketts HJ, Spencer MP: A new Doppler flowmeter system and its operation with catheter mounted transducers. In: Cardiovascular application of ultrasound (ed. RS Reneman). Amsterdam/London/New York: North-Holland/American Elsevier, 1974, 183-192.
11. Reneman RS, Hoeks A, Spencer MP: Doppler ultrasound in the evaluation of the peripheral arterial circulation. Angiology, 30:526-538, 1979.
12. Baskett JJ, Beasley MG, Murphy GJ, Hyams DE, Gosling RG: Screening for carotid junction disease by spectral analysis of Doppler signals. Cardiovasc Res 11:147-155, 1977.

13. Reneman RS, Spencer MP: Local Doppler audio spectra in normal and stenosed carotid arteries in man. Ultrasound Med & Biol 5:1-11, 1979.
14. Spencer MP, Reid JM: Quantitation of Carotid stenosis with C-W Doppler ultrasound. Stroke 10:326-330, 1979.
15. Barnes RW, Bone GE, Reinertson J, Slaymaker EE, Hokanson DE, Strandness DE: Noninvasive ultrasonic carotid angiography: prospective validation by contrast arteriography. Surgery 80:328-335, 1976.
16. Giddens DP, Mabon RF, Cassanova RA: Measurements of disordered flows distal to subtotal vascular stenoses in the thoracic aortas of dogs. Circ Res 39:112-119, 1976.
17. Sandmann W, Peronneau P, Schweins G, Bournat J, Hinglais J: Turbulenzmessung mit dem Doppler-Ultraschallverfahren: Eine neue Methode der Qualitätskontrolle in der Arterienchirurgie. In: Ultraschall-Doppler-Diagnostik in der Angiologie (ed A Kriesmann, A Bollinger). Stuttgart: Georg Thieme Verlag, 1978, 77-81.
18. Coughlan BA, Taylor MG, King DH: On-line display of Doppler-shift spectra by a new time compression analyser. In: Cardiovascular applications of ultrasound (ed RS Reneman). Amsterdam/London/New York: North-Holland/American Elsevier, 1974, 55-66.
19. Spencer MP, Brockenbrough EC, Davis DL, Reid JM): Cerebro-vascular evaluation using Doppler C-W ultrasound. Ultrasound in Medicine 3B:1291-1310, 1977.
20. Spencer MP, Reid JM, Davis DL, Paulson PS: Cervical carotid imaging with continuous-wave Doppler flowmeter. Stroke 5:145-154, 1974.
21. Spencer MP, Reid JM, Paulson PS: Diagnosis or carotid artery disease and cerebral vascular insufficiency with Doppler angiography and ophthalmic artery sonography. In: Cardiovascular applications of ultrasound (ed. RS Reneman). Amsterdam/London/New York: North-Holland/American Elsevier, 1974, 249-266.

11. THE PERIORBITAL COLLATERAL ARTERIES

EDWIN C. BROCKENBROUGH, M.D.

Obstruction to blood flow through the internal carotid artery invokes collateral blood supply from the Circle of Willis and from reversal of flow in the ophthalmic artery. These collateral pathways serve to ameliorate the effects of the restricted carotid blood flow. In addition they provide a simple means by which the diagnosis of carotid obstruction may be suspected. Using a Doppler ultrasonic velocity detector, flow in these vessels may be examined and the presence or absence of functioning collateral pathways may be determined. The technique for this examination has been developed over a period of years and has proved to be a reliable method of screening for significant carotid obstruction.

Our first experience in this area began in 1967 with the advent of the early commercial models of the Doppler velocity detectors [1]. The concept of the supraorbital Doppler test for carotid obstruction was developed in conjunction with another diagnostic technique for carotid disease which we called *Ocular Plethysmography* [2]. Both of these tests were based on the principle of compressing collateral vessels feeding the ophthalmic artery as a means of recognizing the abnormal flow patterns associated with internal carotid obstruction. The Doppler test became more refined when direction capability was added to the instrument in 1968. As our experience grew, it became apparent that the frontal, supraorbital, and angular arteries were each important to an understanding of the vagaries of collateral circulation, hence the more descriptive term *periorbital* Doppler examination.

A number of other investigators have made observations similar to ours and produced their own contributions in this area. Maroon and his collaborators independently described 'Ophthalmosonometry' in 1969 [3]. Müller expanded on this concept in 1972 and stressed the importance of retrograde flow in the frontal artery as a diagnostic sign for internal carotid occlusion [4]. Machleder and Barker utilized the periorbital test in 1972 and emphasized its usefulness in recognizing unsuspected carotid obstruction [5]. More recently, Barnes and Wilson have contributed a very comprehensive treatment of this subject, adding many of their own observations as well as reviewing in detail the principles involved [6]. The following is a status report on the periorbital test: the anatomy and principles on which the test is based, the technique of the examination, what information can be derived, and the role of the test in the spectrum of non-invasive diagnostic tests of the cerebrovascular system.

1. ANATOMIC BASIS OF THE PERIORBITAL EXAMINATION

Blood flow through the internal carotid artery is distributed almost entirely to intracranial vessels. The one exception to this is the ophthalmic artery. This artery passes into the orbit, gives rise to a number of intra-orbital branches, and then terminates in three branches which surface on the face. These are the nasal, frontal and supraorbital branches (Figure 1). The nasal artery becomes the angular artery, which descends along the lateral border of the nose and communicates with the facial branch of the external carotid artery. The frontal and supraorbital arteries turn upward and pass into the subcutaneous tissue of the forehead where they communicate with branches of the superficial temporal artery. These communications serve as collateral pathways in the event of internal carotid obstruction. Other communications between the ophthalmic artery and branches of the external carotid artery occur through the ethmoid and lacrimal branches. Although these are not

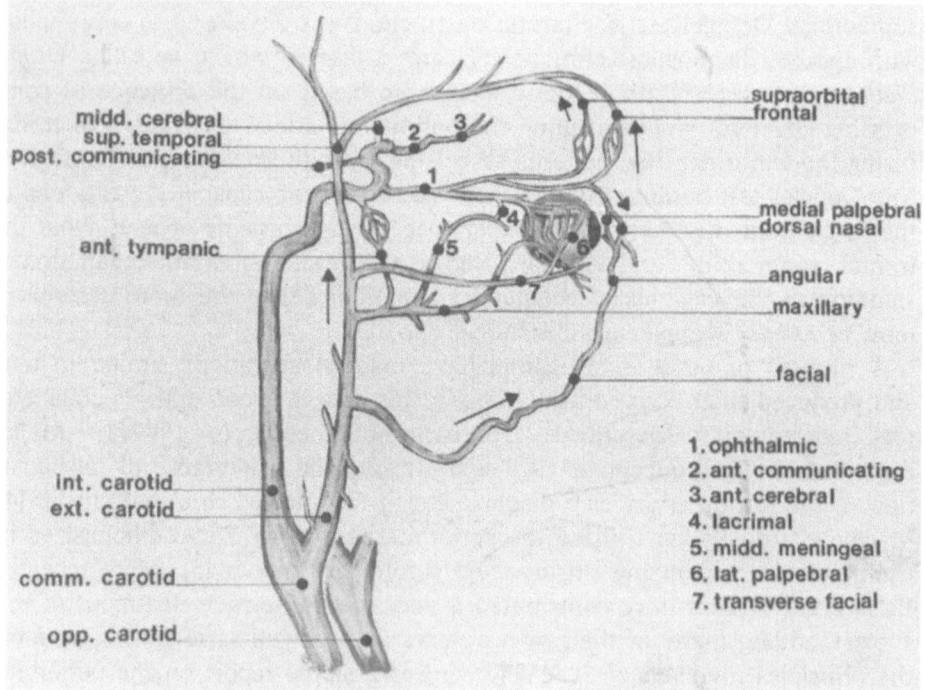

Figure 1. Arteries of significance to the periorbital Doppler test. Normal flow pattern.

accessible for Doppler examination, they need to be considered because of their contribution to the collateral blood supply. In addition to the periorbital anastomoses, the other major collateral pathway is the anterior communicating artery of the Circle of Willis. It is through this pathway that 'crossover' circulation occurs from the opposite internal carotid artery.

2. TECHNIQUE OF EXAMINATION

The examination consists of detecting flow in the periorbital vessels, noting the quality and direction of the velocity signals, and determining the response of these signals to compressions about the face and neck.

The Doppler equipment for the examination should have directional capability and the probe should be small enough to permit separate examination of each of these vessels. The examination is begun with the patient in the supine position and the eyes gently closed. The probe is then placed at the inner canthus of the eye and the maximum flow signal identified. It is then moved along this signal toward the rim of the orbit. This is the point of examination of the frontal artery. The probe is then moved laterally to the supraorbital notch where the supraorbital signal is identified. The angular artery may be located over the lateral aspect of the nose. It is the smallest of the three vessels and usually accompanied by a large vein (palpebral), making examination more difficult than the preceding vessels. Furthermore, this vessel is often absent in patients whose eyeglasses rest on this portion of the nose. For these reasons, examination of the angular artery is reserved for the patient in whom the frontal and supraorbital flow signals are abnormal.

If the Doppler probe is held in the proper angle, the direction of flow can usually be determined reliably. In some instances, however, a tortuous artery may alter the geometry of the probe angle in relation to the vessel and the observed direction of flow may be reversed. Compression techniques help to minimize errors of this sort.

During the examination it is important that the examiner hold the probe in a steady position, facilitated by resting the hand holding the probe on the patient's forehead and bridge of the nose. It is also important that the probe be held lightly because even a modest pressure from the tip of the probe can obliterate flow in these small vessels. In this regard the examiner must resist the tendency to press with the probe at the same time he is compressing the temporal or facial vessels with the opposite hand.

After the examiner has located the frontal and supraorbital arteries and noted the direction and quality of the flow signals, he compresses the superficial temporal artery in front of the ear, just above the zygoma. In most patients there will be slight augmentation of the frontal and supraorbital signals but in some normal individuals there will be no change. If the signals are diminished or obliterated by temporal artery compression, the flow may be assumed to be retrograde. The facial artery is then compressed along the lower border of the mandible and the effect of this compression on the frontal artery is noted. These maneuvers are then repeated on the opposite side.

Finally, common carotid compression is performed in order to identify crossover circulation. This compression is accomplished low in the neck, well away from the carotid bifurcation, and is maintained for only one or two heart beats. During this compression the probe is usually held at the inner canthus of the eye where the maximum flow signal is located.

Normally the signal at this point is obliterated or greatly diminished by ipsilateral carotid compression and is not effected by contralateral carotid compression. With the ipsilateral carotid compressed, the residual flow signals on both sides should be about the same. While there is undoubtedly some inherent risk of dislodging an embolus during carotid compression, the risk is low if the compression is brief and gentle. We have not recognized any complications in over five thousand patients in whom the compressions have been carried out.

3. PATTERNS OF COLLATERAL BLOOD FLOW

There are a variety of patterns of collateralization seen around the orbit in the presence of internal carotid obstruction. The following representative examples will be considered:

3.1. Dominant periorbital collaterals (Figure 2)

This is the most common pattern of collateralization, constituting over 90% of all abnormal examinations. This pattern is usually associated with high-grade stenosis or total occlusion of the internal carotid artery. The examiner first notices that there is asymmetry between the two sides. The signal on the obstructed side is dampened and has only a single component, or it may be loud and continuous. The direction indicator on the Doppler instrument shows that the direction of flow in the periorbital vessels is reversed. Furthermore, the periorbital signals are obliterated or diminished with temporal and facial artery compressions. In some instances a reversed signal may be converted to a normal directional signal by these compressions. Finally, there is usually some evidence of crossover flow with common carotid compression. Ipsilateral common carotid compression results in a prominent residual signal which may be either antegrade or retrograde, depending upon whether the dominant collateral supply is via the opposite internal carotid or the opposite

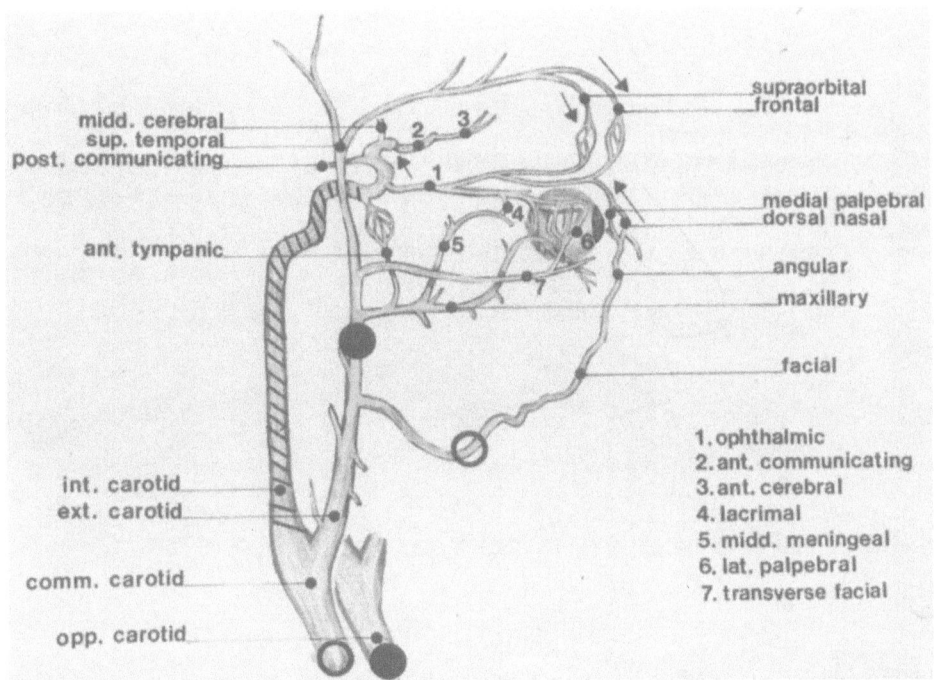

Figure 2. Carotid occlusion or high-grade stenosis: dominant periorbital collaterals. This is the flow pattern seen in over 90% of patients with this condition.

external carotid artery. Compression of the contralateral carotid artery will usually increase the retrograde flow in the periorbital vessels.

3.2. Dominant crossover collaterals (Figure 3)

This is the next most common condition and is usually seen in patients with long-standing occlusion on the internal carotid artery or in patients with a common carotid artery occlusion. The examiner first notices asymmetry between the two sides and usually detects an abnormal signal on the affected side. The flow is noted to be coming from within the orbit, but with compression of the common carotid artery on the affected side, there is augmentation of the periorbital flow signals in a normal direction. The diagnosis is confirmed with contralateral common carotid compression, which eliminates the crossover supply and usually produces a reversal of flow in the periorbital vessels.

148

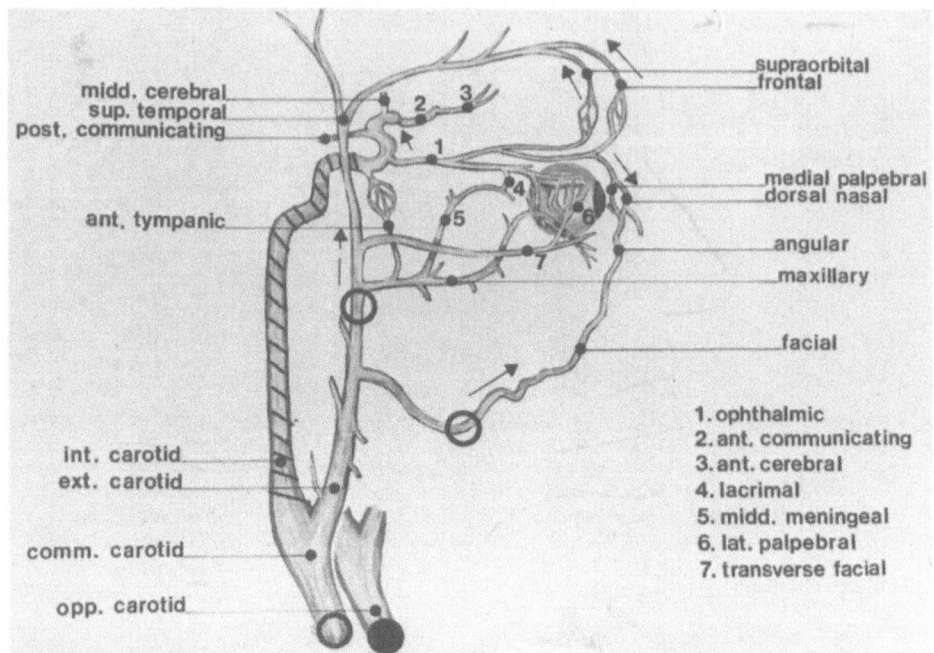

Figure 3. Carotid occlusion or high-grade stenosis: dominant crossover collaterals. Sometimes seen in a long standing carotid obstruction. The key diagnostic maneuver is contralateral carotid compression.

3.3. *Dominant facial artery collateral (Figure 4)*

This is a variant of the pattern seen in Figure 2, in which the facial artery not only supplies retrograde flow to the angular artery, but also supplies flow to the frontal, and sometimes the supraorbital vessel. This results in normal directional flow in the latter vessels so that the response to temporal artery compression may be normal. The diagnosis is made by compressing the facial artery and noting that it diminishes or obliterates the frontal and supraorbital signals, as well as the angular signal.

3.4. *Dominant intraorbital collaterals*

Occasionally communications within the orbital may provide sufficient flow to produce normal directional signals in the periorbital vessels. These anastomoses probably occur between the orbital branches of the ophthalmic (anterior and posterior ethmoid, lacrimal) and branches of the internal maxillary (sphenopalatine, middle meningeal). This variant has been observed on several occasions in patients with long standing internal carotid artery occlusion. It is

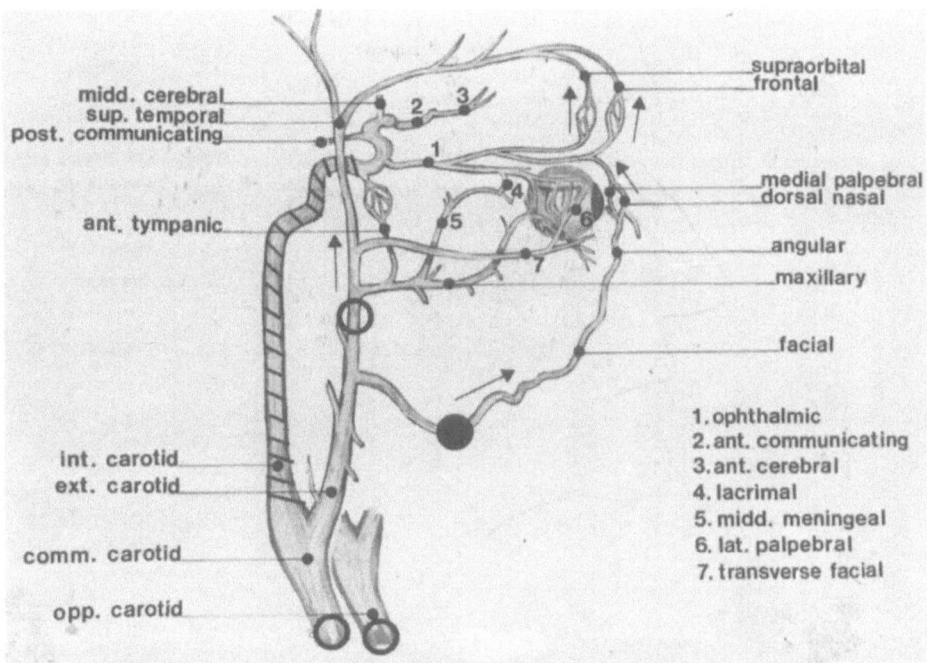

Figure 4. Carotid occlusion or-high-grade stenosis: dominant facial artery collateral. A variant of the pattern in Figure 2. The key diagnostic maneuver is facial artery compression.

fortunate this is a rare condition since the compression techniques may suggest normal blood supply. If suspected, the diagnosis can be made by selective compression of the external carotid artery, which will obliterate or diminish the periorbital signals. With a little practice, this compression can be accomplished satisfactorily, while monitoring the temporal artery with the Doppler probe for completeness. (Figure 5)

3.5. *Balanced internal carotid / external carotid artery supply*

This is usually a sign of early hemodynamic obstruction of the internal carotid artery and occurs in patients in whom the stenosis has not progressed to the point of producing complete reversal (Figure 6).

The examiner first notices asymmetry between the two sides. The signal on the affected side will be in a normal direction during the systole and reversed in late diastole. In this balanced state small changes in collateral flow or in peripheral resistance may shift the periorbital flow direction in either direction. Compression of the contralateral common artery, for example, may result in periorbital flow reversal. Nitroglycerin, if administered sublingually, will produce a progressive reduction in the normal directional component and

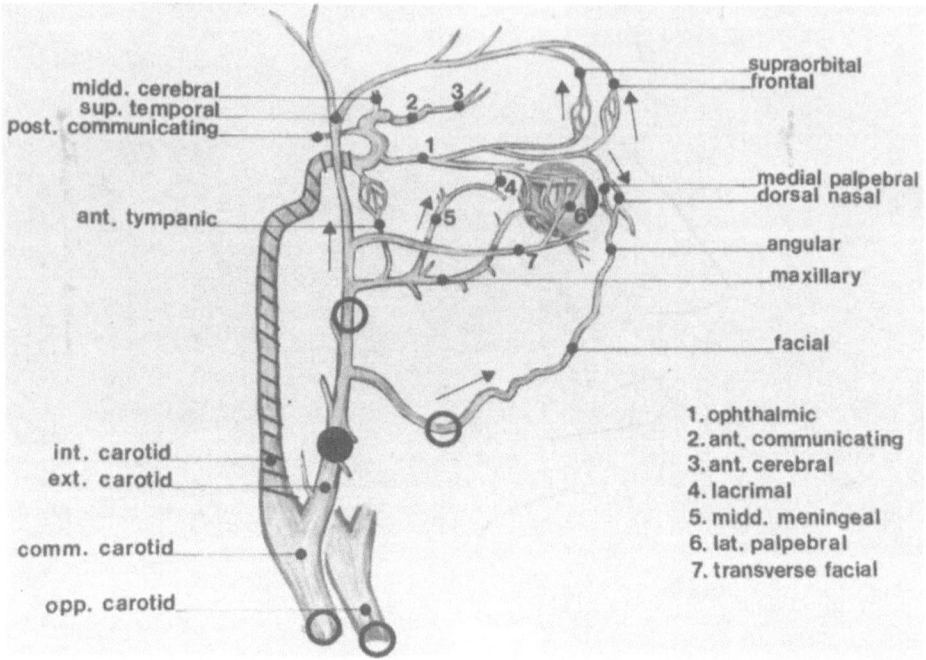

Figure 5. Carotid occlusion or high-grade stenosis: dominant intraorbital collaterals. A rare cause for diagnostic error. The key diagnostic maneuver is selective compression of the external carotid artery.

progressive increase in the reversed component. Occasionally this balanced state is produced by stenosis of the external carotid artery as well as of the internal carotid artery, or by a stenosis in the common carotid artery at the bifurcation (Figure 7). In either of these situations, however, there is usually evidence of collateralization from the opposite side which may be demonstrated with contralateral carotid compression.

4. DIAGNOSTIC CRITERIA

From the observations made during the periorbital Doppler examination, one can be reasonably confident about the presence or absence of collateral blood flow. If collateral circulation is present, the diagnosis of carotid obstruction may be inferred. However, no distinction can be made between total occlusion of the carotid and high-grade stenosis; and it must be emphasized that clinically significant, but non-obstructing, lesions cannot be detected by this method.

Collateralization around the orbit can usually be recognized when the diameter of the internal carotid is reduced by 65% to 70%. This corresponds

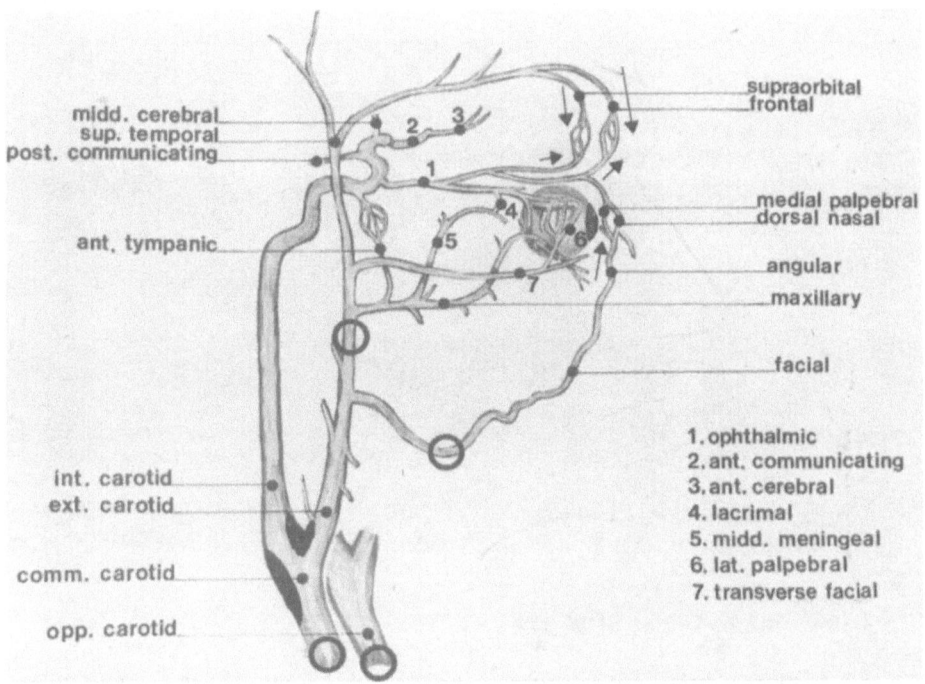

midd. cerebral
sup. temporal
post. communicating

ant. tympanic

int. carotid
ext. carotid

comm. carotid

opp. carotid

supraorbital
frontal

medial palpebral
dorsal nasal

angular

maxillary

facial

1. ophthalmic
2. ant. communicating
3. ant. cerebral
4. lacrimal
5. midd. meningeal
6. lat. palpebral
7. transverse facial

Figure 6. Carotid stenosis: critically balanced flow in the periorbital vessels. Bidirectional flow may be identified.

to a two millimeter or smaller channel as seen on the angiogram. We prefer to quantitate the obstruction in terms of the diameter at the narrowest point, since this is the measurement obtained most easily and agreed upon most readily.

The most reliable signs of collateralization are *retrograde flow* from the temporal and facial arteries, and evidence of *crossover flow* from the opposite carotid artery. Doppler changes which are not diagnostic, but strongly suggestive, include *asymmetry* between the two sides, *dampened* velocity signals, and change from a normal two-component signal to either a *systolic* signal or a *continuous* signal.

Retrograde flow. This is recognized from the direction indicated on the Doppler instrument, as well as from compressing the facial and temporal arteries. Occasionally the periorbital vessels will be supplied from the contra-lateral temporal and facial arteries, which must be compressed to confirm the source.

Crossover flow. Abnormal supply via the anterior communicating artery is diagnosed by compressing the contralateral common carotid artery. If there is *normal directional* periorbital flow, the Doppler signals will be diminished or

152

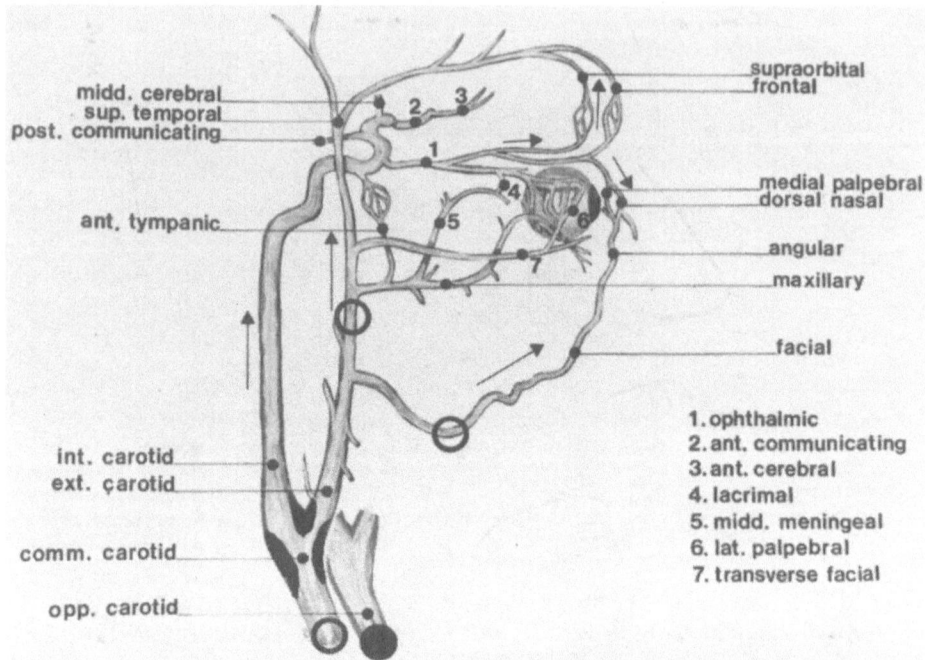

Figure 7. Combined internal and external carotid stenosis: normal directional periorbital flow may be present. The key diagnostic maneuver is contralateral carotid compression.

will become reversed by this maneuver. Likewise, compression of the ipsilateral common carotid artery will not obliterate the periorbital signals and may augment them.

If there is reversed periorbital flow, opposite carotid compression will augment the reversed flow. Compression of the ipsilateral carotid causes the periorbital flow to become normal directional.

Asymmetrical signals. While asymmetry between the two sides is not diagnostic, it is suggestive of abnormal flow and tips off the examiner to look carefully for other signs of collateralization. The asymmetry is caused by one of the following signal abnormalities.

Dampened flow signal. Whether normal directional or reversed, the periorbital signals on the side of an obstructed carotid will be less brisk than on the opposite normal side.

Single-component flow signal. As an obstructing lesion begins to reduce flow in the internal carotid artery, one of the first Doppler changes that one observes is elimination of the diastolic component of the periorbital signal.

Bidirectional flow signal. With further progression of the stenosis, the flow signal becomes bidirectional, with reversed flow detectable at the end of diastole. In this balanced state, changes in peripheral resistance may shift the flow in either direction. This can be demonstrated by administering sublingual nitroglycerin to the patient. Over a period of a minute or two the antegrade component will diminish and the retrograde component will increase. Flow can be completely reversed by this technique, which may be useful as a provocative test for lesions of borderline significance. This response is considered to be a result lowering the peripheral resistance in the intracranial distribution more than the resistance in the external carotid distribution.

Continuous flow signal. Occasionally a nearly continuous signal will be heard in the periorbital vessels, resembling the sound of an arteriovenous fistula. This is often observed in the presence of an acute internal carotid occlusion and suggests that a high pressure gradient exists between the external and internal carotid arteries.

5. DIAGNOSTIC ACCURACY

The purpose of the periorbital Doppler examination is to recognize functioning collateral pathways around the orbit and, by inference, hemodynamically significant carotid obstruction. We feel that an accuracy of 95% or better is realistic and readily achieved by a careful, reasonably astute examiner. Using essentially the same method of approach, Barnes and Wilson recently reported a 98.7% overall accuracy of diagnosis in a series of 76 patients undergoing angiography[6]. These investigators had two false-negative diagnoses (five %) in a group of 38 carotid arteries with occlusion or stenosis of 75% or better.

There are a number of possible sources of error in the examination and the examiner should be aware of these if he is to obtain the highest degree of accuracy. It is important that the anatomy of the periorbital vessels be well understood and that at least the frontal and supraorbital vessels be identified in each examination. The flow signals should be located just beneath the rim of the orbit and that the probe be angled toward the direction of flow so that a correct direction assessment can be made. The probe must be held steadily, particularly when the compressions are performed. It is essential that the examiner avoid pressing too firmly with the probe and obliterating the flow signal.

Anatomic variant which might lead to diagnostic errors have been illustrated. Occasionally normal individuals will exhibit a reversed flow in the supraorbital artery, even when care is taken to identify the vessel in the supraorbital notch. The reason for this is not certain, but this single abnormality should not lead to an error of interpretation if the remainder of the examination is normal. The lateral palpebral artery may sometimes be misidentified as the supraorbital artery, and since this arises from a branch of the temporal artery, a false positive compression response may result.

In interpreting the results of the examination, it is important for the examiner to resist the temptation to give a precise anatomic diagnosis. The observed data are concerned with collateralization about the orbit and the basis for this collateralization can only be inferred. While most patients with periorbital collateralization will have carotid obstruction in the neck, obstruction at the level of the carotid siphon or of the ophthalmic artery will also produce positive findings. In fact, as it has already been pointed out, the distinction between total occlusion of the internal carotid and high-grade stenosis cannot be made with these data. It must also be emphasized that the diagnosis is almost never based on a single abnormal finding. There are usually two or more abnormalities and these abnormalities must be consistent with one another. If there is an unexplained finding, or if the findings are inconsistent, the examiner should persist with compressions, i.e., contralteral, facial or temporal compressions, until the collateral pathways are delineated.

6. ROLE OF THE PERIORBITAL DOPPLER EXAMINATION

The primary advantages of the periorbital Doppler examination are that it is a relatively simple examination that can be performed with portable equipment at the bedside or in the office. It is inexpensive and involves minimal risk. We have found it to be a valuable adjunct to carotid surgery. It is particularly reassuring in the recovery room to find that the previously abnormal signals have reverted to normal in your postoperative patient. The patient may later be followed on an outpatient basis and the continued patency of the vessel confirmed on subsequent visits.

It must be re-emphasized that fewer than one-half of the patients with *clinically significant* atherosclerotic disease at the carotid bifurcation will have Doppler signs of collateralization about the orbit. For this reason a normal periorbital examination, by itself, should not be relied upon to rule out disease in a symptomatic individual who might be a candidate for carotid surgery. Our primary use of the periorbital examination, therefore, is as a component of a comprehensive non-invasive cerebrovascular evaluation. We have designed a technician-administered study which begins with a pertinent history and physical examination and includes audio and analogue recordings of the vertebral signals, the ophthalmic artery signals in the posterior orbits, and Doppler imaging of the carotid bifurcation [7]. As a part of this study, the periorbital examination helps to distinguish obstructing from non-obstructing lesions and to estimate the size of the lumen at the stenosis site. The periorbital Doppler findings should be consistent with the other findings and serve to increase the confidence by which the diagnostic interpretation is made. During the past three years, approximately 2800 patients have been examined in this manner. This combined approach provided an overall diagnostic accuracy of 98%, when compared with angiographic stenosis of 50% or better [7]. As a result of the experiences gained from Doppler imaging of the carotid bifurcation and analysis of the Doppler signal characteristics along these vessels, we have found it possible to derive considerable information from a direct examination of the bifurcation area with a simple hand-held Doppler probe. The internal and external carotid artery signals can usually be recognized with confidence and signal abnormalities, such as the increased frequency seen with stenosis, can be readily identified. The significance of this is that using the same relatively simple directional Doppler equipment with which the periorbital exam is performed, the examiner may carry out a reliable screening examination of the carotid bifurcation.

7. CONCLUSIONS

The periorbital Doppler test is a relatively simple method by which functioning collateral pathways around the orbit may be identified. The presence of carotid obstruction may be inferred from these findings. Using the techniques described, the correlation between the Doppler evidence for collateralization and the angiographic evidence for significant obstruction should be 95% or better. The periorbital Doppler test does not detect non-obstructive lesions which may be of clinical significance and, for this reason, is utilized to best advantage as a component of a more comprehensive non-invasive cerebrovascular evaluation. In this setting the periorbital Doppler information distinguishes between obstructing and non-obstructing lesions and adds to the confidence of the overall diagnostic interpretation. The periorbital Doppler test, by itself, is useful as an office or bedside screening test for carotid obstruction and is valuable for serial follow-up on patients following carotid surgery.

REFERENCES

1. Brockenbrough EC: Screening for the prevention of stroke: use of a Doppler flowmeter. Information and Education Resource Support Unit, Washington/Alaska Regional Medical Program, 1969.
2. Brockenbrough EC, Lawrence C, Schwenk WG: Ocular phlethysmography: a new technique for the evaluation of carotid obstructive disease. Rev Surg 24:299, 1967.

3. Maroon JC, Pieroni DW, Campbell RL: Ophthalmosonometry, an ultrasonic method for assessing carotid blod flow. J Neurosurtl, 30:238, 1969.
4. Muller HR: The diagnosis by directional Doppler sonography of the ophthalmic artery. Neurol 22:816, 1972.
5. Machleder HI, Barker WF: Stroke on the wrong side: use of the Doppler ophthalmic test in cerebral vascular screening. Arch Surg 105:943, 1972.
6. Barnes RW, Wilson MR: Doppler ultrasonic evaluation of cerebrovascular disease. University of Iowa, 1975.
7. Spencer MP, Brockenbrough EC, Davis DL Reid JM: Cerebrovascular evaluation using Doppler c-w ultrasound. Proc of the World Federation of Ultrasound in Medicine and Biology Meeting, San Francisco, August, 1976.

12. ULTRASONIC DETECTION OF THE NON-STENOTIC PLAQUE

MERRILL P. SPENCER, M.D.

One of the goals of non-invasive carotid examination is to define signals associated with non-stenotic lesions and to make the diagnosis of ulcerated plaques. At the present time, there is no Doppler ultrasonic signal which is diagnostic of ulceration. There is, in fact, no clinically applicable technique which will non-invasively identify areas of denuded intima. It is true, however, that a deep crater-like indentation in the wall of the carotid artery, when associated with TIA's, frequently represents the site of ulcerated intima. X-ray angiography cannot, however, actually resolve the presence of denuded intima and the term 'ulceration' is a misnomer when what is actually seen is cratering or wall roughening. Radio isotope techniques provide a method of disclosing adherent blood elements which are more pertinent. Developments may in the future disclose ulceration and adherent blood elements.

This chapter is intended to disclose the present state of Doppler art in identifying non-stenotic plaques and the signals representing calcium deposits in the artery wall as well as irregularities in the wall surface. In the future, we may find certain combinations of Doppler ultrasonic signals which will show a high correlation with ulcerated intima in a similar way that the presence of craters on an angiogram is often associated with an ulcerated intima.

1. CLINICAL EXPERIENCE

1.1. The asonic gap

The first evidence (Spencer et al. 1973) that Doppler could detect a non-stenotic plaque appeared in the images shown in Figures 1a and 1b.

Doppler imaging of the right bifurcation disclosed an asonic gap at the origin of both the external and internal carotid arteries. The carotid signals above and below this gap in the common external and internal 'were normal in quality. On the left side a similar asonic gap was seen across the bifurcation but in addition on the internal carotid downstream from the bifurcation a section of weak but very high frequencies was found diagnostic of a stenosis. The angiograms confirmed the presence of the stenosis and also demonstrated

158

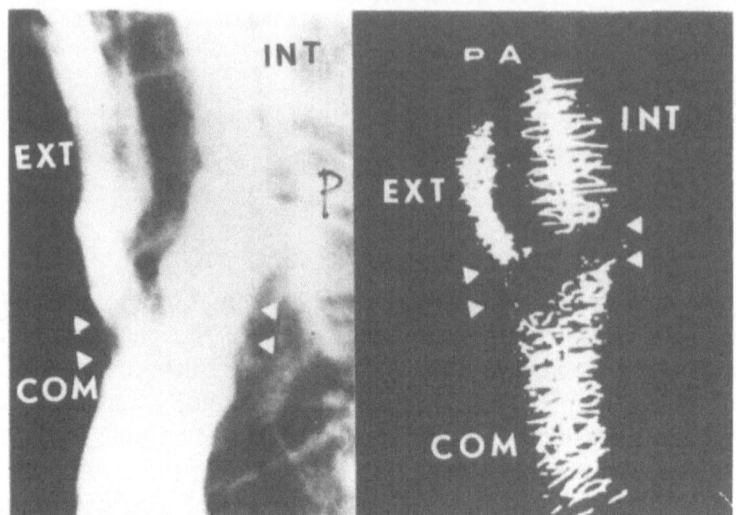

Figure 1a. Doppler bifurcation image with angiogram from a patient with a non-stenosing calcified plaque across the carotid bifurcation which appears as an asonic gap in the Doppler image.

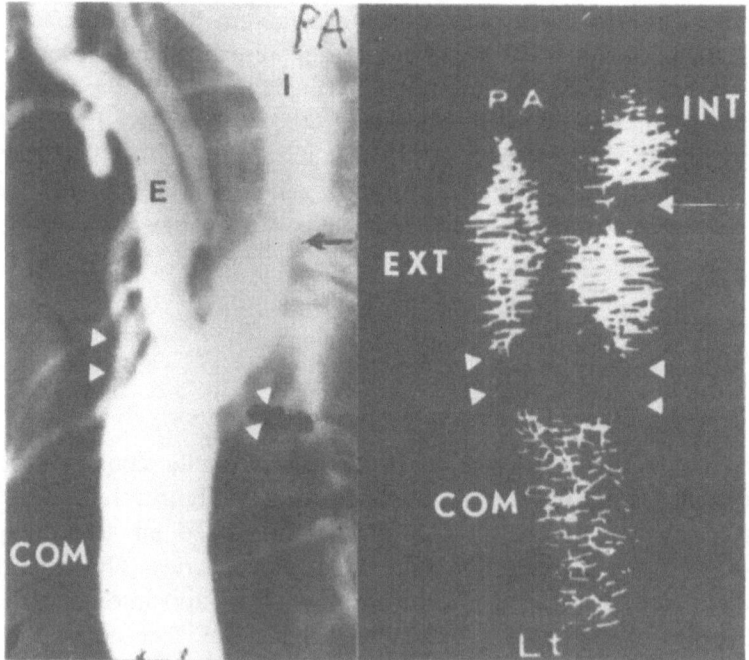

Figure 1b. Doppler image with angiogram in the mid-internal carotid. DOP-SCAN image and angiogram from opposite side of same patient shown in Figure 1a. Asonic gaps are shown at the bifurcation and on the internal where high frequencies of stenosis were also found (arrow).

severe luminal wall irregularities around both bifurcations. Carotid endarterectomy at the left bifurcation disclosed a very hard arterial wall in which much calcium was deposited and proven by xeroradiography of the endarterectomy specimen.

Our continuing experience with Doppler demonstrates asonic gaps on the carotid image, though less frequently since the Doppler signal-to-noise ratio in the electronics has improved, are rarely present in such localized areas of non-imaging blood flow. Sections of comparitively weak signals are, however, still found in association with calcium deposits but weak amplitude alone is not considered sufficient to make the diagnosis of calcified plaque. Rarely does the presence of isolated segments of very weak or asonic gaps impede the detection of stenosis. (Spencer et al. 1977 and Spencer 1977)

A series of 20 carotid endarterectomy specimens were xeroradiogrammed. All but one disclosed dense amorphous calcium deposits similar to that seen in Figure 2. The specimen without calcium deposits was determined to represent arterial fibromuscular dysplasia. (Barriga et al. 1976)

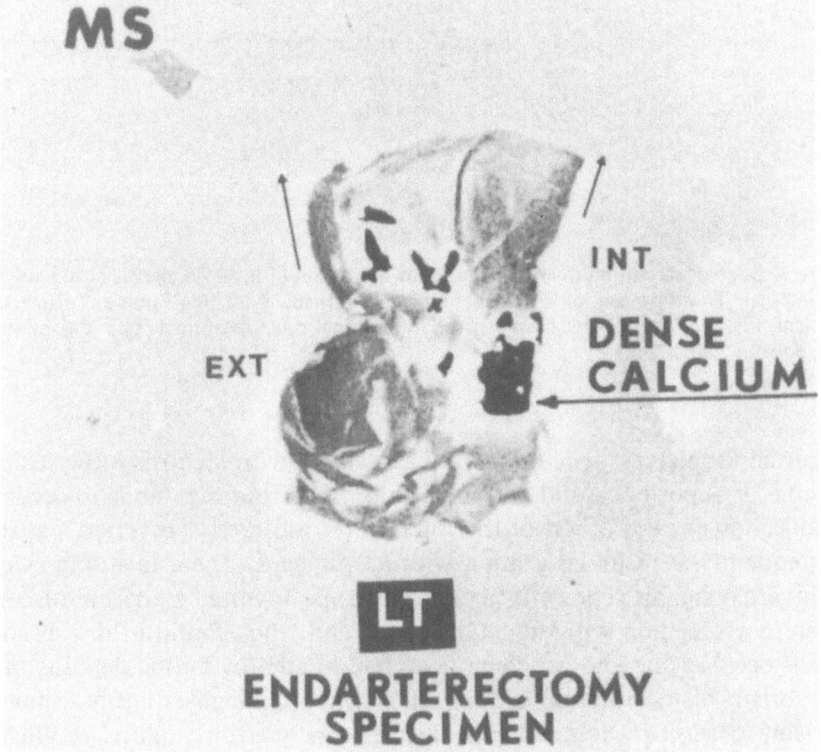

Figure 2. Xeroradiogram of a carotid endarterectomy specimen removed from a patient's internal carotid in surgery. The scattered dark regions are dense calcium deposits which cause asonic images and inverted Doppler flow signals.

1.2. The inverted signal

Another Doppler characteristic associated with non-stenotic plaque is the 'inverted' signal appearing in isolated segments (Figure 3).

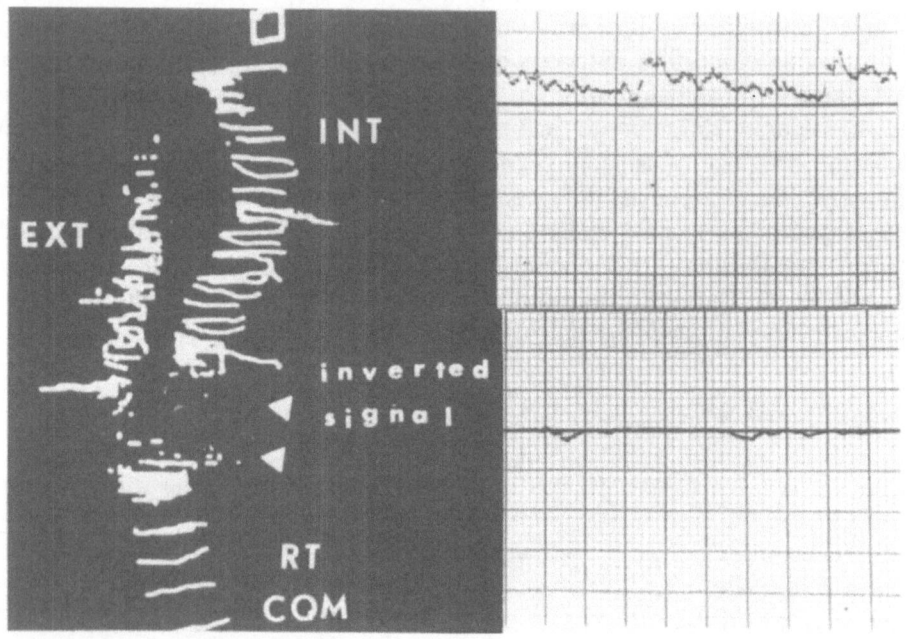

Figure 3. Doppler carotid bifurcation image showing region of inverted signals on the origin of the internal. The diagnosis of non-stenotic plaque is made from this finding. To image the segment, the inverted signals shown on the lower panel must be turned 'up-right' by means of a polarity switch.

Like the asonic gap, it is frequently associated with stenosis or occlusion on the same or opposite carotid and its location, like stenosis, tends to occur with a predilection for the origin of the internal carotid artery. Inverted signals are also frequently seen in association with asonic gaps. There is strong evidence that inverted signals represent calcium deposits. Inverted signals are frequently seen in association with stenotic plaques and when found in the absence of stenosis occur at the site generally favorable to atherosclerotic deposits, namely the origin of the internal carotid artery. Inverted signals are not, however, invariably observed when calcium deposits are present. Figure 4a illustrates how the non-stenotic calcified plaque produces the inverted spectrum on bidirectional spectral displays. The inverted analogue signal of Figure 3 occurs when the Doppler energy is primarily in the inverted spectrum.

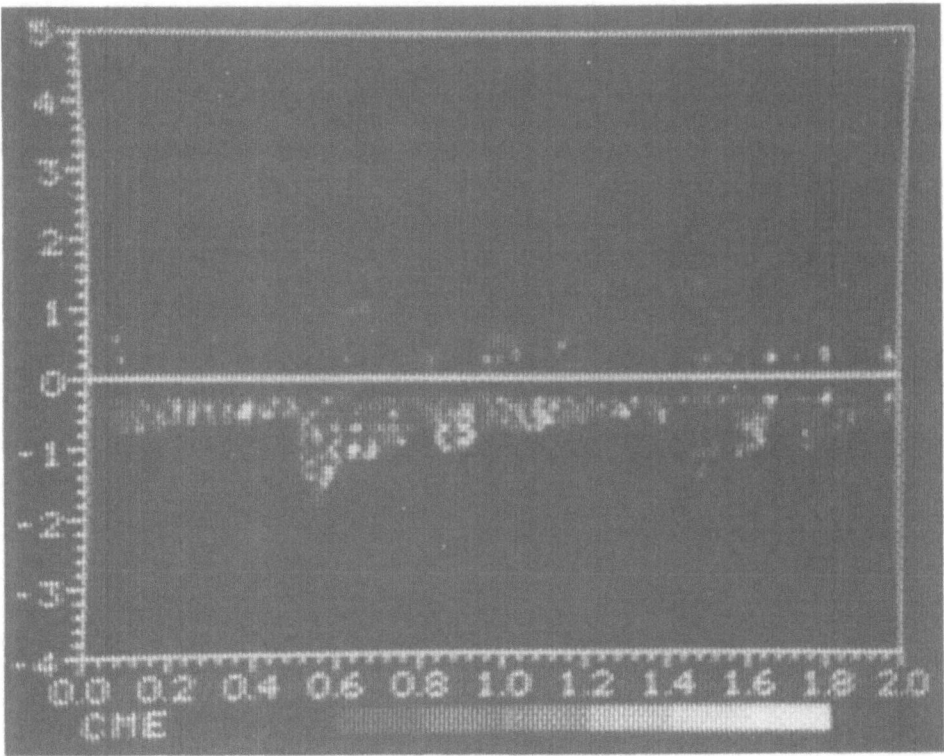

Figure 4a. Bidirectional spectral display of inverted spectrum from a carotid calcified non-stenotic plaque. The preponderance of energy in the inverted spectrum also produces an inverted analogue signal. See Chapter 15 for explanation of spectral display.

1.3. Other signals associated with non-stenotic plaque

Other Doppler signals, each of which alone is insufficient to establish the diagnosis of plaquing may, when present in combination, suggest the presence of plaque. 1) 'Coarseness,' somewhat a wastebasket term used to indicate that the sound is not smooth and does not seem normal, but also does not represent fluttering or gruffness of turbulence. Spectral analysis of such signals demonstrates spectral widening with relatively even distribution of amplitude over the frequency range of the spectrum, Figure 4b. 2) Low frequencies at the origin of the internal carotid are sometimes associated with plaquing, though the normal internal carotid, because it is usually wider at the take off, can also produce low frequencies. There is, of course, normally a progression of increasing frequencies as the Doppler beam is moved along the internal from the bulbous origin towards the angle of the jaw. 3) Systolic qualities in isolated positions along the internal carotid are suggestive of plaquing when the major part of the internal length visualized contains the

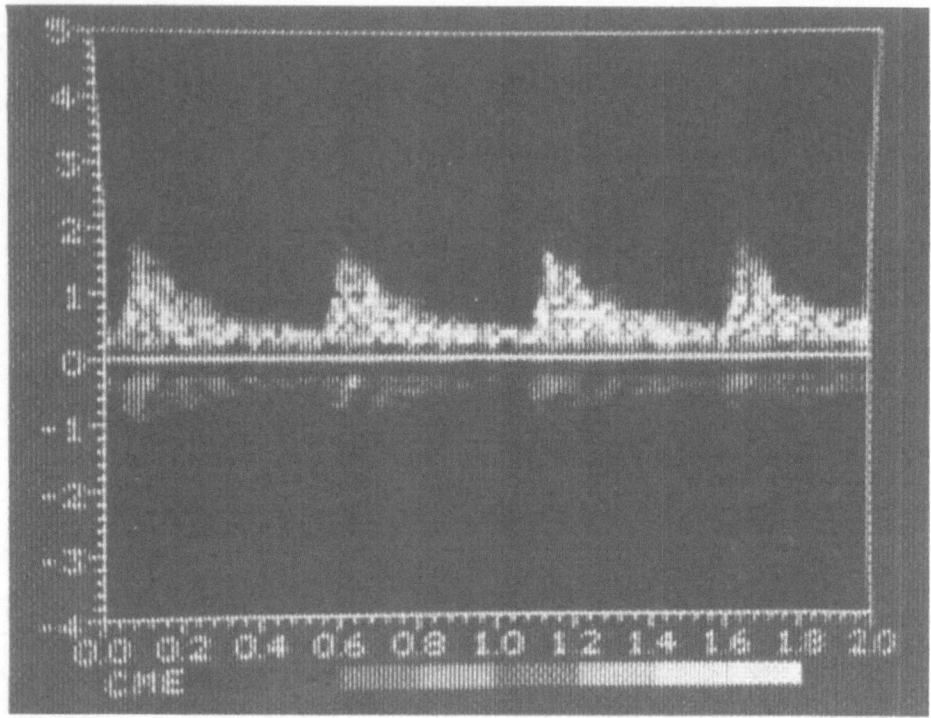

Figure 4b. Bidirectional Doppler signals from a carotid non-stenotic plaque demonstrating spectral broadening and an inverted spectrum 'ghost' of the normally directed signal. See Chapter 15 for explanation of the display.

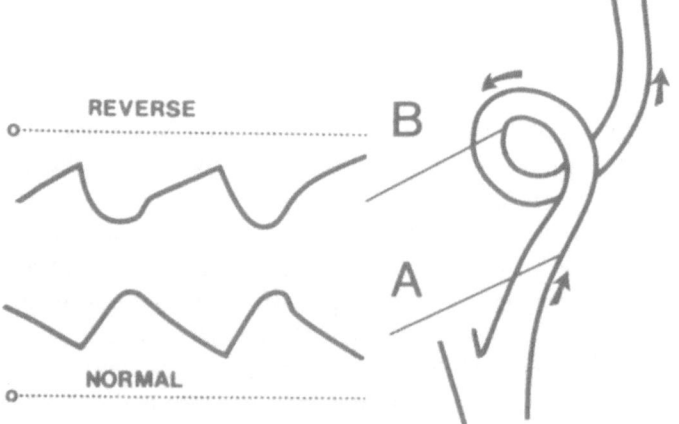

Figure 5. Diagramatic representation of how an arterial loop can produce an apparent change in direction of flow. The normal sense is shown at 'A' where flow is in the direction of the transmitted sound beam. At 'B' the flow direction is against the sound beam, producing an inverted signal.

normal diastolic flow characteristics of the normal internal. 4) Biphasic signals which display an apparent change in direction within the same heart cycle may represent a variant on the inverted signal which is also associated with non-stenotic plaquing. The combination of any three of the above signals when present together appear sufficient to establish a diagnosis of plaquing. We recommend that the diagnosis in this situation be made conservatively.

Caution should be exercised when coiling or kinking of the carotid is suspected because these conditions also can cause inverted signals. Figure 5 diagrams the situation in which inverted signals can be produced in the presence of the carotid loop by reversed direction of the blood flow.

The audio qualities of the inverted signals generally include the range of audio qualities otherwise found in normal and diseased carotid arteries.

1.4. The flutter signal unassociated with high frequencies

Fluttering associated with stenosis is discussed in detail in Chapters 1 and 13. Audio signals displaying the fluttering quality of turbulence represents a third highly diagnostic characteristic of non-stenotic plaque. This quality is believed to represent irregularities in the lumen wall which break up the laminar flow into turbulent eddies. The irregularity of the intimal lumen is, of course, a frequently observed characteristic of atherosclerosis by direct observation and also on the angiogram. If any of the three foregoing conditions: asonic gaps, inverted signals, or fluttering without the high frequency are present alone, the diagnosis of non-stenotic plaque can be made. Of course, calcified plaque can also be diagnosed in the presence of stenosis when either asonic gap or an inverted signal is present with the high frequency and other stenosis characteristics.

2. ULTRASONIC THEORY OF PLAQUE SIGNALS

In order to explain the cause of the abnormal Doppler signals obtained from carotid arteries with overlying plaque, we have developed a working hypothesis which is based on the assumption that progressively increasing amounts of calcium deposited in an amorphous manner within the plaque and artery wall produces a progressively greater amount of scattering of the sound. Where dense sonically opaque calcium deposits occur, an edge effect occurs which bends most of the sound beam to a direction against the flowing blood rather than with the flowing blood. Figure 6 illustrates the expected results of these theoretical considerations.

If the undisturbed ultrasonic sound beam is visualized passing through the normal artery wall and reflecting back along the same source path, we obtain

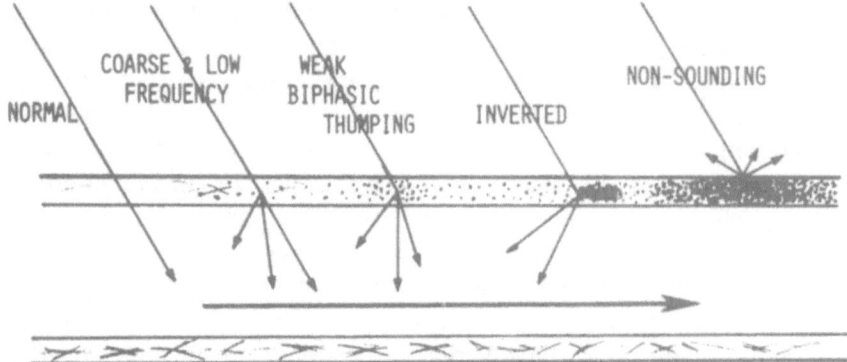

Figure 6. Representation of how increasing density and concentration of calcium granules in an artery wall can influence the quality, frequency, direction and amplitude of the returning Doppler shifted signal.

a smooth 'laminal flow signal.' If, however, the sound beam is broken into multiple pathways by distortions caused by deposits of calcium granules, there are multiple pathway returns from the blood. Thus, the earliest detectable signs of plaquing consisting of the coarse low frequency quality is a result of spectral broadening because of the multiple pathway signal. As deposits further increase, much of the soundbeam is absorbed or deflected and does not enter the blood producing weak flow signals. These are often accompanied by biphasic thumping qualities which represent accentuated artery wall motion signals. This biphasic thumping quality is often seen in minimal plaquing where the artery wall retains a relatively great amount of elasticity and expansile motion.

As the calcium deposits become more dense, the soundbeam reflects from the edge of such a deposit so that the return Doppler ultrasonic signal appears to the electronics as if the transducer was pointed in the opposite direction, against the flowing stream. The same effect can be caused by bending of the soundbeam at the downstream edge of the dense calcium deposit. This effect produces an inverted analogue signal.

Finally, when the calcium deposit is so dense that the soundbeam cannot enter the blood vessel because of total absorption and total reflection, no blood flow Doppler signal is returned to the instrument. In this manner an asonic gap is produced in the image.

Though this theory has not been tested in its entirety, the clinical observations mentioned in the previous section are consistent with the hypothesis and our experimental results. Bidirectional spectra of the clinical signals also support the hypothesis. It is possible that other components of the plaque also influence the soundbeam such as cholesterol crystals and fibrous tissue but in all probability these produce a much lesser effect than calcium deposits.

3. EXPERIMENTAL RESULTS ON THE EFFECTS OF CALCIUM DEPOSITS

Our experimental approach to testing the above theory of non-stenotic plaque consisted of examination of diseased arteries from human subjects obtained from autopsy. The arteries principally used were external iliac arteries. They were xeroradiogrammed to locate areas of calcium granules which then were marked for visual identification with india ink (Figure 7).

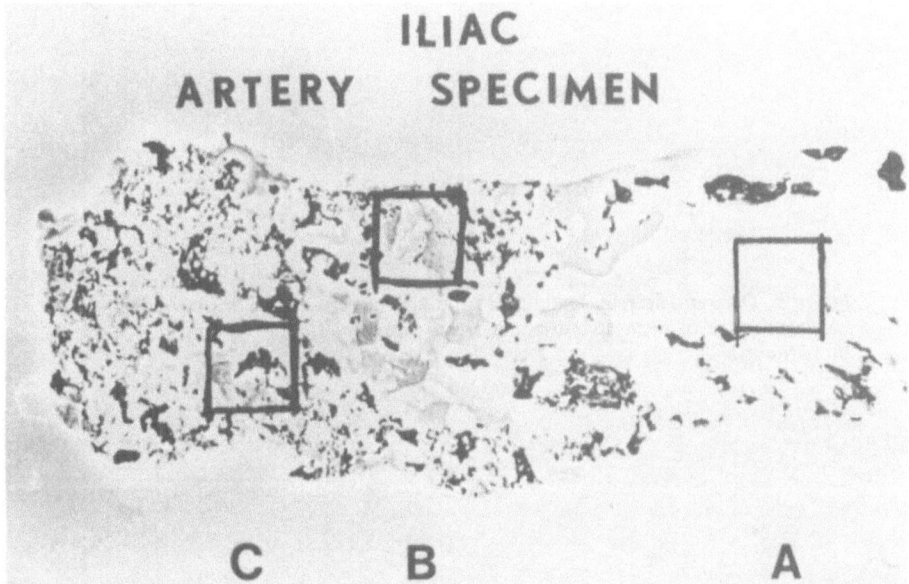

Figure 7. Xeroradiogram of an excised human aorta showing calcium granule deposits. The squares indicate the areas A, B, and C that were tested for ultrasonic scattering and attenuation in the apparatus of Figure 7. Square A represents the control area in which no calcium granules were found. B and C include plaques with calcium deposits.

3.1. Quantitative scattering studies

The tagged specimens were then opened with a longitudinal incision and stretched on a special holder for examination with an ultrasound beam. The testing was performed in a water bath with two special transducers, one for transmitting and one for receiving placed on either side of the sample tissue (Figure 8).

Normal artery sections, without calcium granules, did not display angular dependence (Figure 9). When areas of calcification were examined and the angle of the tissue with the sound beam was rotated through known angles, the attenuation of the sound beam was found to vary greatly with the angle of incident (Figure 10).

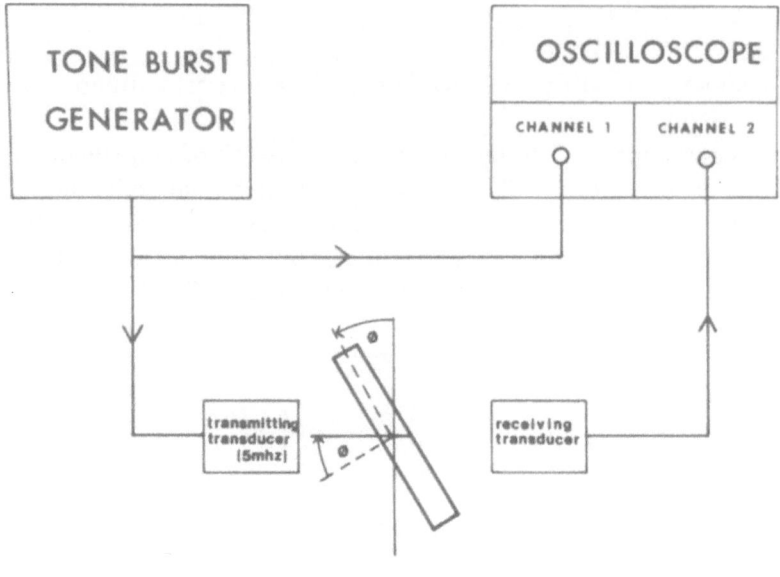

Figure 8. Diagramatic representation of the apparatus used for testing the angular dependence of ultrasonic attenuation in plaque and control areas of excised human aorta.

Ultrasonic Characterization of Control Tissue (no. 1)

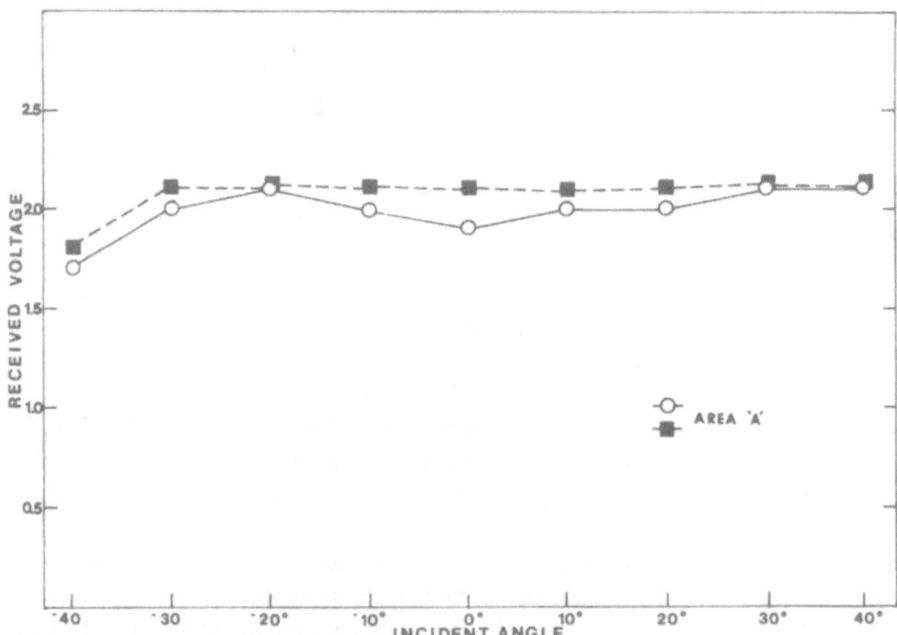

Figure 9. Plot or received signal voltage and its small angular dependence from the non-calcified plaque of area A, Figure 6.

Ultrasonic Characterization of Plaque Area (no.1)

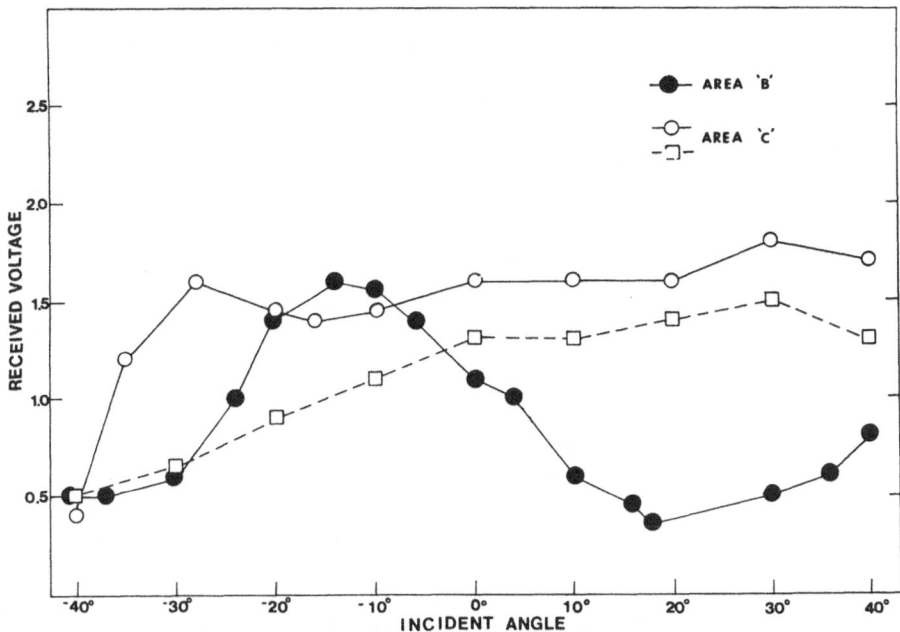

Figure 10. Plots showing great variations in angular dependence when a sound beam of 5 MHz is passed through calcified plaque areas B and C of Figure 6.

3.2. Doppler imaging studies

Blood flow studies through unopened iliac arteries containing severe plaquing with calcium deposits were examined by means of Doppler imaging. Figure 11 discloses the in vitro experimental arrangement in which whole blood was passed through the arterial segment with the Doppler probe lowered into the surrounding bath. The results demonstrated both non-sounding segments and inverted signals in the region of calcium deposits. In arteries without calcium deposits these effects were not found.

4. CONCLUSION

It is apparent that ultrasound is more sensitive to the presence of calcium deposits than x-ray angiography and Doppler signal itself is influenced considerably by plaquing abnormalities on the artery wall. Clinical and experimental results confirm the justification of Doppler diagnosis of non-stenotic plaquing when asonic gaps, inverted signals and fluttering signals are found.

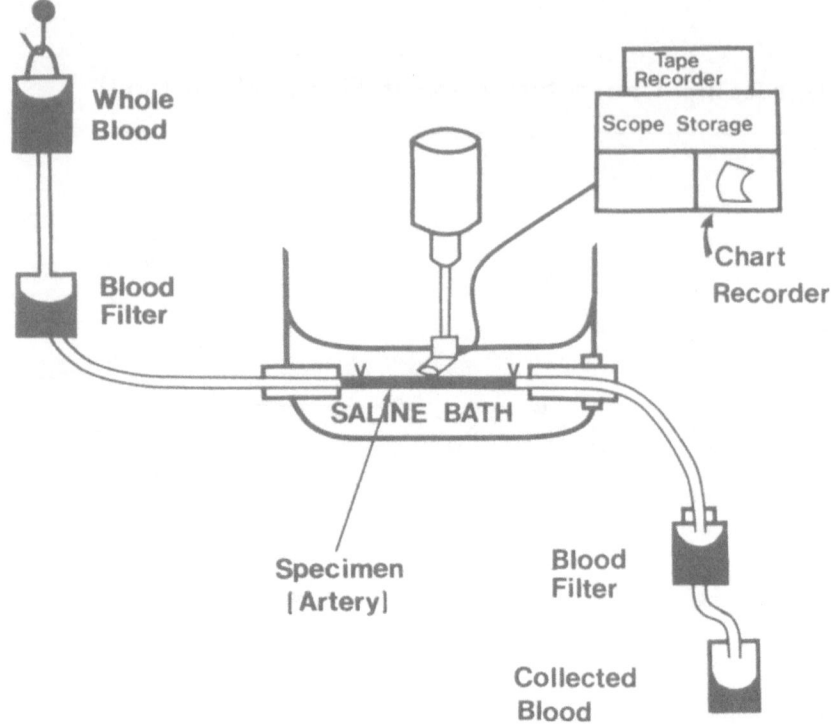

Figure 11. Diagramatic representation of the method of performing Doppler imaging in excised arteries in vitro.

The diagnosis of plaquing may also be justified where subtle abnormalities are present in combination including coarseness, low frequency, biphasic and systolic qualities.

No Doppler signals to date have been proven to be associated with ulceration of the intima, but it is proposed that the presence of fluttering with inverted signals may represent craters associated with severe plaquing. A great need exists in the area of stroke prevention for a non-invasive technique which will identify platelet and fibrin adherances at the site of ulcerations.

REFERENCES

1. Spencer MP, Reid JM, Davis DL, Paulson PS: Cervical carotid imaging with a continuous-wave Doppler flowmeter. Stroke 5:145-154, 1974.
2. Spencer MP, Brockenbrough EC, Davis DL, Reid JM: Cerebrovascular evaluation using C-W ultrasound. Ultrasound in Medicine 3B:1291-1310, Plenum Press, C White (ed), August 1976.
3. Spencer MP: Doppler ultrasonic imaging and non-invasive cerebrovascular evaluation. International Journal of Neurology 11 (2-3):228-242, 1977.
4. Barriga P, Spencer MP, Turnipseed W: Correlation of a non-sounding area in the carotid Doppler ultrasound. Ultrasound in Medicine 3B:1395, Plenum Press, D White (ed), August 1976.

13. OBSTRUCTIVE LESIONS DIAGNOSED BY DOPPLER ULTRASOUND

MERRILL P. SPENCER, M.D. and GEORGE I. THOMAS, M.D.

Doppler ultrasound examinations occupy a needed position between simple office screening techniques and more costly and invasive procedure of x-ray arteriography. Doppler supplements arteriography by providing functional information not provided by x-ray and serving as a screening procedure to clarify the need for arteriography and surgery. This chapter is intended as a catalogue of obstructive lesions which are surgically correctable or when present with other 'surgical' obstructions can be assessed with Doppler to plan the surgical approach.

Figure 1 provides an overview of stenotic and occlusive lesions which threaten the extracranial arterial supply to the brain.

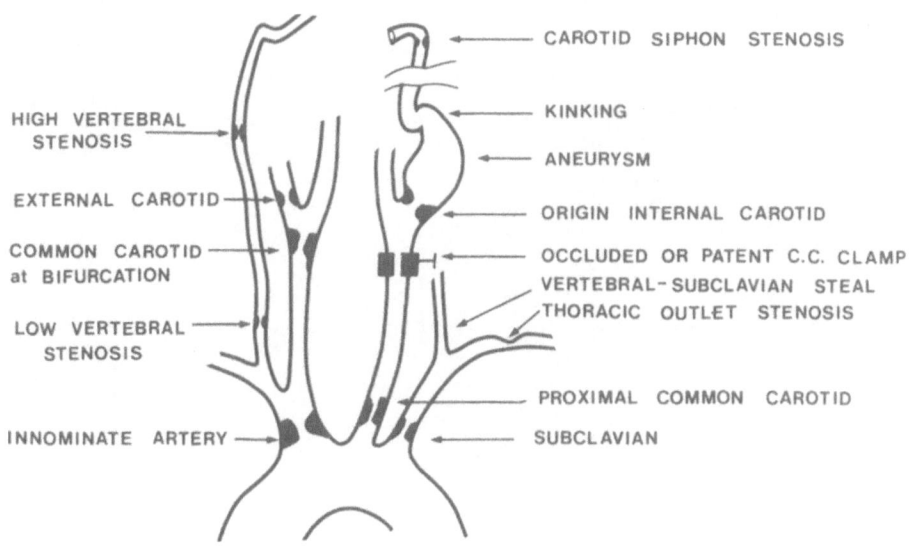

Figure 1. Obstructive vascular lesions diagnosed by Doppler ultrasound which may adversely effect cerebral circulation. 'Obstructive' lesions include both stenosis and occlusions occuring in the aorto-cranial circulation.

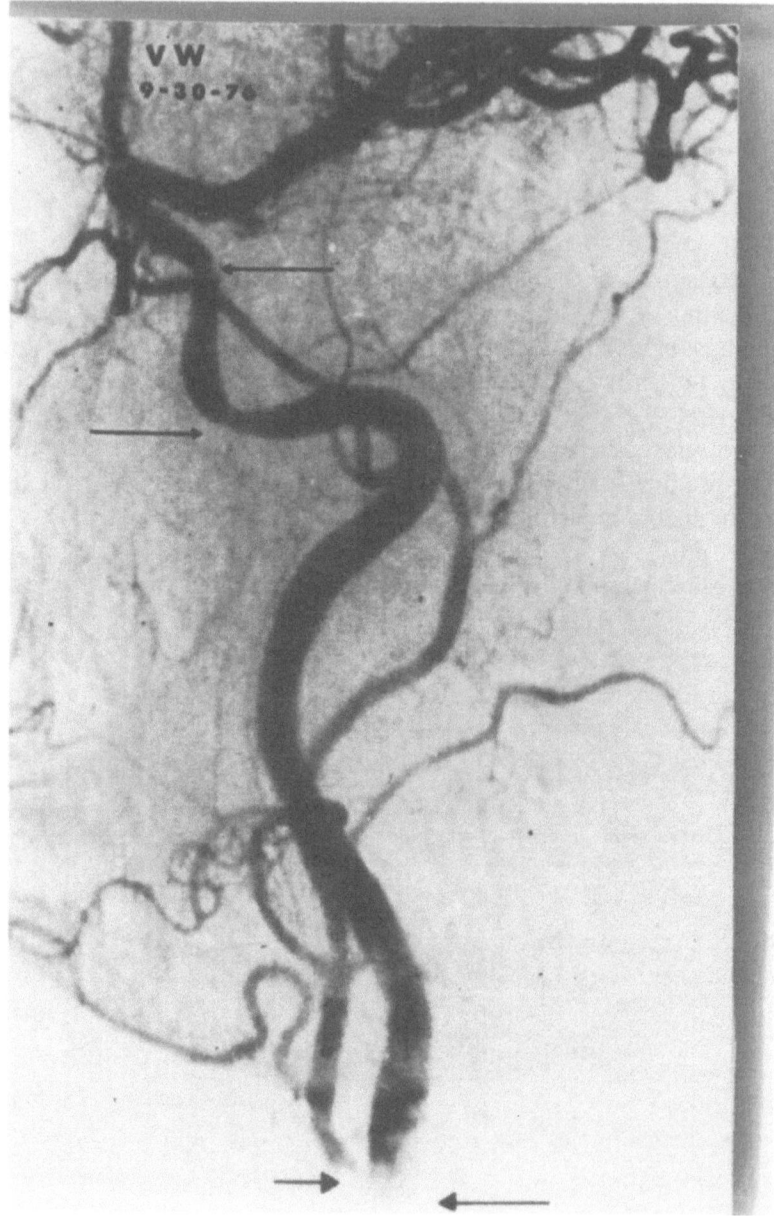

Figure 2. Patient V.W. had a bruit over the left bifurcation region and the left eye. She was diagnosed by Doppler to have bilateral external carotid stenosis, confirmed by angiography but was not operated because both Doppler and angiography indicated that the bifurcation lesions were insignificant as compared to the tandem internal carotid stenosis at the base of the skull.

1. SIPHON STENOSIS

Internal carotid lesion high above the bifurcation, out of reach of the ultrasound beam, cannot be diagnosed directly by Doppler, but the significance of tandem lesions can be evaluated by simultaneous analysis of the carotid audio signals as well as posterior orbital signals. Of particular diagnostic importance, is the presence of a bruit heard over the eyes.

Bruits over the eye lids can be detected by gently placing the bell stethoscope over the eye. Soft Grade I to II low-frequency and often-continuous bruits are easily detected in patients with intracranial siphon lesions which have been ultimately confirmed by angiography. Although surgery at this time does not hold a prominent place in the correction of these symptomatic lesions, antiplatelet medication can be used judiciously and effectively to alter TIA symptoms (Figure 2).

Siphon and carotid lesions frequently co-exist and it is important to suspect these tandem lesions and operate the accessible, more proximal lesion at the carotid bifurcation. Whether or not an associated siphon lesion increases the risk of proximal carotid bifurcation surgery cannot be stated in fact, since no hard data exists on this matter. It has been our experience that there is no greater risk if all of the attendant standards of good carotid surgery are carried out. Oftentimes it is a more suitable technical procedure to shunt the endarterectomy than to depend on the stump pressure, particularly if it is in the lower ranges around 30 to 25 mm of Hg.

2. KINKED CAROTID

The internal carotid artery above the bifurcation can undergo tortuosity, coiling and kinking as a result of congenital, dysplastic, hypertensive or arteriosclerotic forces. The structural alterations can be easily tracked by the Doppler ultrasound probe, and if areas within the redundant vessel are kinked, high-frequency shifts are detected. These redundant and kinked carotid arteries are as potentially dangerous to patients as the common arteriosclerotic stenosis, and surgical repair is mandatory to stop repetitive and dangerous TIA's and stroke. We have detected a number of these interesting lesions by Doppler technique in patients in the sixth and seventh decade of life, most of them resulting from hypertensive elongation of the cervical carotid vessel. The more unusual bilateral, symmetrical and S-shaped coiling of the internal carotid vessels thought to be congenital and seen in young patients have not been diagnosed by our Doppler techniques, probably due to the position of these lesions high up under the mandible.

172

Operative treatment basically consists in straightening out the coiled or tortuous vessel, removing the kink and doing a beveled end-to-end anastomosis of the straightened vessel to the bifurcation with or without the use of a shunt, depending on the stump pressure. As much as 1.0 to 2.0 cm of redundant vessel has been removed from some patients, showing the marked increase in length and tortuosity that can result from hypertension. These operations have proven as successful as carotid endarterectomies.

Figure 3 illustrates the capability of imaging to provide the findings for diagnosis of aneurysm at the origin of the internal carotid artery, accompanied by kinking. This patient, one of the first studied by imaging, was seen during September, 1973 because of a noise he was hearing in the left side of his neck, but was otherwise asymptomatic. There was a continuous, blowing systolic bruit of low frequency at the left bifurcation region. Imaging demonstrated a wide origin to the internal, a non-sounding segment above (a calcified plaque) and an occlusion of the right common carotid artery. Because of the high frequency present at the upper end of the image, and just before the beginning of the non-sounding segment, a diagnosis of stenosis of the

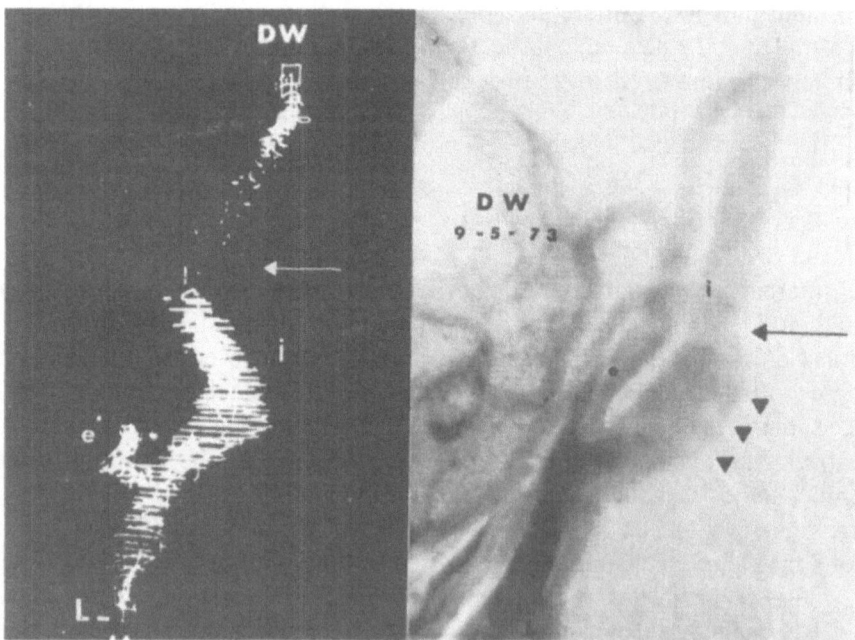

Figure 3. Patient D.W. with aneurysm and stenosis in the origin of the internal carotid artery. The opthalmic flow traces were normal indicating a normal Circle of Willis pressure in spite of the opposite carotid which was found to be occluded.

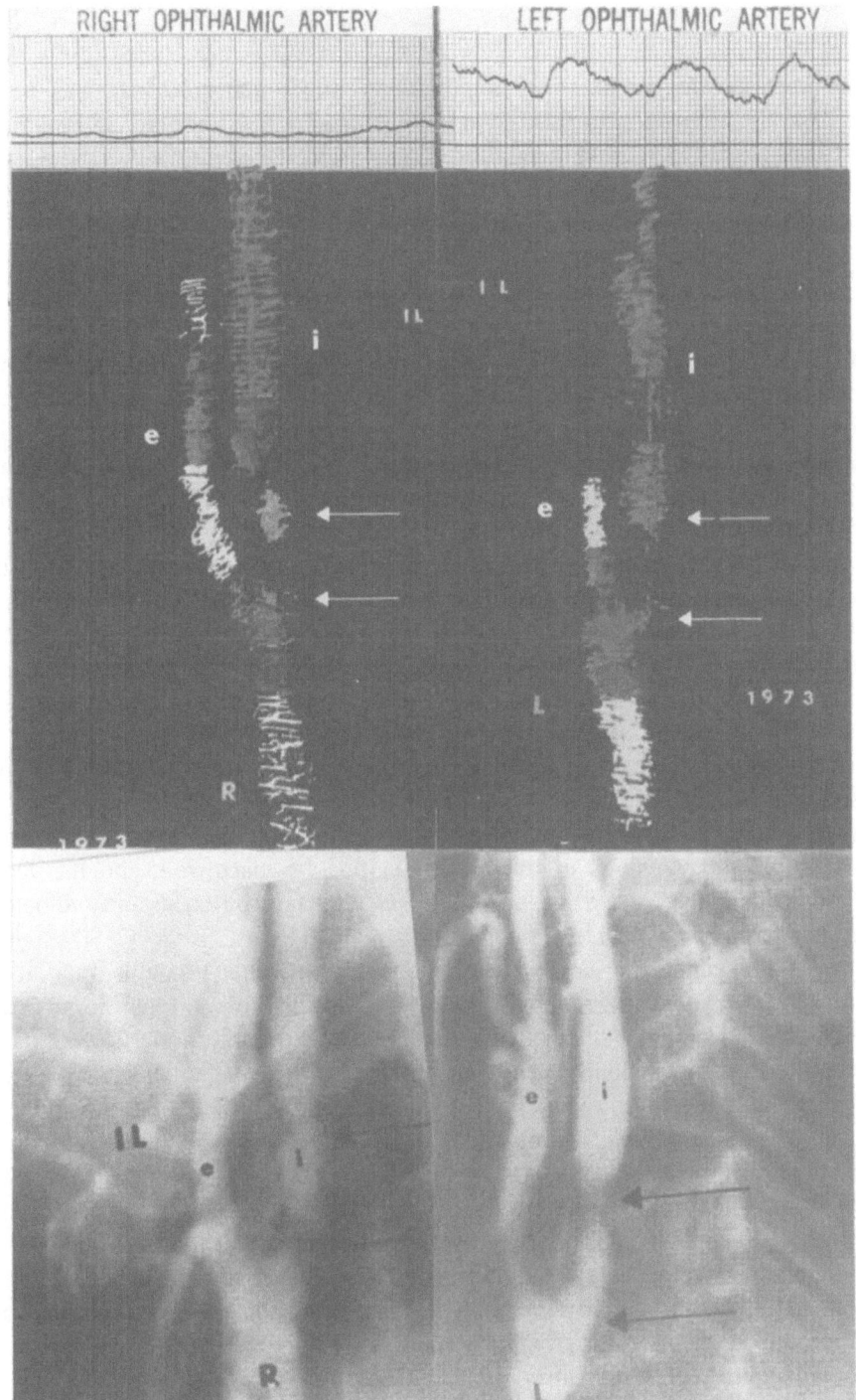

Figure 4. Doppler imaging and x-ray angiogram of bilateral internal carotid artery stenosis. Both ophthalmic artery flow directions are reversed due to lowered Circle of Willis pressure.

internal carotid was made. After angiography and endarterectomy was performed on the internal carotid, blood flow changed from 156 to 260 ml per minute as a result of the surgical repair.

3. INTERNAL CAROTID STENOSIS AND OCCLUSION

Since 1954, when Eastcott et al. performed the first endarterectomy for ischemic attacks and popularized the procedure, the widely accepted assumption over the past two years has been that removal of stenotic lesions and for markedly ulcerated plaques in the internal carotid artery will prevent strokes [1, 2]. Certainly, TIA episodes stop in most patients or diminish in severity on those patients with distal disease after carotid endarterectomy. The source of the stroke in the cervical portion of the carotid artery is generally accepted to be in the neighborhood of 30–40%, and with the operative risk in responsible vascular surgeions' hands of 1–2% with post-operative neurologic deficit, the continued promotion of the procedure is an obvious rational approach to the problem of carotid bifurcation atherosclerotic disease.

The carotid Doppler using bifurcation imaging with the continuous-wave ultrasound probe can define the position of the stenosis in the internal carotid artery. It has a high degree of accuracy in assessing its severity with the greatest accuracy in lesions in the range of 70–95% narrowed, and has less accuracy in lesions in the 20–40% range when turbulence and velocity alteration are minimal to absent.

Figure 4 illustrates the capability of Doppler ultrasonic imaging (mapping) in finding bilateral carotid stenosis and evaluating the hemodynamic significance of each lesion. The upper tracings represent the ophthalmic flow signals in the posterior orbits which in this patient are both reversed, the one on the left strongly so. The middle panels illustrate the right and left DOPSCAN image. The arrows indicate the regions of high frequency in the audio Doppler signals. The internal carotid artery in the imaging always appears to the right side of the image while the external carotid branch is to the left. The gaps in the image just above each arrow on the internal carotid artery represent calcified plaques which are producing stenosis. Color coding of the image illustrates the physiological nature of the image as opposed to morphological image produced by x-ray angiography. The lower panel represents the x-ray angiograms taken of both bifurcation regions and illustrates corresponding narrowing points which correspond to the high frequencies in the Doppler signal. The fact that both ophthalmic flow signals are reversed, flowing away from the transducer, indicates that there is low pressure in the Circle of Willis and that there is compensatory collateral flow in the external carotid arteries.

This patient, one of the earliest studied with the imaging technique, was imaged on July 17, 1973. She complained primarily of general weakness and had angina. On physical examination she demonstrated a long, blowing, almost continuous bruit over both the right and left bifurcations, louder on the right. Endarterectomy was first performed on the left bifurcation with a pre-repair flow of 110 ml per minute in the internal carotid and 110 ml per minute in the external carotid. Post-repair, the internal carotid flow increased to 215 ml per minute while the external carotid flow diminished to 40 ml per minute. Subsequent endarterectomy at the right bifurcation reported flow in the internal carotid of 80 ml per minute before repair, and following repair 410 ml per minute.

From the angiogram alone it would not be apparent which lesion was hemodynamically most significant. The imaging information provided the clue, and was proven correct at the time of surgical blood flow.

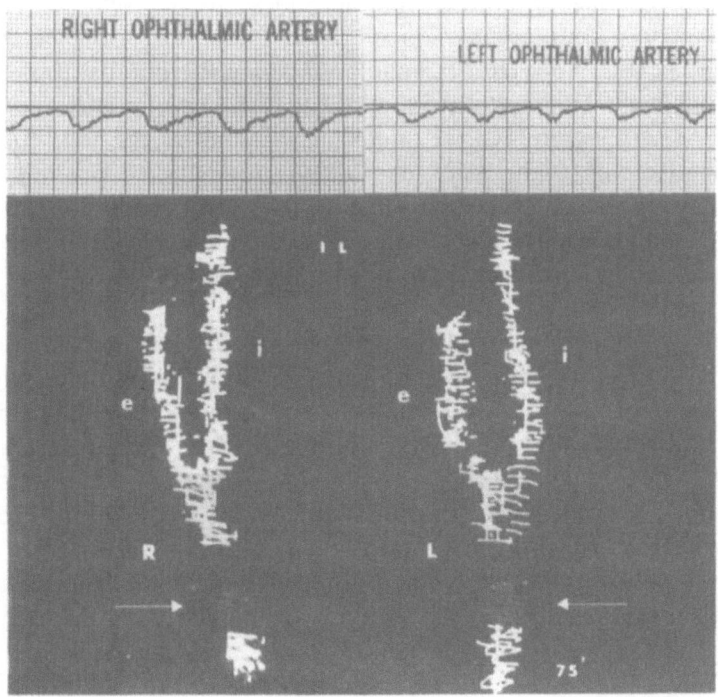

Figure 5. Postoperative imaging on patient, I.L., two years following bilateral endarterectomy at the carotid bifurcation. Minor stenosis and turbulance remains in the common carotids proximal to the endarterectomy sites. Ophthalmic artery flow in both posterior orbits is converted to the normal direction by raising the pressure in the anterior Circle of Willis. See Figure 4 for pre-repair images.

The patient was examined again with imaging two months later and again two years later. Both of the postoperative examinations demonstrated common carotid stenosis (Figure 5) representing residual of the proximal portion of the extensive plaque which could not be reached at the time of endarterectomy. The ophthalmic flow signals in both posterior orbits were changed to the normal anterior direction.

Figure 6 illustrates the ability of the imaging to diagnose total occlusion of the internal carotid artery. In addition, this case dramatically illustrates the large volume of blood flow that may pass through what appears on angiography to be a very narrow lesion. The blood flow through this stenotic region carried 320 ml per minute before repair and was unchanged following endarterectomy. Undoubtedly the large flow was compensatory to the total occlusion on the opposite side.

Figure 7 and 8 illustrate the capability of the Doppler to follow the regression of a stenotic lesion on the origin of the internal carotid artery. This patient (M.L.), first seen at age 34, was taking birth-control medication, and complained of visual dimming, and numbness in her right arm for about 1 minute, with recent progression of these symptoms. Doppler on the left (Figure 7) disclosed very faint systolic puffs along the internal carotid channel of low frequency and systolic-only quality. The left ophthalmic flow was reversed indicating a low Circle of Willis pressure on the left. Angiography demonstrated a very tight lesion on the left internal carotid artery.

Treatment consisted of stopping the birth-control medication and a brief period of steroids. She rapidly improved and repeat Doppler imaging and repeat ophthalmic flow signals showed progressive improvement over the following year (Figure 8).

Virtually all centers involved with simple non-invasive screening of carotid bifurcation disease, whether it is ocular pneumoplethysmography, ocular water plethysmography, carotid compression tonography or simple periorbital Doppler evaluation, know it is important to define who are candidates for screening. We hear from the non-advocates of non-invasive testing this statement: 'If my patient is symptomatic, I get an arteriogram.' We have no argument in this category, but there are categories of patients for screening that extend well beyond this isolated group. Figure 9 is a working model for patients in three major categories, which will be discussed in more detail.

3.1. Symptomatic patients with neck bruit

The patient presenting with a single or previously repetitive classic TIA with a neck bruit is a candidate for Doppler screening, in our opinion. This patient, however, should not be delayed from receiving arteriography. Screening provides a means of expediting this x-ray examination if a significant tight or

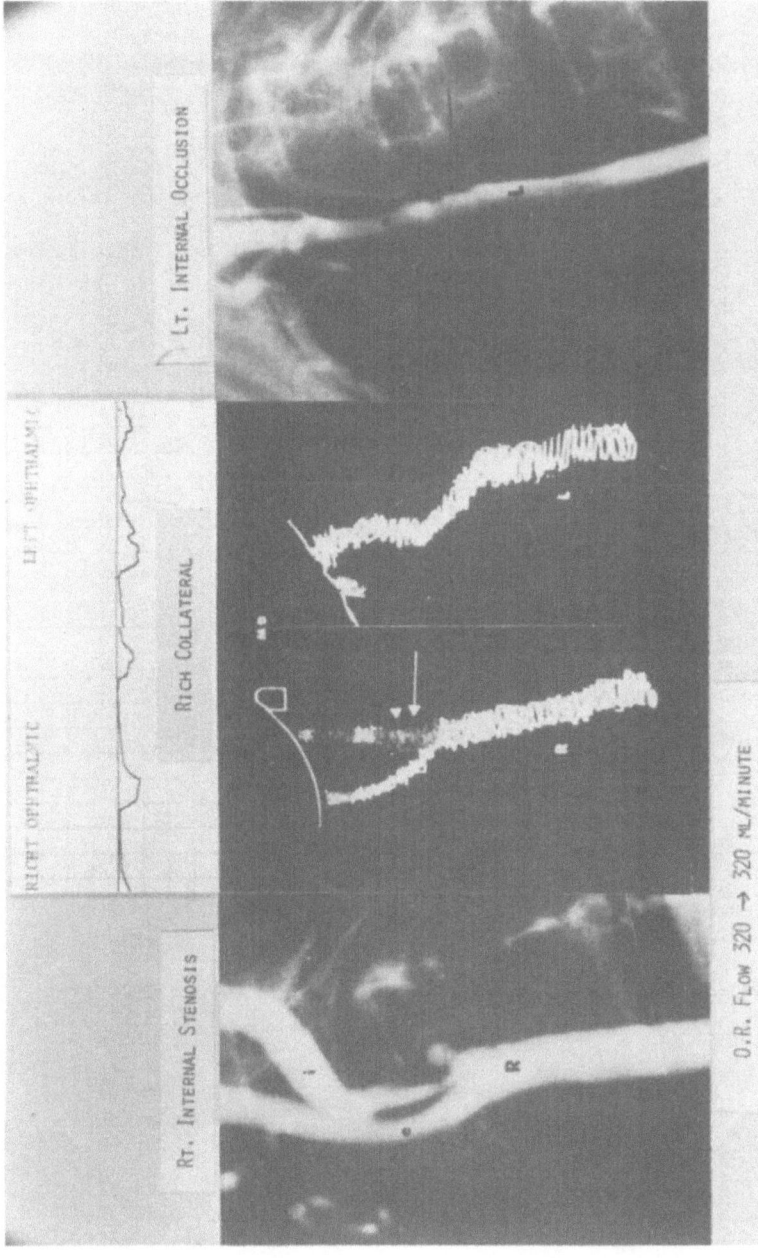

Figure 6. Doppler images demonstrating the ability to diagnose total occlusion of the internal carotid as well as contralateral stenosis and to evaluate collateral circulation. In this patient, the Doppler demonstrated that good collateral circulation to the Circle exists.

178

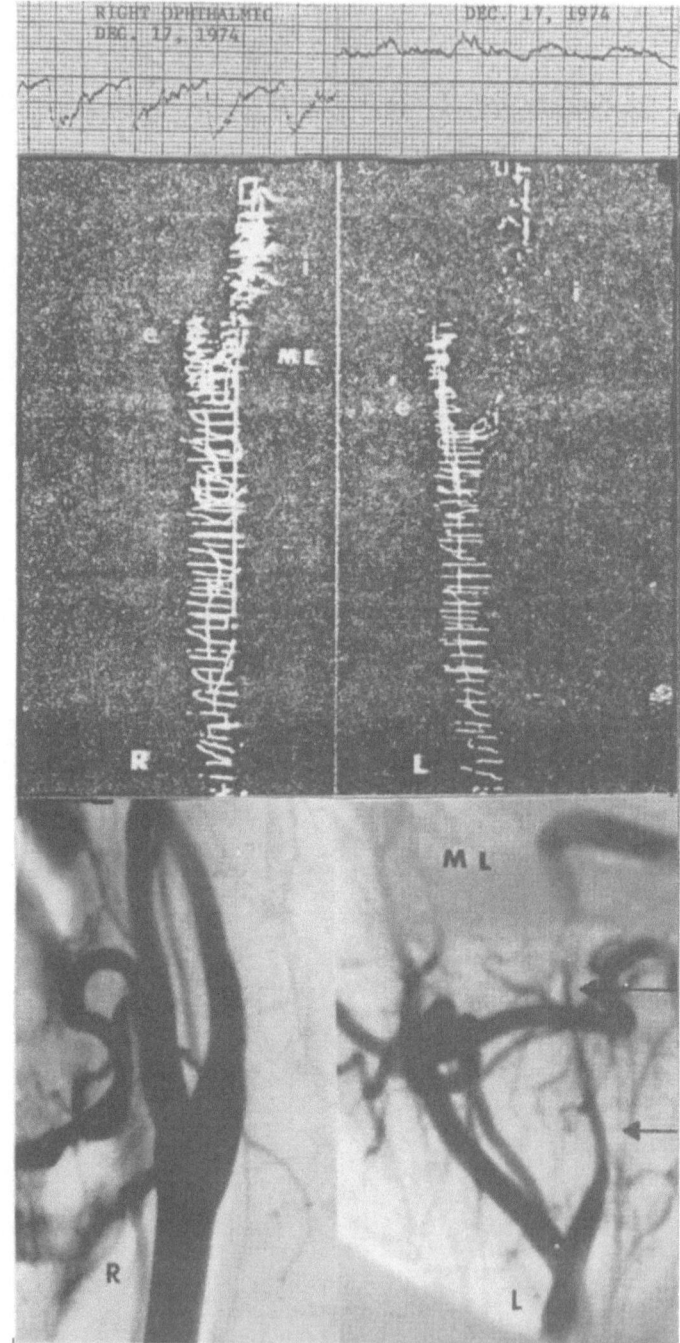

Figure 7. Patient M.L. demonstrating very tight internal carotid stenosis on the left with insufficient collateral support in the left Circle of Willis.

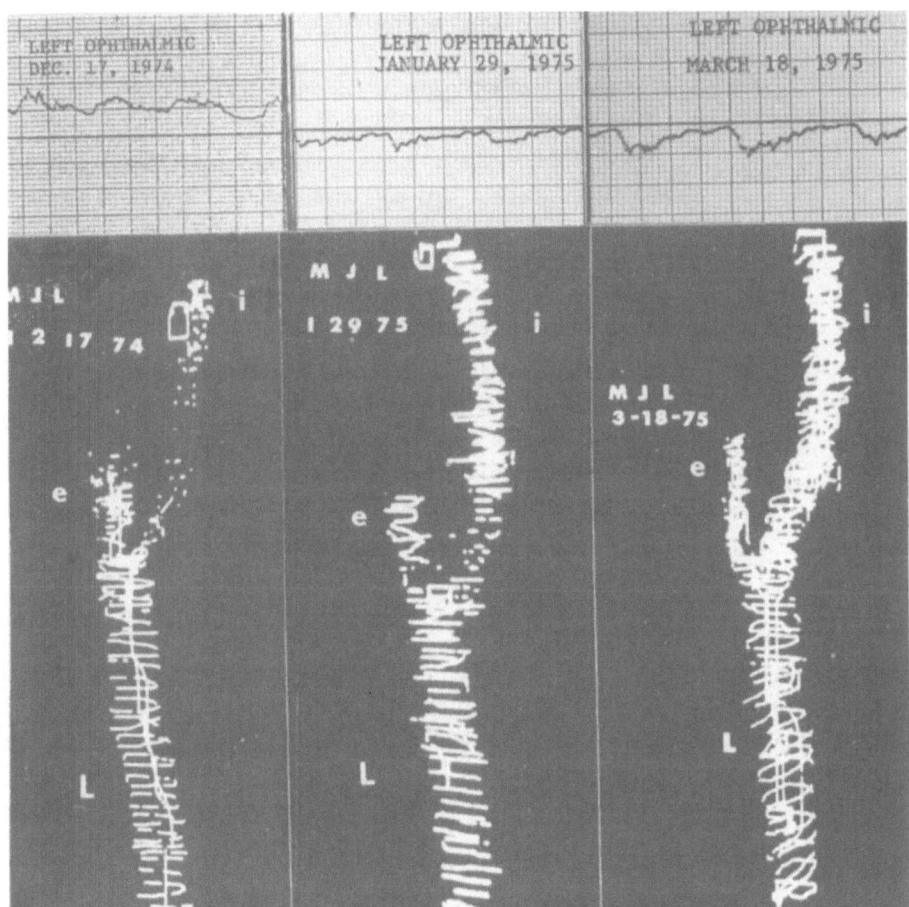

Figure 8. Successive periodic Doppler imaging on patient M.L. following removal from birth-control medication demonstrating progressive improvement in the Doppler signal and change of the left posterior orbital flow signals to normal direction.

severe internal carotid lesion is found. Delays at this point have caused serious strokes, with unfortunate or tragic sequelae (Figure 10).

It is our belief that a postscreening call to the referring doctor facilitates urgent hospitalization and treatment if a very tight stenosis exists. This is particularly true if the clinical course suggests a very early stroke in evolution, a waxing and waning neurologic deficit is occurring or crescendo transient ischemic attacks appear [2]. Again, screening in these cases is not as important as arteriography and the endarterectomy, but when patients with 95% stenotic lesions are found, the process by which definitive treatment is accomplished is usually highlighted and expedited.

Candidates   for   Screen

1. Symptomatic patient <u>with</u> neck bruit
   a. The "bruit" side
   b. The "nonbruit" side

2. Symptomatic patient <u>without</u> neck bruit
   a. No disease
   b. Tight (extreme) 85 – 95% lesion
   c. Total occlusion of internal carotid
   d. Intracranial internal carotid lesion

3. Asymptomatic patient <u>with</u> neck bruit/bruits
   a. Alone, or :
   b. Associated c̄ other main C. V. lesions

      (aneurysm, Leriche   syndrome
      operable   coronary artery disease etc.)

Figure 9. Outlines the range of patients who would benefit
from imaging and Doppler ultrasonic screening.

The 'non-bruit side' further deserves mention. The opposite carotid may be occluded or be so tight that one does not hear a bruit. A finding of this nature compounds the existing symptomatic side, indicating a situation in need of urgent attention. Again, we communicate to the referring physician, with emphasis on our findings.

3.2. Symptomatic patients without a neck bruit

Patients with TIA's or symptoms may present without neck bruits. In this category are many poorly understood areas wherein the diagnosis of hypertensive encephalopathy, diabetic arteritis, migraine equivalents and others have been made. Certainly no disease in the carotid bifurcation may exist. We have mentioned siphon disease entities which present with a bruit over the eyes (Figure 2). One of the problems physicians may fail to realize is that a lesion might be so tight that the pressure drop is great, preventing turbulence and downstream sonic activity. We have seen a number of these patients and it is oftentimes very difficult to determine the patency of the downstream internal carotid artery. Arteriography shows a pinpoint opening and a very small downstream vessel, its size due to low flow and low pressure; but patency is present. The symptomatic patient without a neck bruit, of course, may have a totally occluded internal carotid on that side. Whether or not the TIA's are due to small microemboli traversing through the enlarged external carotid artery, which has been mentioned in the literature, cannot be stated at this time. One may also have a rather delicately balanced

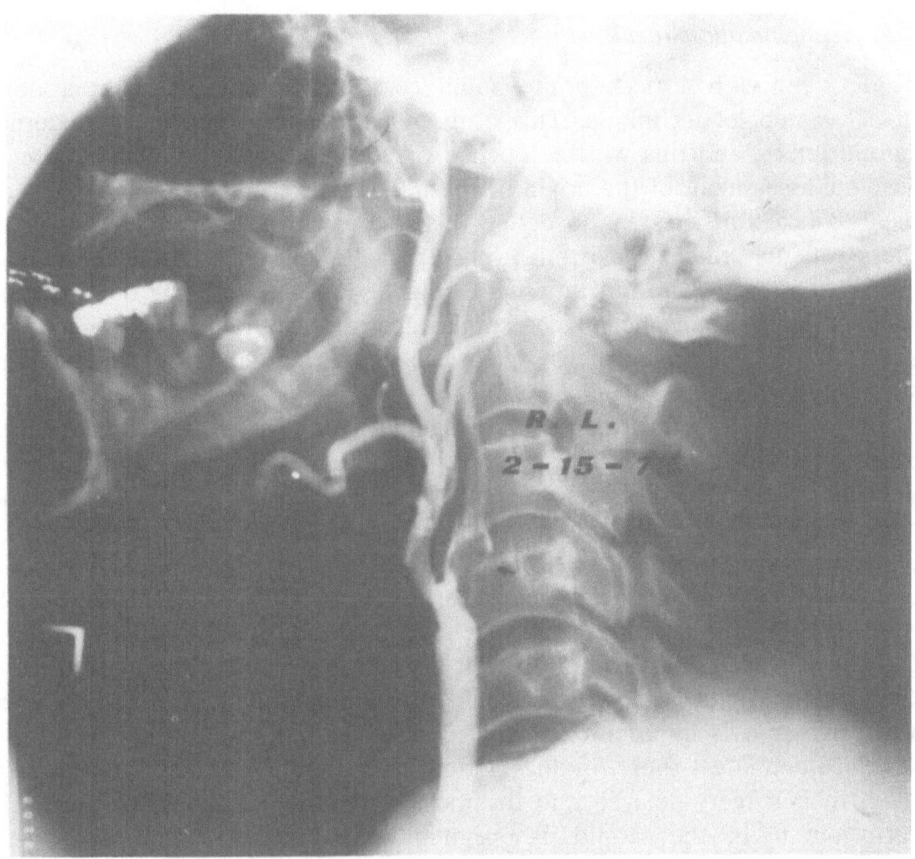

Figure 10. A 40-year-old male with unrecognized TIA followed by severe right hemiplagia, loss of speech. Note large thrombus at origin of left internal carotid artery associated with a stenotic plaque.

collateral circulation and a drop in perfusion pressure with a drop in arterial blood pressure might well produce the cortical TIA episode. These patients can be readily detected by the Doppler probe with an accuracy close to 95%. The false negative that arises is generally due to a large cervical collateral in juxtaposition to where the normal internal carotid should be, and the technician simply picks up this vessel with the probe, indicating on the image and through the tape cassettes that the internal carotid artery is present. There, of course, is no surgical procedure for a chronically occluded internal carotid except those in the clinical research investigative phase, where a segment of the temporal artery is passed intracranically to one of the angular vessels on the cortical surface of the temporal lobe.

3.3. Asymptomatic patient with neck bruit or bruits

The patient with a neck bruit should certainly be screened with a non-invasive Doppler technique. This bruit may have its origin in the external carotid artery, and this will be touched on the next segment. This is a very accurate assessment of the origin of the neck bruit, and in general we do not have to take further steps to define this lesion with arteriography. Many of these patients present for carotid work-up alone, and it has been our experience that if there is a tight internal carotid lesion on either the dominant or non-dominant hemisphere side, surgical correction should be carried out, since the risk is extremely low, again utilizing current sound and meticulous surgical principles.

Many asymptomatic patients are evaluated with neck bruits, who are scheduled for major cardiovascular surgery in other areas. Prominent in this area are those patients with coronary artery disease wherein a delay of either the correction of the carotid lesion or correction of the coronary problem may place the patient in jeopardy. A number of these patients present with elective abdominal aortic aneurysm resections or severe aortoiliac occlusive lesions. If the DOPSCAN indicates a very tight stenosis in the neighborhood of 85–95%, the downstream signals behind the left or right eye may indicate poor flow to the Circle of Willis. With this evidence of collateral build-up around the eye, we feel that it is important to communicate with the physician or surgeon involved and stress these findings. Oftentimes these patients are arteriogrammed, their surgery delayed and the most significant lesion, which generally turns out to be the carotid, is operated upon first. With coronary artery disease, if unstable or severe, the surgery is done at the same time, with excellent results in both the carotid area and the coronary artery area [3, 4]. The carotid endarterectomy procedure is generally done first prior to large-dose body heparization and cardiopulmonary bypass to be sure the vascular bed to the involved hemisphere is wide open and will not suffer from eschemia during bypass.

In summary, we have defined three candidates to screen for internal artery stenosis and have elucidated the philosophy of our group with respect to promoting Doppler non-invasive testing. Each patient, of course, has a different situation, but in brief can fall nicely into these three categories and be handled accordingly.

4. EXTERNAL CAROTID STENOSIS

Hardly a week goes by in our large outpatient Doppler non-invasive screening test wherein a rather prominent bruit is found to lie wholly within the external carotid artery and there is no impediment to flow in the internal carotid artery whatsoever. In these situations it is safe to allow the stenosis to remain, and even if extremely tight and reducing flow to the face, tongue and mouth, no corrective surgery needs to be done. However, if there is an associated obstruction of the internal carotid artery, namely, total occlusion, the external carotid artery may contribute significantly to the periorbital circulation and to the posterior orbital circulation and thence to the Circle of Willis, so that revascularization and endarterectomy of this stenosis is important. The internal and external carotids may be also potential sources of retinal emboli. Since the microemboli may well pass through the 1.0 to 3.0 mm diameter external carotid, collaterals then develop if the internal carotid is occluded [5]. We have performed many of these carotid revascularization procedures on the external in situations like this, and have found rather significant improvement in our symptomatic patients. The TIA's stop and the periorbital collateral build up is impressive. It is a safe procedure because shunting does not need to be carried out during the endarterectomy, although one could easily supply excellent flow downstream by the same technique with the Javid shunt as we do with the internal carotid artery when operated (Figure 11).

5. VERTEBRAL STENOSIS

Figures 12 and 13 demonstrate the capability of imaging to diagnose vertebral artery stenosis near its origin and separate external from internal carotid

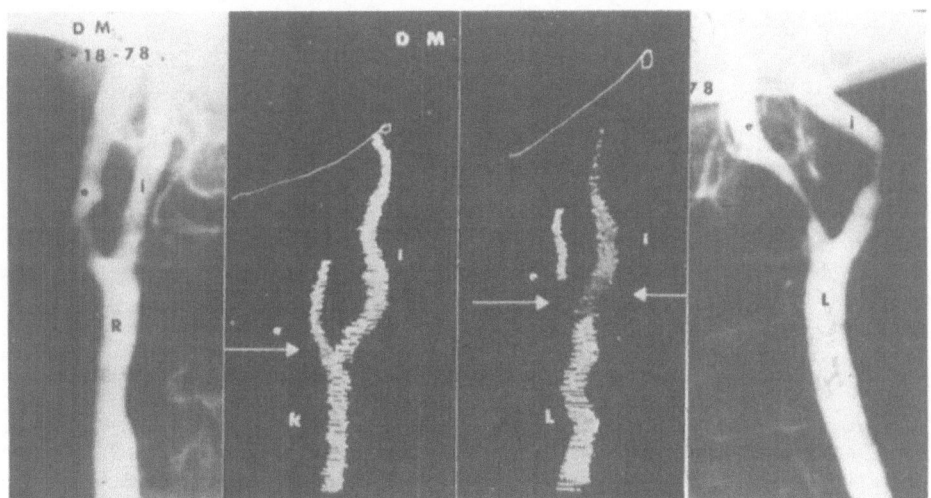

Figure 11. Bilateral external carotid stenosis diagnosed with imaging. Also present is left internal carotid stenosis.

184

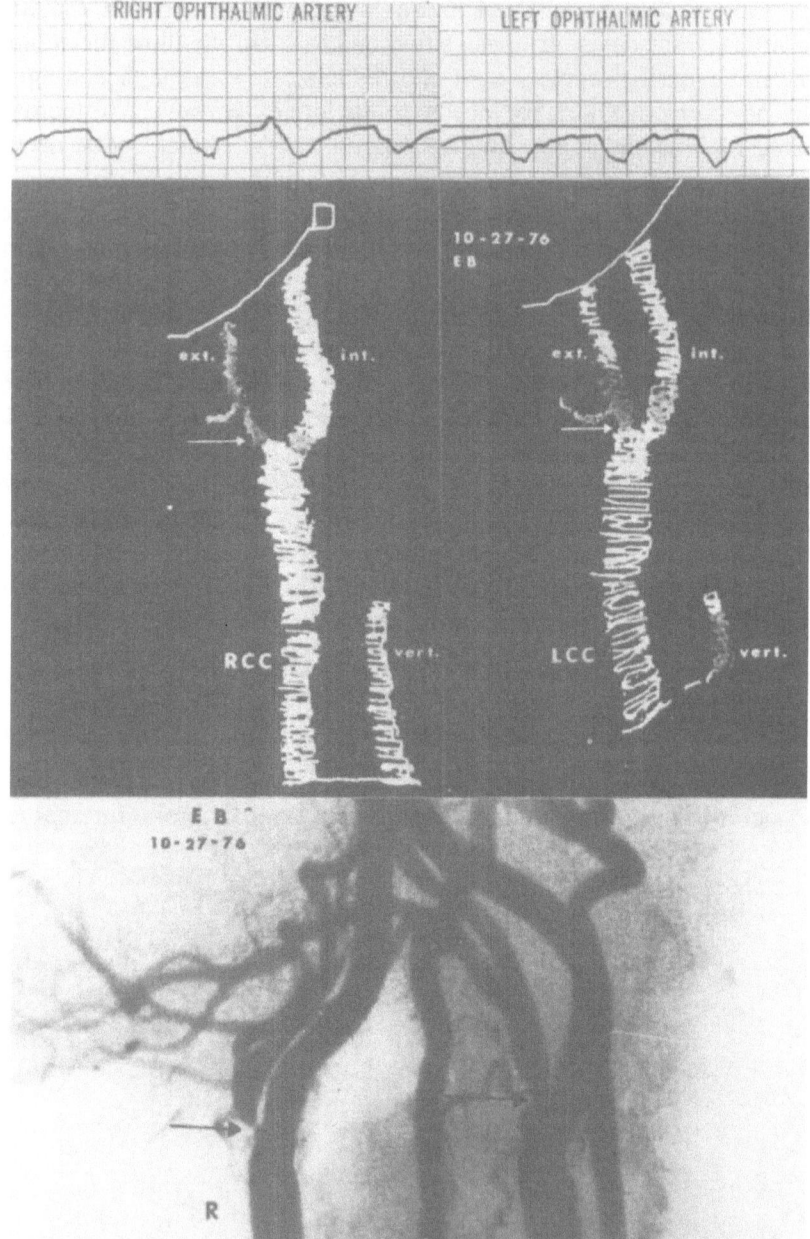

Figure 12. Imaging and ophthalmic flow tracings (patient E.B.), compared to the x-ray angiography, demonstrate the ability of the imaging to diagnose external carotid stenosis to the exclusion of internal carotid stenosis and also to diagnose vertebral artery stenosis at its origin from the subclavian artery.

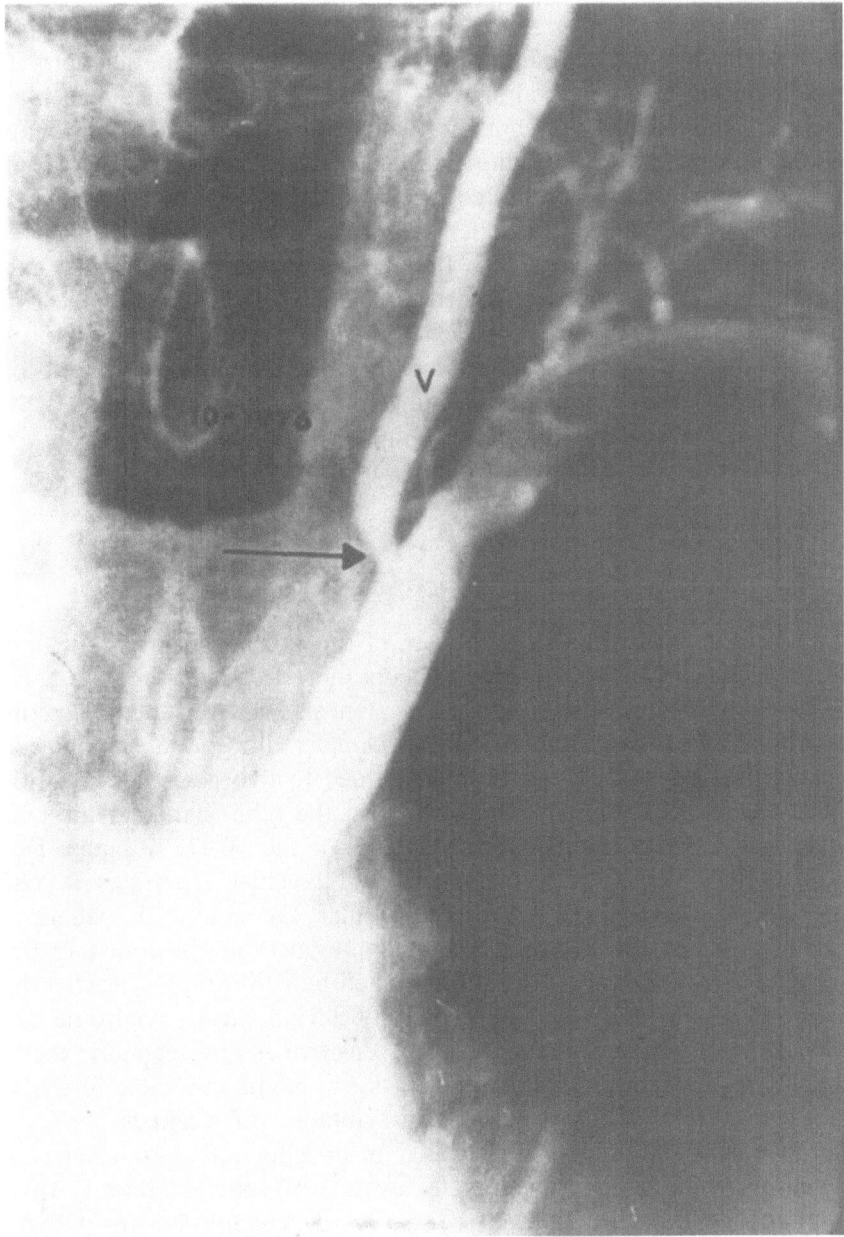

Figure 13. X-ray angiogram showing stenosis at the origin of the proximal left vertebral artery in patient E.B.

stenosis. By means of inverse imaging with the Doppler flow probe directing the sound beam in an inferior direction, 30 degrees from the normal, the common carotid and vertebral arteries are traced to their position behind the clavicle. On the left, the vertebral artery signal demonstrated a high frequency but with flow in the normal direction. The patient was essentially asymptomatic but demonstrated high frequency wheezing quality bruits over both bifurcation regions and a systolic bruit in the left supraclavicular region. Bifurcation imaging disclosed high frequencies on the origin of both external carotid arteries and also demonstrated the occasional capability of the Doppler to find and follow branches of the external carotid just above the bifurcation. Since the internal carotid signals were of good amplitude, stenosis of the internal carotid artery could be eliminated. The diagnosis of left vertebral stenosis was made from the Doppler imaging and was confirmed by x-ray. The patient was not submitted to vascular surgery.

6. SUBCLAVIAN OCCLUSION

Arteriosclerotic narrowing, or occlusion, of the subclavian artery at its origin from the aorta or innominate artery occurs more frequently than is generally appreciated by physicians. Insignificant stenosis which is hemodynamically unimportant is easily diagnosed by the Doppler ultrasound techniques, and we make this diagnosis in an estimated three to five percent of our routine carotid screenings. Significant narrowing, on the other hand, to the point of producing a reduced arm blood pressure is in the 70–75% range. Doppler examination of the subclavian, axillary and brachial arteries is a standard measurement in our Doppler cerebrovascular evaluation. In patients with unequal pressures, the vertebral artery (if present) may be found to flow in the reverse direction and this is substantiated by performing a reactive hyperemia test on the involved side. The 'Subclavian Steal' syndrome is thus confirmed by these maneuvers and is as sensitive as arteriography, the latter, of course, recommended if the patient has symptoms referrable to the vertebral-basilar system or has ischemic arm symptoms of weakness, arm claudication or a cold extremity. The majority of patients with significant subclavian stenosis or occlusion can tolerate reversal of vertebral flow and remain asymptomatic. This situation, of course, is dependent on the presence of pressure, flow characteristics of the opposite vertebral or adequate communication via the Circle of Willis. If these sources of 'collateral' are inadequate, the patients will present with typical vertebral-basilar insufficiency symptoms and surgical correction is necessary.

Two procedures are available to the surgeon in correcting subclavian obstruction. Both are extra-anatomic and both are equal in restoring true

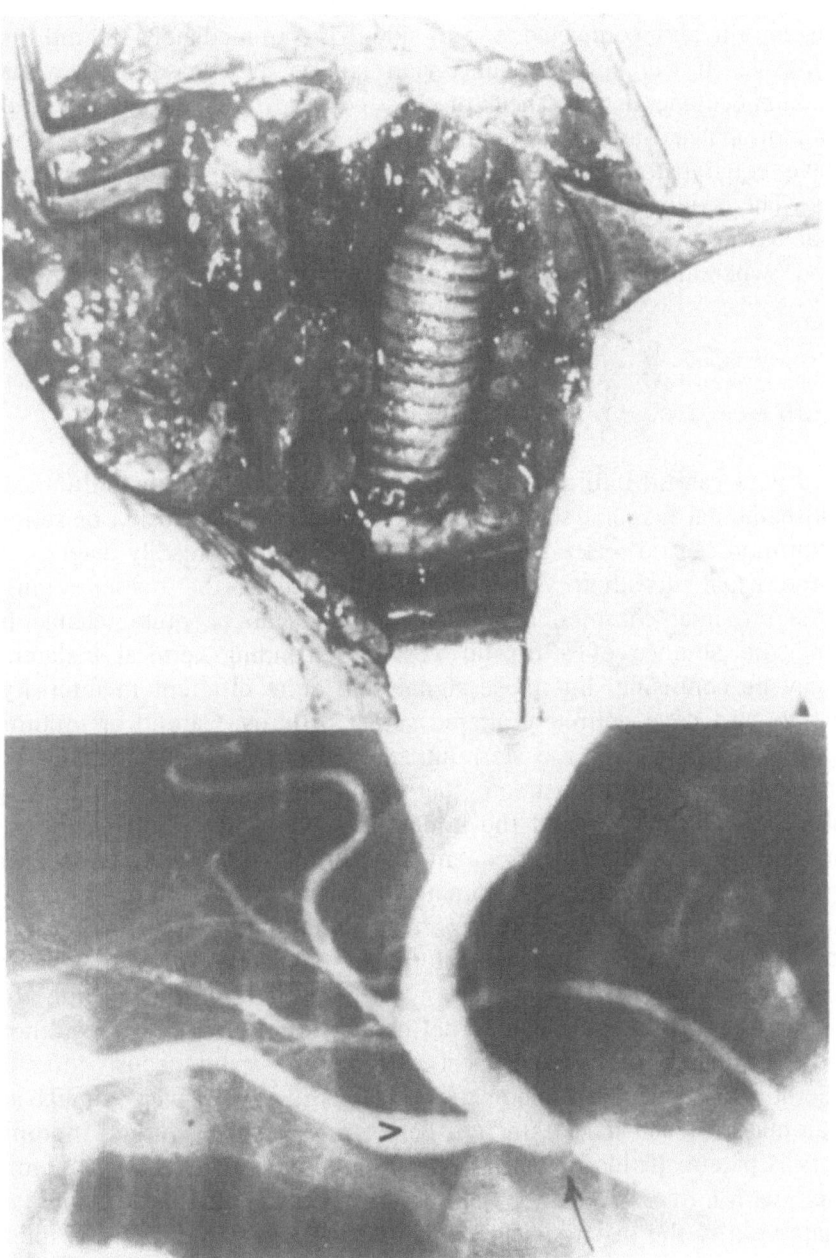

Figure 14. Subclavian stenosis angiogram and surgical repair with carotid-to-subclavian arterial prosthetic graft. Doppler diagnosis is made from abnormal signals in the subclavian artery found above the medial end of the clavicle and in the brachial artery.

systemic pressure and correcting reverse vertebral flow. The first is a carotid-subclavian bypass performed via a small supraclavicular incision on the involved side. A 6- or 8-mm prosthetic graft is sutured end-to-side to the ipsilateral carotid and connected end-to-side lying immediately behind the scalene muscle. If the opposite subclavian is free of disease or proximal occlusion, a subcutaneous cross-neck or chest bypass from the contralateral or subclavian or axillary artery to the ipsilateral partner is constructed. Both grafts have equal patency and long-term follow-up and the choice is the surgeon's. The axillo-axillary procedure is usually recommended over the carotid-subclavian bypass if the donor carotid is diseased proximally or at its bifurcation, wherein a 'carotid steal' syndrome might well result (Figure 14).

7. COMMON CAROTID AND INNOMINATE ARTERY OCCLUSION

Associated with carotid bifurcation disease and as a result of our multiphasic and multisegmental Doppler screening, innominate artery occlusion or stenosis and common carotid artery stenosis or occlusion can be readily diagnosed. Besides the usual auscultatory and palpatory findings, the DOPSCAN fairly images the proximal common carotid vessels and can be quite reliable in diagnosing the absence of a carotid vessel. Ascending cervical collateral trunks may be confusing, but these signals are quite different in intensity, small in size and have definitely altered signal patterns. Carotid or innominate stenosis lying beneath the sternum and below the clavicle boundaries oftentimes have marked downstream coarse and fluttering signals, indicating the post-stenotic turbulence and the nonlaminar blood flow. Surgical reconstruction of these two vessels is frequently performed and there have been a number of successful patients symptomatic with TIA's who have had a reconstruction from the ipsilateral subclavian artery with a venous autogenous graft to the distal external or to the distal internal-external branches which are in continuity with each other. Imaging is very important in establishing the presence of patent distal internal-external carotid arteries when the common carotid has occluded itself, either post-surgically or spontaneously due to arteriosclerotic disease. Innominate artery reconstruction usually entails an extra-anatomic approach if the junction between the subclavian and innominate artery is patent. If this is found to be stenotic or occluded, a sternotomy is required, with a bypass prosthetic graft from the ascending aorta below the innominate vein to the distal subclavian-carotid system. Usually this is tolerated quite well in most patients.

Patient J.R.M., (Figure 15 and Figure 16) demonstrates the ability of imaging to diagnose both common carotid stenosis and subsequent common

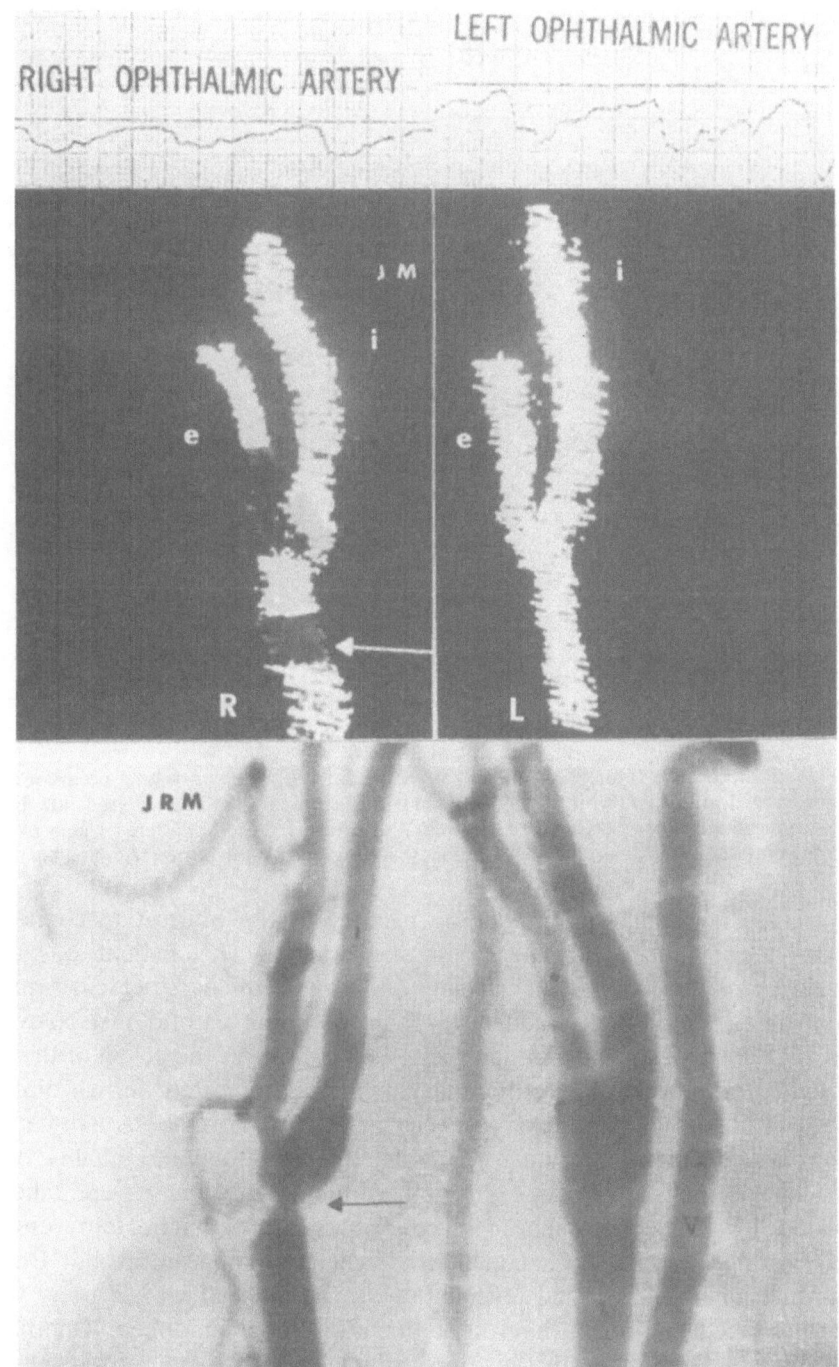

Figure 15. Doppler imaging in patient J.R.M. leading to the diagnosis of common carotid stenosis but with good volumetric blood flow.

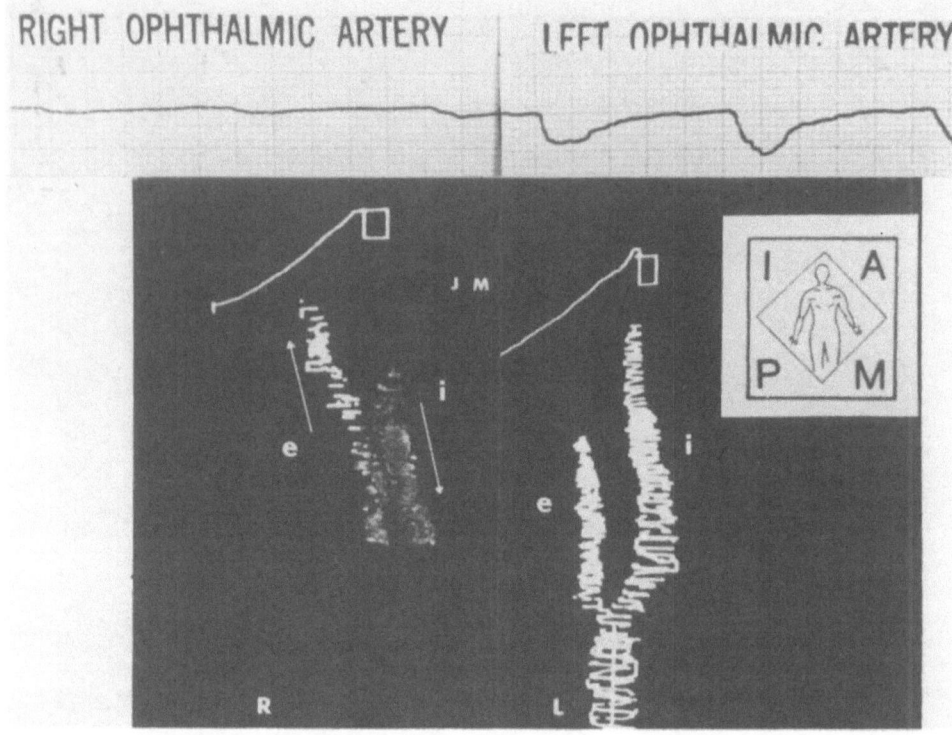

Figure 16. Postoperative bifurcation imaging of patient, J.R.M., demonstrating occlusion of the common carotid artery but with a patent bifurcation diagnosed from the reversed flow internal carotid connecting to normally directed flow in the external carotid. Lowered Circle of Willis pressure is indicated by weak and low frequency and damped right posterior orbital signals.

carotid occlusion but with remaining patency at the bifurcation connection between the external and internal carotid arteries. This patient was a 56-year-old man who complained of sounds in his right ear. DOPSCAN imaging demonstrated slight high frequency in the common carotid just below the bifurcation as well as a nonsounding calcified plaque on the origin of the right external common carotid. Ophthalmic flow traces indicated normal direction but because common carotid stenosis can maintain a normal gradient between the circle and external carotid collaterals, the low frequency quality of the otherwise normally directed right ophthalmic flow signals were taken to indicate a low Circle of Willis pressure. Subsequent endarterectomy unfortunately resulted in total occlusion of the right common carotid, but Doppler imaging clearly demonstrated reverse flow in the internal carotid artery which was interpreted to mean that the bifurcation remained open. Ophthalmic artery signals deteriorated but his only complaint at the time of re-evaluation was one episode of blurred vision, lasting for 30 seconds, which has not recurred.

REFERENCES

1. Eastcott HHG, Pickering GW, Rob C: Reconstruction of internal carotid artery in a patient with intermittant attacks of hemiplegia. Lancet 2:994, 1954.
2. Goldstine J, Moore WS: A new look at emergency carotid artery objectives for the treatment of cerebrovascular insufficiency. Stroke 9:599, 1978.
3. Hertzer NR, Loop FD, Taylor PL, Bevan EC: Staged and combined surgical approach to simultaneous carotid and coronary vascular surgery. Surgery 84:803, 1978.
4. Mehigan JT, Buch WS, Pipkin RD, Fogarty TJ: A planned approach to coexistant cerebrovascular disease in coronary artery bypass candidates. Arch Surgery 112:1403, 1977.
5. Burnbaum MD, Selhorst JB, Harbison JW, Brush JJ: Amaurosis fugax from disease of the external carotid artery. Arch Neurol 34:532, 1977.
6. Thompson JE, Austin DJ, Pitman RD: Carotid endarterectomy for cerebrovascular insufficiency. Ann Surgery 172:663, 1970.

14. CLINICAL MANAGEMENT DECISIONS BASED ON DOPPLER CEREBROVASCULAR EVALUATION

MERRILL P. SPENCER, M.D.

The growth of non-invasive techniques for diagnosis of diseases of the extra-cranial arterial circulation has been questioned on the basis that the physicians are making management decisions on test results without knowing the answers to such important questions as whether or not surgery for extracranial vascular disease actually prevents stroke and because the clinical use of non-invasive studies depends on the bias of the physician. Doppler is indeed making a contribution in understanding the natural history of atherosclerotic lesions and their relationship to stroke but meanwhile physicians and patients need all the non-invasive information available to make rational decisions concerning x-ray angiography, surgery, medical treatment, or for following the patient with no special treatment. Decisions should be based on informed rational consideration of all available diagnostic information and treatment modalities in the hope of preventing stroke and alleviating symptoms of cerebrovascular insufficiency.

The technique of examination and interpretation of imaging and the complete Doppler Cerebrovascular Evaluation including a pertinent history and physical examination has been disclosed in the previous chapters. Our experience with the complete evaluation is based on 6,000 CVE's with patients referred by 500 physicians over a seven year period to three Seattle laboratories. All Doppler data of patients subjected to angiography (approximately 20% of those referred) is analyzed at a weekly conference by a physician medical/surgical group. It is obvious from these case analyses and from the increasing demand for Doppler CVE that physicians in the Seattle metropolitan area are relying on Doppler reports in their clinical practices. The purpose of this chapter is to share our observations on how Doppler CVE is utilized in clinical management decisions.

1. SYMPTOMATIC CATEGORIES

Both symptom categories and Doppler diagnosis classifications are used in this discussion. The percentages of Table 1 were derived from the clinical records of all patients (547) referred during the year 1976 to the Providence

Table 1. Patient cerebrovascular symptom categories.

Category	%
I Asymptomatic cervical bruits	6
II Dizzy, non-focal or not fitting other categories	34
III Vertebral basilar symptoms	9
IV Focal or lateralizing, not clearly TIA	14
V Classical TIA or RIND	22
VI Completed stroke with or without residual symptoms	15

Medical Center Vascular Laboratory in Seattle, Washington and are representative of all the Seattle laboratories.

1.1. Category I and category II patients with carotid bruits

Imaging can disclose the source of a cervical bruit and determine the hemodynamic significance of the lesion. If the external carotid is diagnosed as the source of the bruit, considerable concern is alleviated, (Patient #1, F.J.D.). If a stenosis is found in the internal carotid as the source of bruit, either unilateral or bilateral, and is determined to cause less than 50% reduction in the lumen, angiography and surgery (A & S) is usually not performed but the patient is followed with Doppler at 6 month to yearly intervals for progression of the lesion. If there are some non-focal symptoms of cerebrovascular insufficiency the patient is often treated on a preventive basis with aspirin and Persantine. If DOPSCAN determines that there is an internal carotid stenosis with greater than 75% reduction in the lumen, angiography and surgery is often carried out (Patient #2, A.S.). This procedure is particularly practiced before major surgery such as coronary artery bypass grafting or abdominal laporatomy because it is a widely held opinion that a hemodynamically significant lesion should be repaired before risking hypotension from major surgical interventions.

1.2. Category II and category III patients

One third of our patients are referred for symptoms of cerebrovascular insufficiency but which do not appear to represent embolism of TIA's in the carotid territories. If Doppler demonstrates normal velocities in the carotid and vertebral arteries contrast angiography is not performed. Medications are often prescribed and the patient followed or other diagnostic tests carried out (Patient #3, E.R.B.). This presumes, however, that operable intracranial lesions are eliminated by neurological examination or computerized x-ray tomography. If carotid stenosis is found greater than 80% ($\gtrsim 1$ mm diameter), arteriogram and surgery is a rational course. If, however, total occlusion is found, no special treatment is necessary if there is good collateral supporting the Circle of Willis pressure. This collateral support is indicated by the strength of the collateral signal through the circle and if, for example, there is a normally directed ophthalmic flow signal which is demonstrated by contralateral common carotid compression to be arising from the opposite carotid one may assume that the circle pressure is well supported on the occluded side.

1.3. Category IV patients

Doppler findings are of special value in determining the management plan in patients with focal or lateralizing symptoms not clearly TIA's. If the Doppler findings are negative, angiography and surgery may be eliminated and antiplatelet medication treatment indicated (Patient #4, E.B.).

If a calcified plaque is found, arteriography may be carried out with the hope of finding crater evidence of ulceration but only if surgery is contemplated for such a finding. Antiplatelet medication is an appropriate alternate course with many specialists.

If stenosis is found arteriography may be carried out on the basis that stenosis evidence of ulceration and embolization will be found and an endarterectomy performed.

1.4. The category V patient

Cerebral angiography including 4 vessel arch injections and selective carotid injections is performed in most patients displaying classical TIA's. Doppler, however, is also useful in many of these patients. 1) Often the patient or non-specialist physician is not convinced of imminent danger of a stroke. Imaging, if finding a stenotic lesion on the appropriate artery, encourages the patient and the physician of the necessity for angiography and definitive surgical treatment (Patient #5, L.E.O.). 2) There is a reluctance to angiogram the elderly patient or the patient with other severe debilitating disease such as coronary disease or cancer. Imaging offers an interim test to establish the presence or absence of a stenotic lesion in a surgically approachable region adding information for the management decision. 3) If Doppler reveals no carotid stenosis in a patient with TIA's, anticoagulant or antiplatelet medication offers an appropriate alternative to the angiography and surgery 'route.'

Doppler often assists the radiologist in planning his procedures and offers the dye sensitive patient an alternative for angiography. For the surgeon, imaging performed prior to and following carotid endarterectomy is useful to determine the adequacy of surgical corrections (Patient #6, J.W.G.). The surgical approach itself is assisted by the functional information concerning collateral and deciding whether or not to shunt.

Patients with TIA's may be found with moderate or no stenosis at the bifurcation but at the same time displaying an ophthalmic bruit on the side of the symptomatic hemisphere. In this situation the probability of the stenosis at the siphon, as a source of the symptoms, is highly probable. Relief of the bifurcation lesion may not be appropriate when in tandem with the more severe siphon lesion. Temporal artery bypass might be considered in these patients.

1.5. The category VI patient

Angiography is usually not performed in the patient with a fresh or completed stroke because of the danger of producing an intracranial hemorrhage into the infarcted area or because 'the horse is out of the barn and it is too late to close the gate.' Imaging may, however, disclose an unsuspected severe stenosis at the bifurcation for which an appropriately timed endarterectomy may prevent further embolization and extension of the brain damage. We have found patients on the stroke ward in which Doppler detected an appropriate occlusion coinciding with the involved side to explain the stroke, but with a simultaneous severe stenosis on the opposite internal carotid (Patient #7, E.N.L.).

2. DOPPLER DIAGNOSTIC CLASSIFICATIONS

2.1. Subclavian, innominate and vertebral abnormalities

Doppler CVE has disclosed a surprising incidence of subclavian, vertebral and innominate disease in patients of all symptom categories. Should the Doppler disclose such a lesion, Doppler would assist in answering the difficult question as to whether or not surgical relief by means of bypass grafting or vertebral-basilar insufficiency when hemodynamically significant abnormalities are found, subclavian bypass grafting is often performed or in the case of an innominate obstruction a thoracotomy and endarterectomy may be performed (Patient #8, N.M.C.).

If a vertebral steal is disclosed by the Doppler examination and is affecting flow in the vertebral artery at the base of the skull, the clinical or 'brain significance' can be ascertained at the time of the Doppler examination by observing for exacerbation of symptoms when the steal is exaggerated by the arm cuff reactive hyperemia test. If the symptoms are exacerbated, the likelihood of improvement by surgical relief is enhanced. If they are not produced or exacerbated, bypass grafting will probably not relieve the symptoms.

2.2. Critical carotid stenosis

The Doppler CVE is capable of accurately differentiating the extremely tight stenosis from lesser degrees of stenosis and from total occlusion. The techniques that are especially useful in this important differentiation are discussed in Chapters 6, 9, and 11. Grades III, IV and V stenoses ($\lesssim 1$ mm diameter) are found in patients of all symptom categories. When this diagnosis is made by non-invasive Doppler, many specialist physicians in the Seattle area recommend immediate carotid endarterectomy following angiographic confirmation. If the patient has classical TIA's, endarterectomy is performed on an emergency basis with the rationale that a major stroke may occur, not necessarily from the loss of the small amount of residual blood flow passing through the lesion but rather because large, 'red' fibrin clots are prone to develop downstream to the stenosis and may be dislodged into the cerebral circulation (Patient #9, E.M.C.). Grades IV and V stenosis (0.5 mm) are treacherous lesions because no bruit is heard and they may be found on the side opposite to a carotid bruit or the side opposite the one implicated by lateralizing symptoms.

In the dizzy patient or the patient with symptoms of vertebral basilar insufficiency, in which there are multiple extracranial obstructions, surgical relief of carotid lesion is given priority (Patient #2). This decision is based on the rationale that vertebral-basilar symptoms are caused by reduced flow to the posterior circulation and is less likely to produce a stroke. If Doppler CVE indicated the carotid lesion is not hemodynamically significant, while the vertebral problem is flow significant and symptomatic, subclavian or innominate surgery is often performed.

It is recognized that imaging, except in the hands of the most skilled personnel, may indicate total occlusion of the internal carotid when there is in fact a severe grade stenosis with less than 0.5 mm diameter. Because of this difficulty, angiography should not be deferred in category IV or category V patients on the basis of Doppler diagnosis of total occlusion. When total occlusion is apparent from Doppler CVE findings, the diagnosis should be 'probably' total carotid occlusion and if the patient displays focal symptoms related to the apparently occluded side, carotid angiography should be performed on the possibility that a thin thread-like opening exists or that an ulcerated crater or stump pouch at the origin of the internal is persisting and dislodging debris to the external carotid.

2.3. Bilateral carotid stenosis

When bilateral internal carotid stenosis is detected, Doppler assists greatly in determining which of the two lesions is of greater significance as far as blood flow is concerned (Patient #5). Many Seattle surgeons operate on the most hemodynamically significant lesion when the symptoms do not clearly implicate one lesion or the other. The rationale is that global ischemia during carotid clamping is less likely if the tightest lesion is operated first. Often, x-ray angiography cannot indicate which stenosis is most significant or may be misleading in this regard. The principle problems of x-ray arise from resolving the cross-sectional area within the stenosis and from vasodilation caused by the contrast material.

3. DIAGNOSIS OF INTIMAL ULCERATION

The term 'ulceration' should be reserved for a condition of denuded endothelium. At present there are no Doppler ultrasonic signals which are diagnostic of ulceration of the intima but the future may provide Doppler signals, such as turbulence accompanied by signals of calcium deposits, or associated with craters in the artery wall. The presurgical diagnosis of ulcerated intima with adherent thrombi is poorly diagnosed by either Doppler or x-ray angiography. X-ray angiography also does not specifically diagnose ulceration and the presence of indentation in the luminar wall should be termed 'crater' rather than ulcer because an intact endothelial lining may cover its surface. While it is true that the crater formation seen on angiography is sometimes associated with symptoms of embolization, TIA's often occur without the finding of crater or wall roughening and cratering often occurs without embolic symptoms. In fact, stenosis rather than crater is more often associated with embolic symptoms. A technique for specific diagnosis of wall adherent fibrin and platelets is urgently needed in the field of stroke prevention. Such a diagnostic test may arise from the field of nuclear medicine.

4. ENDARTERECTOMY WITHOUT ANGIOGRAPHY

In the present practice of responsible medicine, angiography is a standard requirement in the planning of carotid endarterectomy for surgical relief of any impediments to the extracranial arterial circulation. There have, however, been several occasions in our experience where endarterectomy was performed, without the use of angiography for adequate reason. The criteria for endarterectomy performed without angiography are: 1) the patient displays classical TIA's appropriate to the side where 2) Doppler with imaging provide unquestionable signals of carotid stenosis and 3) in a surgically accessible position at the origin of the internal carotid. Collateral circulation should be checked carefully with Doppler or other non-invasive procedures if shunting is to be considered. Specific patients on whom carotid endarterectomy without angiography have been performed include: 1) the patient who is admitted on Friday afternoon with recurring unstable TIA's when the regular staff of the hospital and department of radiology are not available. 2) Patients have declined angiography but agree to carotid endarterectomy on the basis of DOPSCAN findings and the need for surgical relief. 3) When angiography from months previous had already proven the existence of a carotid lesion and DOPSCAN confirmed the continuing presence of internal stenosis, the patient received an endarterectomy without an additional angiogram.

It has been our observation in one major hospital in the Seattle area that arch studies only are performed on TIA patients. The major justification for angiography in addition to Doppler has been that it discloses the anatomy of the intracranial vessels and establishes the presence or absence of intracranial occlusions, tumors, and aneurysms. In view of the resolution problem of arch studies, DOPSCAN competes well with arch studies alone. We feel that if angiography is performed, intracranial views and selected carotid and vertebral injections should be performed.

5. GENERAL BENEFITS

In addition to the specific clinical values in the decision making process discussed in this chapter, it should be mentioned that there are many general benefits to the availability of Doppler CVE examinations. For example, the expertise of the laboratory personnel is often helpful in clarifying the presence of cervical bruits for the referring physician. The carefully taken history by the laboratory personnel also often brings out symptoms which were not otherwise appreciated. Patient education is enhanced concerning types of symptoms to watch for, as a premonitor of stroke condition.

It is impossible at this early stage in the use of non-invasive testing to prove that the information leads to decisions which prevent cerebrovascular accidents, but it will be clear from the following case histories that the DOPSCAN information does affect management decisions of the referring physicians.

6. PATIENT HISTORIES

Patient #1. A 71-year-old male, F.J.D., was referred to our Vascular Laboratory because of bilateral carotid bruits. Upon direct questioning, he denied all symptoms of cerebral vascular insufficiency. He previously had an axillofemoral shunt for peripheral vascular disease and was admitted to the hospital because of gangrene of his left foot.

Physical examination disclosed blood pressure in both arms equal at 174/82. A scar was seen over the left supraclavicular region and over the right radical artery. Palpation of the pulses disclosed a weak to almost absent right temporal artery pulse but the carotids were palpated normally without the presence of a thrill. On auscultation bruits were found over both bifurcation regions, grade I and of short systolic duration. There was a separate systolic bruit in the left supraventricular region, grade II with a coarse quality.

Hand-held Doppler signals from the posterior orbit and the periorbital arteries were normal. The left axillary signal displayed low frequency and slow acceleration. Doppler imaging of the carotid bifurcation disclosed normal common and internal carotid signals. There was a high frequency Doppler signal detected on the right external carotid artery, about 2 cm above the bifurcation; no high frequency was detected around the left bifurcation. Both vertebral arteries were imaged posterior to the bifurcations.

These findings were interpreted as representing patent common internal channels without stenosis and a normal Circle of Willis pressure. Stenosis of the right external is present and although the source of the bruit at the left bifurcation was not found, it was presumed to arise from a branch of the left external carotid. Flow to the left arm is somewhat impaired by steal to the left axiallary-femoral graft. No significant subclavian stenosis or vertebral steal is present. The weak radial pulse was interpreted as being caused by a previous catherization.

Comment: This patient represents an example of evaluation prior to peripheral vascular surgery where the surgeon required information concerning whether or not a significant carotid lesion was present. Because the common and internal channels were cleared of suspicion and the external carotids were identified as the source of the bruits, angiography was not performed. Revisions to the axillary femoral graft proceeded without special danger to the cerebral circulation.

In addition to this patient, another excellent example of detection of bilateral external carotid stenosis will be found in Chapter 13, Figure 12.

Patient #2. A 57-year-old female, A.S., was first referred to us in 1975 for evaluation of carotid bruits and postural dizzines. She was being treated with high blood pressure medication. One year previously she had a carotid arteriogram which disclosed a 50% stenosis of the left internal carotid at its origin and at that time had abdominal surgery for arterial occlusions.

Physical examination disclosed a 10 mm difference in arm pressure being 136/76 in the right arm and 126/84 in the left arm. There was a delay in the left radial pulse and auscultation revealed a continuous grade II/IV bruit in the left supraclavicular region and a grade III pan-systolic bruit over the axillary artery and the left upper chest. There was also a grade II continuous bruit over the left bifurcation region.

Hand-held Doppler examination detected absence of backflow in the left brachial artery accompanied by low frequency signals. A hyperemia test for vertebral-subclavian steal on the left was negative. Posterior ophthalmic signals were in a normal direction on both sides but on the left they were weak and of slightly low frequency. There were no abnormalities in the periorbital Doppler signals. Doppler imaging of the bifurcation disclosed a high frequency at the origin of the left internal carotid artery accompanied by analog signals which were inverted and biphasic. The downstream internal signals at the angle of the jaw were normal. On the right there was a non-sounding segment on the origin of the internal carotid artery but normal downstream signals were found.

These results were interpreted to represent a calcified plaque producing 60–70% stenosis of the left internal carotid at its origin, of marginal hemodynamic significance. A left subclavian stenosis was present not producing vertebral steal. At that time no special action was taken. The DOPSCAN findings of internal stenosis were consistant with the moderately severe stenosis previously demonstrated by angiography and which was not responsible for the symptoms.

The patient was next seen one year later without symptoms and Doppler indicated slightly higher frequencies and the development of downstream fluttering qualities which represented some progression of the stenotic plaque but not of hemodynamic significance. Stenosis of the left vertebral was suspected and also moderate stenosis of the right external was thought to be developing. Because there were no symptoms and stenosis was not severe, no action was taken at that time.

The patient was seen for the third time one year later; upon direct questioning she admitted to an episode of dimming of the vision in her left eye which occurred several months before her visit. The episode lasted for 5 minutes then cleared completely and no other symptoms suggestive of cerebrovascular insufficiency could be elicited. The 10 mm difference in pressure between the arms persisted as did the abnormal left subclavian-axillary signals but again no vertebral-to-subclavian steal was found. Periorbital signals remained normal although the left posterior orbital signal persisted with a low frequency and damped waveform.

The third DOPSCAN imaging disclosed a further increase in the audio frequency in the left internal carotid and the diameter of the stenosis was judged to be 70% or 1.5 to 2 mm in diameter. These findings were interpreted to represent progression of the stenosis and because of the one episode of the

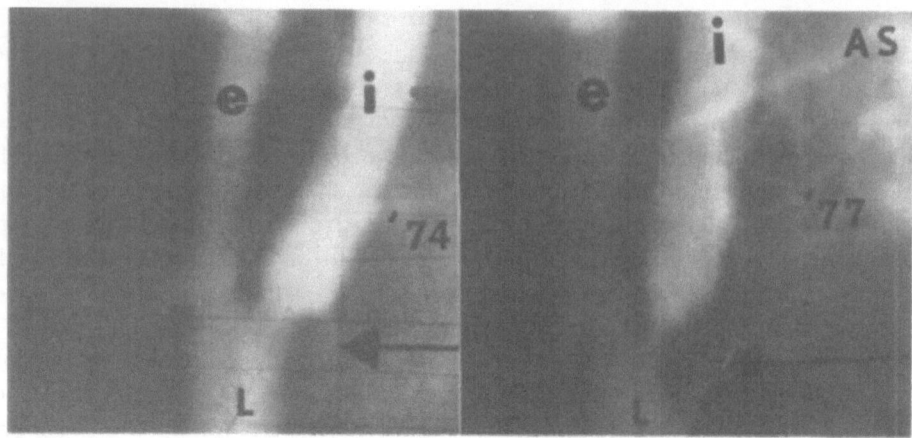

Figure 1. The Doppler spectrum obtained at the site of progressing stenosis quantitated a doubling of the frequency representing a doubling of the severity of the original lesion over a two-year period.

left eye blurring, she was referred for her second angiography. Figure 1 disclosed the progression of the carotid lesion between 1974 prior to our first examination and in 1977 after our third examination. Angiography confirmed the stenosis on the left and an endarterectomy was performed without complications.

Comments: 1) Regular follow-up of 'asymptomatic' bruits may bring out symptoms which represent a TIA. 2) DOPSCAN can be used to follow the progress of stenosis to detect increasing severity. 3) Carotid surgery is given first preference over subclavian surgery and Doppler CVE can diagnose both and clarify the source of carotid or subclavian bruits.

Patient #3. A 71-year-old male, E.R.B., was referred for Doppler CVE because of a bruit in his neck and symptoms suggestive of cerebrovascular insufficiency. He stated that he had 'strokes' in the past which were apparently episodes of blurred vision in both eyes and associated speech disturbances. He said he had numbness and tingling 'all over' and on the day of the examination he had a headache with dizzyness. Angiography had been recommended but was not performed because of sensitivity to contrast material. The patient arrived on a stretcher and demonstrated slow but clear speech, was rather lathargic but demonstrated no gross abnormalities of the face or motion of the extremities.

The findings from physical examination revealed pressure equal in both arms at 126/70 mmHg with normally palpated radial, temporal, and carotid pulses. Auscultation revealed a grade II/IV bruit in the right supraclavicular region radiating widely but no separate bifurcation bruits were identified.

Normal vertebral Doppler signals were detected at the base of the skull as well as anterior along the spine and the posterior orbital signals and the periorbital signals were normal without evidence of collateralization. DOPSCAN imaging of the carotid bifurcations demonstrated patent common external and internal carotid arteries. Abnormalities on the origin of both internals were detected consisting of inverted signals and on the left, downstream, fluttering. The distal internal signals were normal and no high frequencies were detected. Special 'down' imaging detected fluttering signals in the low right common carotid behind the clavical.

The findings were interpreted to represent evidence of intramural calcification in the proximal portion of both internal carotid arteries with irregularity of the left internal carotid lumenal surface producing turbulence. There was no evidence of significant stenosis or restrictions of flow and both vertebrals were patent to the base of the skull. The patient's bruit was thought to be arising from the innominate artery but without sufficient obstruction to produce a difference in the arm pressures.

It was concluded from the interpretation and history that one could not definitely rule out the possibility of microembolization arising from either carotid bifurcations but it was felt that this was unlikely. Angiography was not recommended even though at this point it was discovered that the patient was in fact not sensitive to contrast material.

Comment: This patient's history illustrates: 1) Doppler is an alternative to the dye sensitive patient. 2) The patient with a bruit and questionable symptoms of TIA's can be screened with Doppler to rule out obstructive disease. 3) on the basis of Doppler a decision can be made concerning angiography.

Patient #4. A 64-year-old female, E.B., was referred because of a right carotid bruit and transient blurring occurring in the right eye on several occasions; the most recent episode being three months past. She also described some *right* arm weakness and numbness with tingling which also was occasionally present in the *right* leg. She states she had one fainting spell about two years past but no other symptoms were associated with that problem. She is known to have high blood pressure and claudication. Her medications consist of apresoline, indural, lasix, and ismelin. She had undergone aortic arch arteriograms previous to our examination which were not available at the time of this examination. A later report on these disclosed a bilateral external carotid stenosis with minimal arteriosclerotic irregularity in the right internal carotid and a moderate plaque with possible simple ulceration on the origin of the left internal. Also determined at the time of angiography was a tight stenosis of the left renal artery.

The physical examination revealed wheezing high frequencies at both bifurcations, pan systolic on the right. The right bifurcation presented a slight thrill. There was also a wheezing soft systolic bruit over the right eyelid. There was weakness in the right temporal artery pulse. The blood pressure in both arms was 215/85 mmHg.

The DOPSCAN image is seen in Chapter 13, Figure 12, along with the arch arteriogram and bifurcation projections. Posterior orbital and periorbital signals demonstrated no abnormalities.

Because of the findings of external carotid stenosis the patient was discharged to await renin assays and possible repair of the renal artery. A later follow-up disclosed that renal assays were indeterminate.

Angiographic interpretation of ulceration based on the presence of a small crater at the site of the left internal lesion is a good case in point that such morphology is often not associated with the TIA's in this case being on the symptoms wrong side to assume that there was ulceration in the crater.

Comments: 1) Doppler if performed prior to angiography could have eliminated the necessity for angiography. 2) The patient might well have been treated with antiplatelet agents on the basis of Doppler studies and the presence of an ophthalmic bruit which strongly suggests a siphon stenosis. 3) The skill of the Doppler technician and the routine of listening over closed eyelids can often assist the referring physician in providing a more complete physical examination and could well have been used to direct this patient to anticoagulant therapy years or months previously.

Patient #5. A 59-year-old gentleman, L.E.O., was referred by a general practitioner for an episode occurring eleven days previously in which the patient describes 'my left eye went out for ten minutes'. About four months previous he started seeing spots in this left eye, one or two times per week, each episode lasting only a few seconds. They increased in number recently to the point of several each week. He also describes these episodes as if a curtain came down over his vision. He has had no episodes since the last episode of amaurosis fugax. Upon direct questioning, he denied all other symptoms of cerebrovascular insufficiency. His only medication consisted of daily multivitamins.

Physical examination revealed a blood pressure of 140/80 mmHg in both arms, and no gross abnormalities of speech, face or extremities. There were bruits over both bifurcation regions, both grade II, long systolic, and extending into diastole with a moaning quality on the right.

Doppler examination disclosed abnormalities in the posterior and periorbital signals. Both posterior orbital signals displayed low frequencies; the right one of low amplitude. The left one was bidirectional but the reversed signal was stronger than the normally directed signal. Both supraorbital signals were greatly diminished in amplitude and frequency by ipsilateral temporal artery compression. Both frontal flow signals were low frequency and weak, and the one on the right was reversed. Vertebral Doppler signals were detected with normal quality at the base of the skull on both sides.

Carotid bifurcation imaging disclosed very high frequencies on the origin of both internal carotid arteries. Frequencies were higher on the left than on the right. Downstream signals in the internal displayed roughness and fluttering to the angle of the jaw on both sides. There was a whining quality in the right internal carotid signal similar to that heard with the stethoscope.

These findings were interpreted to represent very tight stenosis of both internal carotid arteries estimated to be 70 to 80% reduction in the lumen on the right and 80 to 90% reduction on the left. Both signals were considered severe enough to elicit collateralization around the eyes. The findings were concluded to explain the symptoms on the basis of probable ulceration at the site, the left stenotic lesion probably shedding emboli to produce the symptoms.

The written Doppler report (marked urgent) and the telephone conversation provided the referring physician with statements that the patient was in danger of a major stroke.

He was seen by a vascular surgeon five days after the initial Doppler and telephone report which recommended 'four vessel arch studies to be accomplished as soon as possible with the feeling that he should have carotid endarterectomy, probably the left side first, followed in about one week or ten days by the opposite side.'

Cerebral arteriogram one week after Doppler demonstrated 'ulcerated stenoses in both internal carotid origins, most severe on the left.' A left carotid endarterectomy was performed on the following day when he was found to have a very tight calcified ulcerating lesion in the left bifurcation extending three to four cm up the internal carotid artery. A right carotid endarterectomy was performed 19 days later. Ulceration was not observed at the site of the right lesion.

Comments: This patient's history demonstrates several points concerning the value of Doppler imaging 1) it encourages both the patient and the non-specialist physician to move rapidly for angiography and endarterectomy. Once the patient reached a surgical specialist, this plan was expedited. It is significant that this particular referring physician did not begin the patient on antiplatelet or anticoagulant therapy in the case of clear amaurosis fugax by the time of the Doppler examination though this is generally the practice of the community for males over age 50. 2) Doppler could determine that the left lesion was hemodynamically most significant when bilateral stenosis was present.

Patient #6. A 62-year-old male, J.W.G., was referred to us because of lightheadedness, balance problems, 'swishing' sounds on the left ear and seeing heat waves in both eyes. Approximately 3 years previous, he had an episode of slurred speech and left arm and left face numbness. He is also known to have a left common carotid bruit and fluctuation blood pressure.

Upon physical examination blood pressure in both arms was found to be 160/90 mmHg and there was a grade II soft moaning bruit at the left bifurcation. Doppler and imaging findings were interpreted as representing stenosis of the left internal carotid, occlusion of the right internal carotid with collateral from the left internal to the right hemisphere. These findings were based primarily on the high frequencies detected on the origin of the left internal carotid at the time of imaging and a non-sounding internal carotid in the right. Evidence of collateral was demonstrated when compression of either the right or left common carotid artery decreased the right posterior orbital signal which at all times was weak, low frequency with slow acceleration. The left posterior orbital and periorbital signals were normal. Ten days later an angiogram confirmed the Doppler finding and a left carotid endarterectomy was performed. As a result of endarterectomy internal carotid blood flow, measured with the electromagnetic flowmeter, decreased from 195 to 175 mm/min while the external carotid flow decreased from 135 to 115 mm/min. Five months after endarterectomy, a repeat Doppler was performed which demonstrated persistent stenosis of the left internal judged to be tighter than before the endarterectomy but still carrying a large flow. This judgement was made easily by comparing the audio tapes from the first and second examination. Five days after the repeat Doppler a second angiogram confirmed severe stenosis of the left internal and a left carotid patch angioplasty was performed. Blood flow was not measured at the second operation.

Nine months following the second carotid surgery, the third Doppler disclosed slightly high frequencies but only residual fluttering in the left internal carotid. The Doppler at this time was interpreted as demonstrating no significant stenosis. The slight high frequencies were consistant with compensatory flow to compensate for the right occlusion. The right circle pressure was considered to remain low but with increased collateral from the left external carotid.

A fourth Doppler performed 11 months following the second surgery demonstrated normal left internal signals with slight residual turbulence. The right ophthalmic was in the normal direction but with persistent low frequency and slow acceleration.

Comments: 1) Doppler is useful in post-surgical follow-up to determine the hemodynamic outcome of surgery. Repeat angiography is not necessary to confirm the follow-up Doppler findings. 2) In the patient with non-focal symptoms and a carotid bruit, Doppler can identify lesions which represent a perfusion defect. 3) Doppler examination is useful in assessing the collateral circulation.

Patient #7. A 78-year-old male, E.N.L., was hospitalized because of left-sided paralysis and to begin physical therapy in the stroke ward. He was referred for DOPSCAN imaging for reasons that are not clear, but possibly because the test procedure had just been introduced into the hospital.

Physical examination revealed no bruits and Doppler diagnosis disclosed a right internal occlusion and severe left internal carotid stenosis judged to be approximately 1 mm in diameter. Angiograms verified the Doppler findings. After a few days consideration for healing of the brain infarct a left carotid endarterectomy was performed.

Comments: This patient provides an excellent example of how imaging with Doppler can identify an additional threatening carotid lesion in a patient with an already completed stroke to allow an approximately timed angiography and surgery. An additional superimposed stroke may be prevented and brain perfusion increased.

Patient #8. A 52-year-old female, N.M.C., was referred to us by a cardiologist because of dizziness, falling, and bilateral visual problems which consisted of difficulty focusing. She said she had a stroke 2 months prior affecting her vision causing her to lose sight in both eyes and with an equilibrium problem associated. She said she has had right hand numbness occasionally which she thought might be caused by an old neck injury. She said that she has had an off-balance feeling 2 to 3 times per week since her stroke. She has had surgery on her hip and walks with a slight limp. She had angiography 6 months prior but the films were unsatisfactory for a definitive reading.

Her cardiologist stated that he referred the patient to us to clarify whether she was having vertebral-basilar or carotid problems. He had already noted a blood pressure difference in the two arms being 20 mm lower on the right than on the left and that she had bilateral cervical bruits and a slow rising pulse in the right carotid.

The physical examination revealed no gross abnormalities of speech, face, or extremities except that she walked with a slight limp. Palpation of the pulses revealed weak right carotid and radial pulses. The right temporal pulse was not palpable. On the left the pulses were normal. The blood pressure in her right arm was unobtainable with stethoscope but a Doppler systolic pressure was indicated at 100 mmHg. On the left the Doppler systolic was 130 mmHg and the auscultatory sounds indicated 122/70 mmHg. A grade II high frequency, blowing, pansystolic bruit at the left bifurcation was found which appeared to radiate posterior up as far as the base of the skull. On the right, the normal heart sounds were faintly heard over the carotid. There were no bruits over the eyes or upper chest.

Vertebral Doppler signals were detected on both sides at the base of the skull but on the right they were abnormal systolic only without diastolic runoff. The right anterior vertebral signal was reversed. On the left the posterior vertebral displayed a high frequency coarse and gruff quality. The left anterior signal was in the normal headward direction. The right subclavian artery demonstrated Doppler abnormalities consisting of a systolic, low frequency velocity pulse without normal backflow. These qualities carried also into the right brachial flow signals demonstrated normal backflow in both subclavian and brachial. A reactive hyperemia test for vertebral steal proved positive on the right.

The ophthalmic flow signals in the right posterior orbit were abnormal demonstrating low frequency and slow acceleration signals but with good amplitude and directed in the normal anterior direction. Upon *left* common carotid compression, the *right* posterior orbital signal decrease in strength and amplitude. The left periorbital signals demonstrated no abnormalities but on the right the frontal artery signals were low frequency, biphasic, and compression of the left facial artery changed the direction of the right frontal signal and augmented its amplitude. On the left, there were no abnormalities in either the posterior, orbital or the periorbital signals.

Imaging on the right visualized one blood vessel being one long channel from the clavical to the angle of the jaw. The signal qualities in this vessel were low frequency, with a low diastolic flow throughout with slow acceleration with a damped quality. There was also a diminished pulsitility in these signals Doppler imaging on the left demonstrated generally high frequencies throughout the common-internal flow channels but still normal range.

These findings were interpreted to represent occlusion of the right innominate artery with a low circle pressure on the right and collateralization from the left external carotid across the face and also intracranial from the left internal. A vertebral steal was present on the right with compensatory flow up the left vertebral artery where some slight kinking near the base of the skull produced the bruit.

On the basis of these findings, a cerebral arteriogram and arch aortogram were performed. The impression of the radiologist upon reading the films was 1) moderately severe and irregular stenosis at the origin of innominate artery with anti-grade filling of right carotid and vertebrals from this vessel and 2) bilateral ulcerations in the common carotid artery bifurcations.

Later review of the aortic arch films by the vascular laboratory personnel and the angiographer confirmed late fill and reverse flow in the right vertebral artery from above, downward. The angiographers accepted these revisions of their interpretation. The angiographic films also demonstrated an unusually large left vertebral.

The patient successfully underwent an innominate endarterectomy. The patient was reportedly doing well two months later at the time of an office visit.

Comments: This unusual but not rare situation in our experience demonstrates several items of interest. 1) Innominate obstruction is diagnosable by Doppler and can be successfully relieved by surgery. 2) Doppler can clarify the location and significance of carotid bruits in patients with vertebral-basilar symptoms' and clear the carotids of suspicion of significant stenosis. 3) Doppler can diagnose vertebral steal which is occasionally misinterpreted by the angiographer as an occlusion. 4) Craters seen on the angiogram should not be interpreted as representing ulceration and do not necessarily mean that the symptoms are arising from embolization.

Patient #9. A 57-year-old man, E.M.C., was examined with Doppler CVE in June of 1977. At that time he was complaining of headaches over the right eye which were followed by double vision lasting 24 hours. He had weakness on the right side of his body from poliomyelitis in his youth. He denies other symptoms of cerebrovascular insufficiency upon direct questioning. He had a history of hypertension and may have had heart disease. Physical examination revealed the blood pressure equal in both arms at 135/80 mmHg. The pulses palpated normally. On ausculatation, a grade II short, soft systolic bruit was heard over the right mid-neck at the bifurcation region but no bruits were heard on the left. Vertebral Doppler signals were detected anterior along the spine flowing in the headward direction. The left posterior orbital ophthalmic signal was normal but the right one was weak and its direction was indeterminate. The periorbital examination demonstrated evidence of collateralization about the right eye with flow from the mandibular to the frontal artery and from the temporal to the supraorbital artery. On the left the periorbital signals were normal.

Doppler imaging of the carotid bifurcation on the left was completed satisfactorily with a slight signal weakness in the proximal 3 cm of the internal carotid artery. On the right, imaging failed to disclose an internal carotid artery and a high frequency zone was detected in the single branch visualized.

These findings were read by the interpreting physician as possible total occlusion of the right internal carotid with stenosis of the proximal right external. There was non-obstructing plaquing in the left internal carotid. The technician, however, reported that she had detected some very low frequency but continuous type signals which could be consistent with the low velocity in the internal carotid artery but which signals were not of sufficient strength to produce an image with Doppler examination.

Thirteen days later, the patient was angiogrammed demonstrating: 1) 98% narrowing at the origin of the right internal carotid with probably recannalization and/or clot within a markedly hypotensive vessel. Though contrast material was seen at the site and level of the carotid siphon, frank patency of the internal was not conclusively demonstrated. 2) 95% stenosis at the origin of the right external carotid artery.' Computerized tomography scan of the brain, electroencephalagram and lumbar puncture were reported as negative.

He was admitted to the hospital with the intention to explore the right bifurcation and open the *external* carotid if in fact the internal was completely occluded. At the time of surgical exposure, a sterile Doppler probe was used to evaluate the flow in the right carotid bifurcation. In the O.R. the technician assisted with the Doppler examination and when the probe was applied over the internal the Doppler technician called attention to signals similar to the ones she had heard in the scan room and convinced the surgeon that there was patency. The right internal carotid was opened and a large red clot flowed back into the incision retrograde from the internal. (Pathological examination of this specimen later demonstrated 'fibrin and fresh as well as old blood clot.') Backflow bleeding was continued until the traction tape was reapplied and the arteriotomy closed. Re-establishment of good velocity in the internal carotid artery was confirmed with the sterile Doppler probe.

The patient recovered from the surgical procedure satisfactorily and was again seen in the vascular laboratory 1 year later without symptoms of cerebrovascular insufficiency. He stated that his headaches disappeared. Hand-held and Doppler examination of the posterior orbital signals was normal with good anteriorly directed flow and no evidence of collateralization. These findings were interpreted to represent excellent surgical results with patent carotids and no significant narrowing.

Comments: This patient represents: 1) Non-invasive Doppler with imaging in the hands of a highly skilled technician can detect 'pre occlusive' grade V stenosis of the internal carotid when even angiographic evidence of patency is questionable. 2) Sterile Doppler probes are useful in the operating room to examine the carotid bifurcation both pre- and post-arteriotomy. 3) Large, red fibrin, clots are prone to develop in the internal carotid downstream to extremely tight stenosis before occlusion which may produce a major stroke if large segments are dislodged by the remaining small flow and embolized to the intracranial arterial circulation. 4) Doppler is useful for post-surgical follow-up of endarterectomy.

15. FULL CAPABILITY DOPPLER DIAGNOSIS

MERRILL P. SPENCER, M.D.

In spite of the great amount of physiological and diagnostic information available in Doppler non-invasive evaluation of the circulation, the use of Doppler has spread slowly within the medical field. Only a few physicians willing to learn the necessary skills and understand its basic physiological principles have benefited from its availability. Undoubtedly the limitations for many is related to the difficulties in understanding the audio presentation of the findings when most physicians are visually oriented. As a parallel example, audio information such as auscultation of the heart has traditionally been regarded as 'soft' information and has been difficult to teach.

Recent availability of bidirectional color spectral display, the video format and binaural dual-direction audio signals provides the availability of a composite audio-visual display of all c-w Doppler characteristics simultaneously in dynamically reproducible format. Simultaneous seeing and hearing of all the characteristics of Doppler in video format is now possible and high quality records can be made. The purpose of this chapter is to disclose a composite audio-visual display which presents all of the information available in c-w Doppler in a video format available for replay and objective interpretation.

1. FUNDAMENTAL DOPPLER CHARACTERISTICS

The range of useful c-w Doppler audio characteristics of blood flow may be categorized according to location, amplitude, frequency, directionality, and pulsations. The *location* from which the Doppler signal is obtained is highly specific to a given vessel segment and with pulsed Doppler may be refined to velocity profiles. The success of the Doppler imaging technique demonstrates the usefulness of precision in this characteristic.

The *amplitude* of the Doppler signal is the least reliable characteristic because in the transcutaneous mode it depends on many factors which do not relate to blood velocity or blood flow such as the distance of the blood vessel from the transducer and intervening ultrasonic obstructions such as air bubbles in the coupling jelly as well as the ultrasonic opacity of intervening tissues. Amplitude is useful, however, when used in conjunction with other abnormalities and when comparing symmetrical arteries of the body.

The *audio frequencies* or more precisely, the frequency spectrum of the Doppler signal is the single most useful characteristic, particularly when following the signal along the axis of vessels running parallel to the body surface or comparing symmetrical arteries on opposite sides of the body and in following changes in frequency within the same artery and from one examination to the next. The spectral distribution carries information concerning mean and maximum velocity, turbulence, and plaquing.

The *direction* of blood flow is usually identified by direction-sensitive circuitry. Direction can change within the heart cycle and can be in both directions simultaneously in both normal and turbulent conditions. Pitfalls are occasionally caused by curvature of the artery direction or nearby bony structures. Bony structures or the presence of calcified plaquing within the artery wall may sufficiently scatter the sound beam, that is reflected, to produce inverted signals making the blood flow direction falsely appear reversed.

Pulsations of the frequency spectrum within the cardiac cycle carry a great deal of physiological information for the interpreter who recognizes the underlying hemodynamic causes. The pulsatility index reflects the relative amount of diastolic runoff present and is related to the resistance of the outflow vasculature and arterial wall elasticity. Changes in the systolic acceleration of the blood flow provides a relatively unexploited characteristic. Slow otid and temporal artery compressions have become a significant part of the complete periorbital and posterior orbital Doppler examination. The effect of carotid compression on vertebral signals at the base of the skull has only recently been devised in our laboratory to evaluate the collateral between the carotid and vertebral circulations. See chapter 6, Figure 1b.

2. AUDIO VISUAL PRESENTATIONS

Many audio visual presentations of Doppler signal characteristics are available to assist the interpreter. These include listening, spectral display, analog tracings, and imaging. Utilizing the human hearing mechanism by listening directly to the signal qualities, even without recording, is the single most useful method of analyzing and interpreting Doppler signals because all signal characteristics are represented including direction, if stereo speakers are used. The exact location of the signal, of course, is visible to the examiner. For clinical purposes the human hearing-analysis mechanism exceeds electronic means of recognition of most characteristics. Instrumentation assists listening by selecting and quantitating special characteristics such as mean velocity and velocity profiles as well as dual-directionality of the signal. The advantages and disadvantages of listening as well as the other methods of presentation are outlined as follows:

1. Listening — All characteristics present
    Advantages
        — Exceeds most electronic means for clinically significant features
        — Faster interpretation
    Disadvantages
        — Subjective and requires great skill
2. Spectral Display — All characteristics present
    Advantages
        — Objective, training aid, quantitative
        — Makes the best of weak signals
    Disadvantages
        — Costly and important qualities may not be recognized
3. Analogue Signal Tracings
    Advantages
        — Selected features objectively quantitated
    Disadvantages
        .— Sensitivity limited to strong signals
        — Discards useful information
4. Doppler Imaging
    Advantages
        — Location of signal objectively quantitated allowing careful search of important vessel segments
        — Temporal and spatial differences in all other characteristics quantitatable
    Disadvantages
        — Requires more training and more examination time

3. COMPOSITE DOPPLER DISPLAY

The composite full capability audio-visual display system utilizes a bidirectional spectrum, bidirectional audio signals and Doppler imaging or other representations of the signal source (Figure 1). The bidirectional color spectral display was developed by Dr. Ron Hileman and Joe Cairo of Carolina Medical Electronics and utilizes a micro processor single-board computer and FFT with a 5 milliseconds updating time. It operates on the phase difference between signals generated from motion toward the ultrasond source and motion away from the source. Blood velocities away from the probe are represented by frequencies above the zero base line while blood velocities towards the probe are represented by frequencies below the base-line. Two selectable frequency scales are available including 0 to 5 KHz positive and 0 to 4 KHz negative or 0 to 10 KHz positive and 0 to 8 Hz negative. Three time bases are available including full sweeps of 1, 2 or 10 seconds. The amplitude of the audio frequencies are represented by color coding. The amplitudes are represented on a thermal scale with red representing the lowest amplitude and white the

214

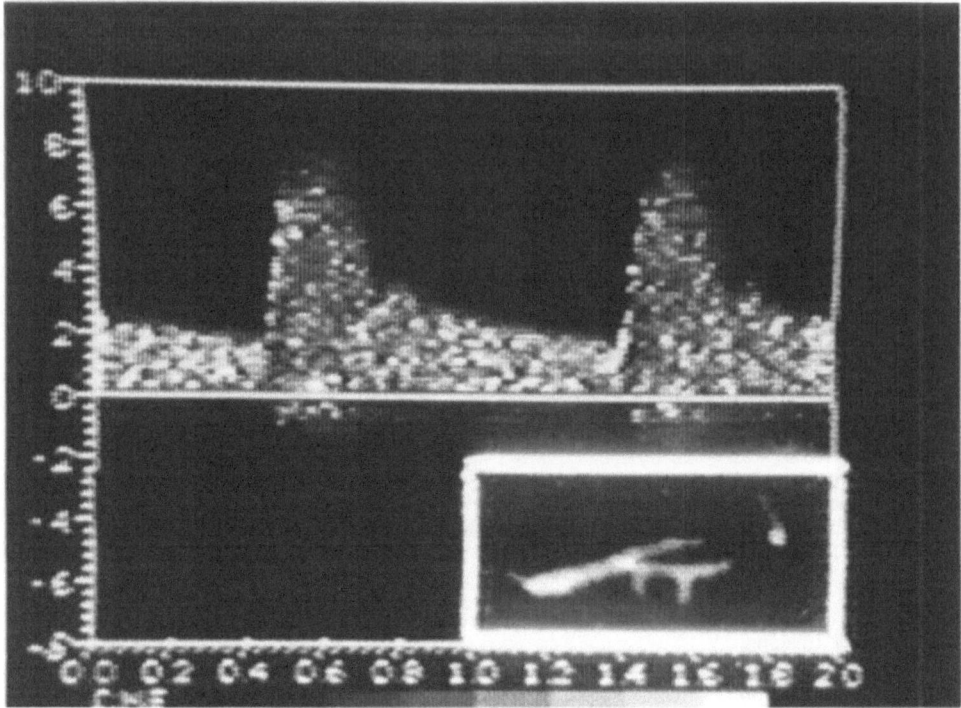

Figure 1. Composite format to display the bidirectional audiospectrum and the Doppler image of the carotid bifurcation. Signal source from the common carotid is indicated by a cursor on image. Frequencies greater than 10 KHz represent severe stenosis. 'Negative' frequencies represent turbulence.

greatest amplitude. Oranges and yellows represent the middle ranges. This color spectral display is presented in a video signal directly displayable on a video monitor and recordable on a VTR. Figure 2 represents the directional and amplitude capability of this spectral display of signals recorded from the femoral artery of a normal human subject.

Dual direction audio signals from bidirectional Doppler are produced by use of the circuitry of Nippa which cleanly separates forward flow (away from the transducer) from reverse flow (towards the transducer). The separate directional audio signals are recorded on stereo channels of a video tape recorder and also presented on stereo speakers mounted on either side of the spectral display. Stereo listening combined with spectral viewing provides a powerful combination, especially for recognition of: backflow phases, Figure 2; reversed flow, Figure 3; venous contamination, Figure 4; turbulence, Figure 5; and non-stenotic plaque scattering of the beam, Figure 6. Voice annotations by the examiners are mixed with the forward flow signal. To preserve clean separation of the directional audio signals the technician performs the

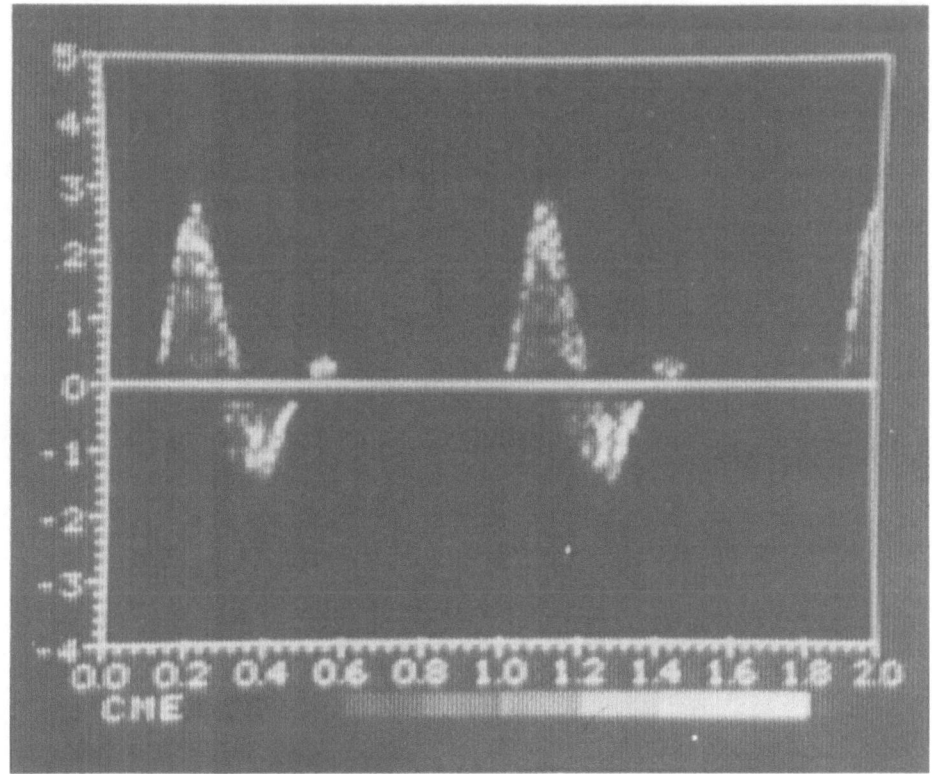

Figure 2. Bidirectional Doppler spectrum of normal femoral artery using 5 MHz probe. Backflow during early diastole is clearly shown.

examination with either a throat microphone or head sets to listen to the Doppler signals on the voice channel.

By means of an insert window on the spectral display the Doppler image of the carotid bifurcation is displayed, Figure 1. This may be accomplished by a TV camera focused on the imaging oscilloscope and, through a split screen device, sharing of the video channel. The exact position of the Doppler probe and the source of the audio signals is continuously provided for the interpreter. This probe position is indicated by a bright spot normally produced by the Doppler signal in image development. The bright spot serves as an automatic cursor for the source of the video displayed Doppler signals and the stereo speaker sounds.

From the video format, the maximum frequency is measured at any point in the heart cycle and can be used to determine the degree of stenosis by the methods previously disclosed. In addition, the acceleration of the velocity pulsed can be measured from the leading edge of the spectral display. This

216

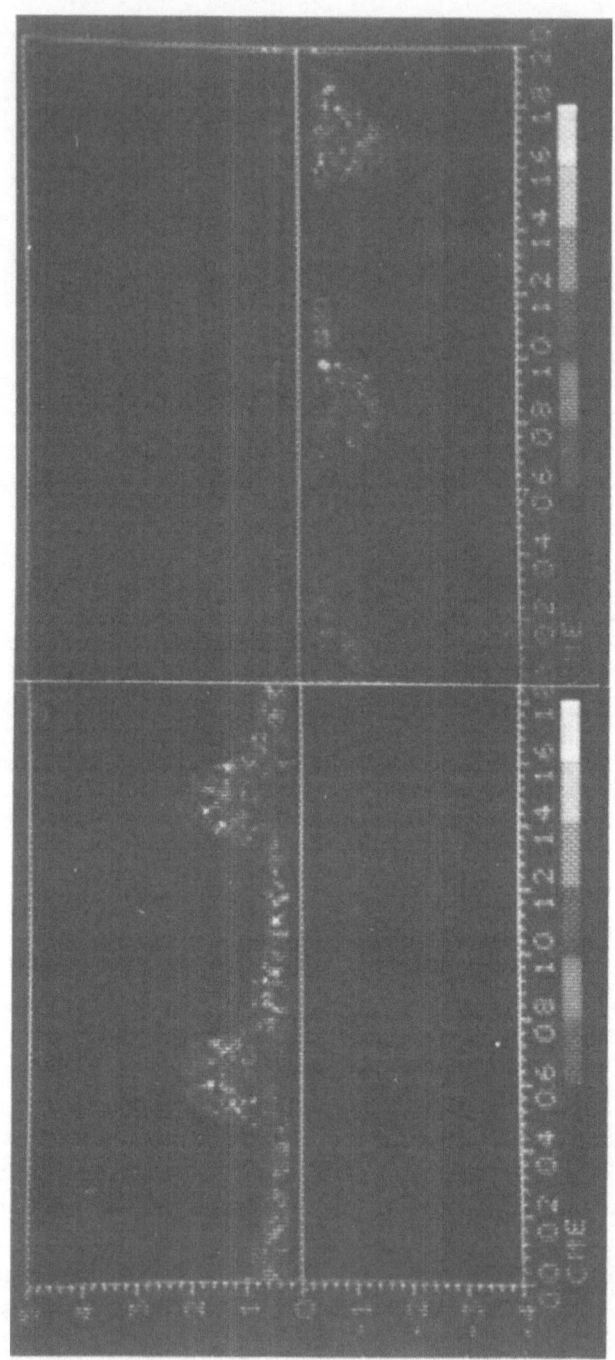

Figure 3. Spectra of opthalmic artery signals from the posterior orbits of a patient with hemodynamically significant stenosis of the right internal carotid. Left hand panel represents reversed flow (away from transducer). Right hand panel signals from the unobstructed side demonstrating the normal flow direction (towards the transducer).

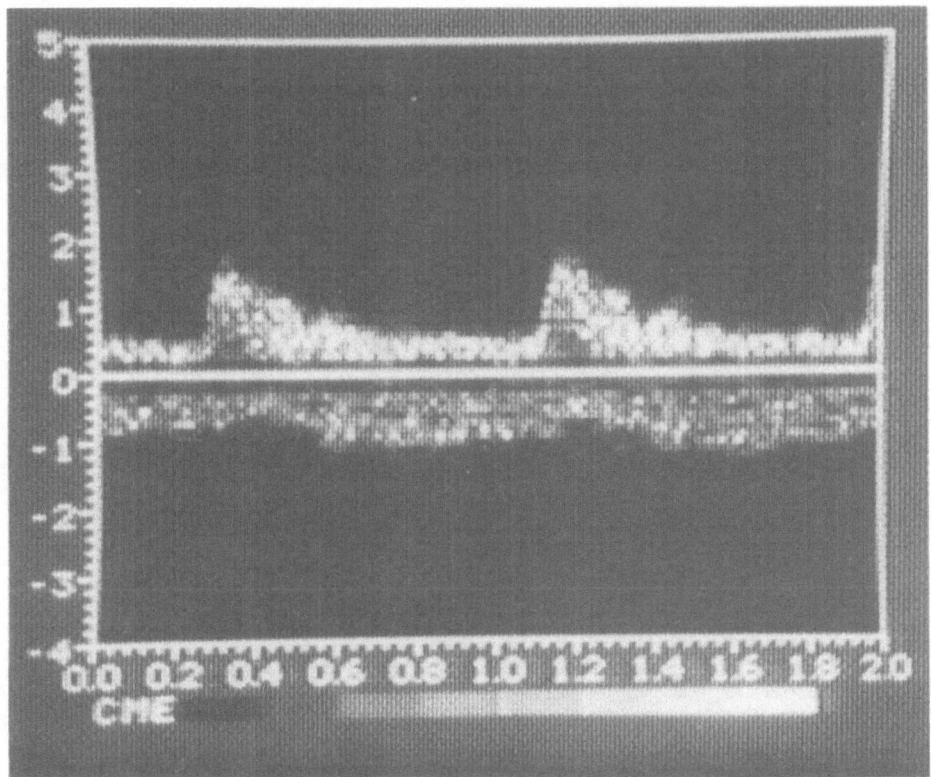

Figure 4. Bidirectional spectrum of normal common carotid signal with negative frequencies representing venous flow in the opposite direction caused by superposition of vein and artery. Typical differences in pulsations of vein and artery is apparent.

acceleration index can be measured in units of KHz/sec convertible to cm/ sec. This measurement is accomplished from a straight line drawn tangent to the maximum slope of the velocity pulse. The acceleration is most accurately accomplished when the spectral sweep is in the fast mode. Differences in acceleration between symmetrical signals from each side of the body is an index of the degree of the damping of the signal.

4. EVALUATION

Evaluation of the new composite full capability display was performed on routine patients passing through two of this Institute's Vascular Laboratories in Seattle, Washington and on normal volunteers. Also, audio tape recordings of patient examinations at a second vascular laboratory were 'played' through

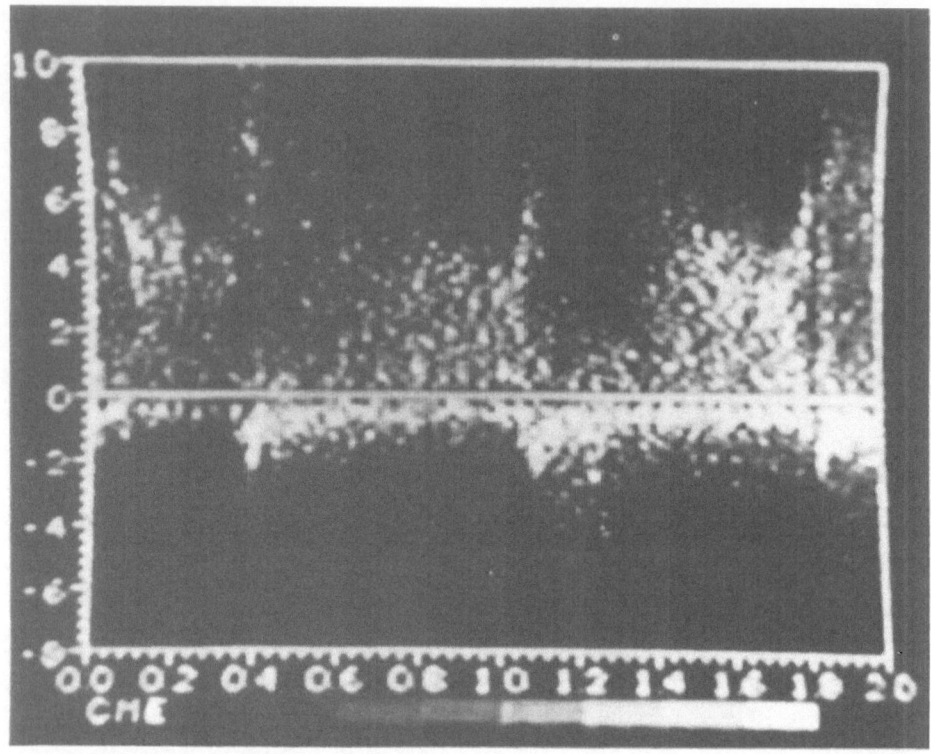

Fig. 5. Spectrum of high frequency stenosis signals from internal carotid demonstrating strong, low, negative frequencies caused by wall vibration and turbulence.

the spectral analyzer for further experience. The evaluation led to several conclusions, establishing the desirability of routine clinical use of the full capability display.

The value of simultaneous display of all c-w Doppler characteristics: 1) increases precision of signal localization by indicating more accurately where the Doppler signals arise, (previous imaging techniques grossly correlated the source of the signal by voice annotations from the technician). This increased resolution: A) increases separation of internal from external signals at the origin from the common carotid and increases accuracy in designating whether high frequencies of stenosis arise from the external, internal, or common carotid; B) indicates to the interpreter the thoroughness with which the technician has searched the bifurcation area for diagnostic signals; C) improves the morphological and physiological representations such as the length of the stenotic segment and details of flow signals upstream and downstream to the stenotic lesion. Of special interest is the future possibility of visualizing

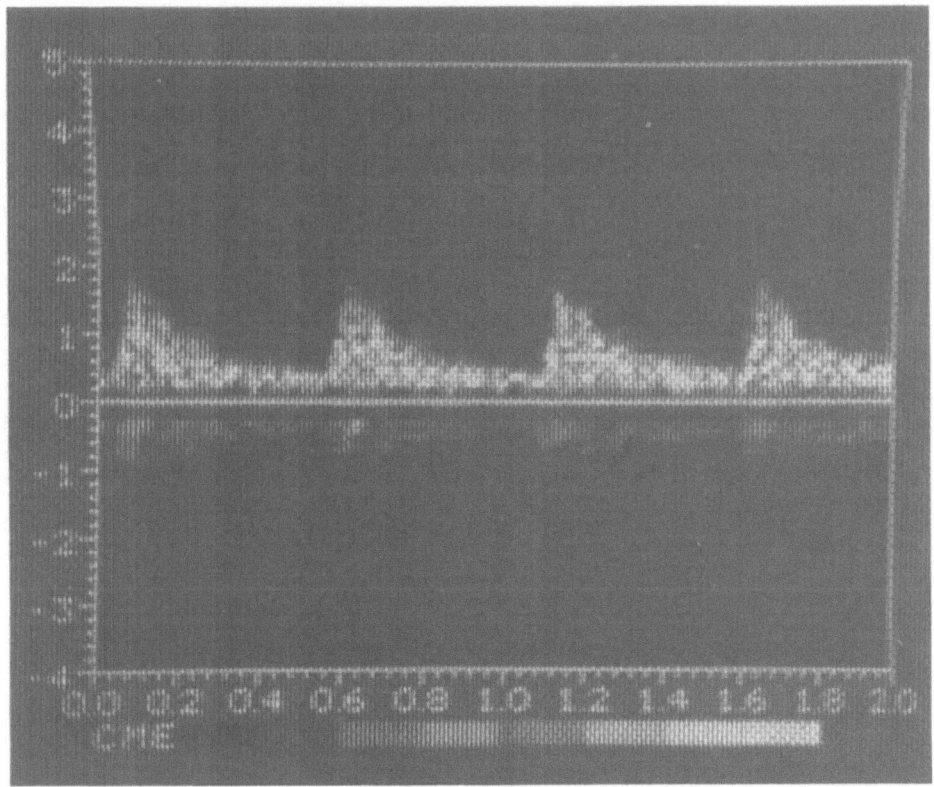

Figure 6. External carotid signals with negative frequencies caused by plaque scattering of the sound beam.

'craters' in the arterial wall by identifying stable vortices; D) improves the differentiation of total occlusion of the internal from grade IV and grade V stenosis. 2) Improves the quantitation of stenosis by: A) indicating to the technician where the highest frequency is located and specifies its exact value. The maximum frequency, not always audible, is further apparent on the real-time spectrum display visually indicating to the examiner when and where the maximum frequency occurs. B) The maximum frequency can be immediately quantitated for accurate on-line diagnosis of the degree of stenosis using the established correlations of the single frequency within the stenosis diameter. C) The f/f frequency ratio method of measuring the percentage of stenosis is improved in accuracy. 3) Encourages new clinics to utilize the capabilities of Doppler by: A) simplifying the examination and interpretation techniques and; B) by providing training concerning the understanding of the audio signals.

Future additions to full capability presentations of Doppler may include automatic triggering of the spectral sweep from the R-wave of the electrocardiogram. This addition will allow comparisons of phase lags between signals. Also useful will be the inclusion of the ear pulsed on the spectral screen when carotid compression is performed in order to confirm the adequacy of the compression. A probable future addition to the video presentation will be monitoring of the patient and hand-held probe position, in the location window.

In the future, the combined advantages of c-w and pulsed Doppler as well as real-time imaging may be accomplished by the Infinite-Gate Pulse-Doppler. The IGPD provides velocity profiles of all vessels in its path at a rate of thousands of profiles per second. By providing both long and short time interval gates, the received signal can allow both the ease of vessel finding inherent in c-w and high resolution of pulsed Doppler, Figure 7. By means of beam deflection techniques, sector scans can also be provided to accomplish

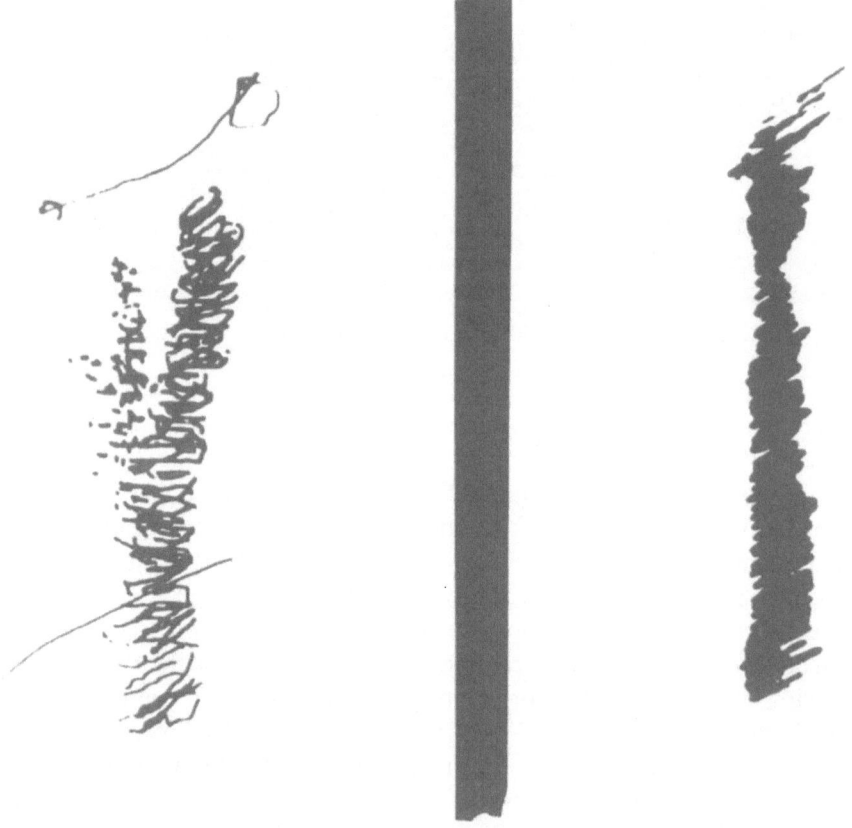

Figure 7. Right hand panel: Infinite-Gate Pulse-Doppler display of common internal channel. Left hand panel: c-w image of same carotid bifurcation which guided IGPD display. IGPD display automatically indicates angle of sound beam with the vessel axis.

real-time imaging. These multiple uses of the pulsed require time sharing or other technology not yet applied to ultrasound.

Non-invasive detection of intimal ulceration and platelet and thrombus adherences to the artery wall is a great present need in prevention of stroke. X-ray angiography, though it sometimes identifies deep craters, cannot specify denuded endothelium. The angiographic interpretation of 'ulceration' is often dependent on clinical signs of TIA's. Also craters are often seen on the asymptomatic side when bilateral carotid angiography is performed. The greatest need exists for non-invasive identification of adherent thrombus, intimal flaps and other 'flagging' tissue threads within the artery lumen. The ultrasonic resolution necessary for these diagnoses may be near but not now present in commercial units generally available. A likely approach to non-invasive thrombus detection might use radioisotope tagging techniques. These have found some usefulness in venous thrombosis but they have not been developed for arteries.

DOPPLER CEREBROVASCULAR REFERENCES

OPHTHALMIC OR PERIORBITAL DOPPLER

Adjodani B, Martin M, Fiebach O, Muller-Wiefel H, Knieriem HJ: Doppler ultrasonic measurement for diagnosing carotid occlusions and stenoses (authors' transl.). Aktuel Gerontol 9(5):211-216, May 1979.

Ardouin M, Urvoy M, Herve C: Doppler effect and the ophthalmic artery. Bull Soc Ophthalmol Fr 76(12):1099-1102, Dec 1976.

Ardouin M, Urvoy M, Sabouraud O, Hany Y, Herve C: Doppler effect: what information can it give the ophthalmologist? Bull Soc Ophthalmol Fr 75(1):91-100, Jan 1975.

Baker WH, Barnes RW: The cerebrovascular Doppler examination in patients with non-hemispheric symptoms. Ann Surg 186(2):190-192, Aug 1977.

Barnes RW, Reinertson JE, Slaymaker EE, Heintz SE: Predictive value of noninvasive screening tests in identifying symptomatic candidates for carotid endarterectomy. In: Noninvasive cardiovascular diagnosis, Diethrich EB (ed). Baltimore: Univ Park Press, 1978, 19-28.

Barnes RW, Garrett WV, Slaymaker EE, Reinertson JE: Doppler ultrasound and supraorbital photo-plethysmography for noninvasive screening of carotid occlusive disease. Am J Surg 134(2):179-182, Aug 1977.

Barnes RW, Russell HE, Bone GE, Slaymaker EE: Doppler cerebrovascular examination: improved results with refinements in technique. Stroke 8(4):468-471, Jul-Aug 1977.

Baskett JJ, Beasley MG, Murphy GJ, Hyams DE, Gosling RG: Screening for carotid junction disease by spectral analysis of Doppler signals. Cardiovasc Res 11(2):147-155, Mar 1977.

Bettelheim H, Grabner G: Experiences with Doppler ultrasonography of the orbital vessels for ophthalmological vascular diagnosis (authors' transl). Klin Monatsbl Augenheilkd 173(6):829-835, Dec 1978.

Bettelheim H, Till P: Diagnosis of orbital circulatory disturbances with the aid of ophthalmodynamography and the echo-orbitography (author's transl). Klin Monatsbl Augenheilkd 164(2):159-172, Feb 1974.

Bone GE, Slaymaker EE, Barnes RW: Noninvasive assessment of collateral blood flow of the cerebral hemisphere by Doppler ultrasound. Surg Gynecol Obstet 145(6):873-876, Dec 1977.

Bone GE, Barnes RW: Clinical implications of the Doppler cerebrovascular examination: a correlation with angiography. Stroke 7(3):271-274, May-Jun 1976.

Bone GE, Barnes RW: Limitations of the Doppler cerebrovascular examination in hemispheric cerebral ischemia. Surgery 79(5):577-580, May 1976.

Bono G, Nappi G, Poloni M: Importance and limitations of directional Doppler ultrasonography (DDS) in neuroangiological diagnosis. Boll Soc Ital Biol Sper 51(15-16):929-933, Aug 1975.

Brisman R, Grossman BL, Correll JW: Accuracy of transcutaneous Doppler ultrasonic in evaluating extracranial vascular disease. J of Neurosurg 32(5):529-533, 1970.

Brockenbrough EC: Screening for the prevention of stroke: Use of a Doppler flowmeter. Information and Education resource support unit, Wash/Alaska Regional Medical Program, 1976.

Budingen HJ, Hennerici M, Voight K, Kendel K, Freund HJ: Diagnosis of internal carotid artery obstructions (author's transl). Dtsch Med Wochenschr 101(8):269-275, Feb 1976.

Buonomini G, Giraldi C, Levorato D: Transcutaneous Doppler ultrasonic in the detection of cerebral blood flow changes. A comparison with angiographic data. J Nucl Med Allied Sci 21(3):103-106, Jul-Sep 1977.

Burger R, Barnes RW: Choice of ophthalmic artery branch for Doppler cerebrovascular examination: advantages of the frontal artery. Angiology 28(6):421-426, Jun 1977.

Carroll RM, Rose HB: Noninvasive vascular testing in clinical practice. Vasc Surg 11(4):201-204, Jul-Aug 1977.

Cohen MM, Skubick DL: Hemicrania in the elderly: suggested use of the directional Doppler flow probe. Ann Neurol 6(2):138-139, Aug 1979.

Duke LJ, Slaymaker EE, Lamberth WC, Wright CB: Results of ophthalmosonometry and supraorbital photoplethysmography in evaluating carotid arterial stenosis. Circulation 60(2 Pt 2):127-131, Aug 1979.

Dyken ML, Doepker JF Jr, Kiovsky R, Campbell RL: Asymptomatic occlusion of an internal carotid artery in a hospital population: determined by directional Doppler. Stroke 5(6):714:718, Nov-Dec 1974.

Englander RN: Doppler ophthalmosonometry letter. Stroke 10(3):348, May-June 1979.

Fischer M, Alexander K: Evaluation of neck bruits by directional Doppler sonography (author's transl). Med Klin 74(28-29):1089-1092, Jul 1979.

Gertner HR Jr: Noninvasive diagnostic techniques in peripheral vascular disease. J Fla Med Assoc 66(10):1070-1074, Oct 1979.

Ginsberg MD, Greenwood SA, Goldberg HI: Noninvasive diagnosis of extracranial cerebrovascular disease: oculoplethysmography-phonoagniography and directional Doppler ultrasonography. Neurology (Minneap) 29(5):623-631, May 1979.

Goldberg RE: Doppler physics and preliminary report of a test for carotid insufficiency. Ultrasonics in ophthalmology, diagnostic and therapeutic applications by Goldberg and Sarin. Appendix I, 1976.

Gross WS, Verta MJ Jr, van Ballen B, Bergan JJ, Yao JS: Comparison of noninvasive diagnostic techniques in carotid artery occlusive disease. Surgery 82(2):271-278, Aug 1977.

Grossman BL, Wood EH: Evaluation of cerebrovascular disease utilizing a transcutaneous Doppler technique. Rad 90:586-587, 1968.

Guell A, Braak L, Barrerre M, Jauzac Ph, Bes A: Correlation between cerebral blood flow modifications and variations in blood velocity as measured by Doppler sonography. In: Cerebral vascular disease 2, Meyer JS (ed). Excerpta Medica, 1979, 93-98.

Gusev EI, Pokrovskii AV, Fedin AI, Kovaneva RA, Kuperberg EB: Ultrasonic flow metering in the diagnosis of occlusive lesions of the extracranial portions of the carotid arteries. Zh Nevropatol Psikkiatr 77(11):1639-1646, 1977.

Hodek-Demarin V, Muller HR: Reversed ophthalmic artery flow in internal carotid artery occlusion. A re-appraisal based on ultrasonic Doppler investigations. Stroke 10(4):461-463, Jul-Aug 1979.

Holleman JH Jr, Raju S: Noninvasive diagnosis of carotid artery disease. J Miss State Med Assoc 20(11):249-252, Nov 1979.

Hyman BN (1974): Doppler sonography: a bedside noninvasive method for assessment of carotid artery disease. Am J Ophthalmol 77(2):227-231, Feb 1974.

Jarrett F: Noninvasive evaluation of the carotid circulation. Can J Surg 21(4):283-284, 1978.

Joyner CR: Transcutaneous Doppler detector in the study of arterial and venous flow patterns. Cardiovasc Clin 6(3):385-399, 1975.

Kaemmerer E: Comparative ophthalmo-dynamographic and Doppler-sonographic examinations (author's transl). Klin Monatsbl Augenheilkd 172(2):150-153, Feb 1978.

Kaneda H, Irino T, Arita N, Minami T, Taneda M, Shiraishi J: Relationship between ophthalmic artery bloodflow and recanalization of occluded carotid artery. Ultrasonic Doppler. Stroke 9(4):360-363, Jul-Aug 1978.

Kaneda H, Minami T, Taneda M, Irino T: The collateral flow via ophthalmic artery in internal carotid arterial occlusions-semiquantitative evaluation. No To Shinkei 29(9):941-947, Sep 1977.

Katz DM, Smith RA, Otis SM, Dalessio DJ: Doppler sonography diagnosis of cerebrovascular disease. Stroke 7(5):439-444, Sept-Oct 1976.

Keitzer WF, Lichti EL: Applications of the Doppler: Common and unusual situations. Angiology 26(2):172-86, Feb 1975.

Keller H, Baumgartner G, Regli F: Carotid artery stenoses and occlusions. Diagnosis by percutaneous ultrasound Doppler sonography at the supraorbital or supratrochlear artery. Dtsch Med Wochenschr 98(37):1691-1698, Sep 1973.

Kempczinski RF: A combined approach to the noninvasive diagnosis of carotid artery occlusive disease. Surgery 85(6):689-694, Jun 1979.

Kindt GW, Youmans JR, Conway LW: The use of ultrasound to determine cerebral arterial reserve. J Neurosurg 31(5):544-549, Nov 1969.

Kriebel J, Schurig E: Directional Doppler-sonography in stenoses and occlusions of the internal carotid artery. Med Welt 26(49):2202-2204, Dec 5, 1975.

Kudrow L: Thermographic and Doppler flow asymmetry in cluster headache. Headache 19(4):204-208, May 1979.

Lieberman A: Directional Doppler in occlusive cerebrovascular disorders (letter). Stroke 8(5):629, Sept-Oct 1977.

LoGerfo FW, Mason GR: Directional Doppler studies of supraorbital artery flow in internal carotid stenosis and occlusion. Surgery 76(5):723-728, Nov 1974.

Lye CR, Sumner DS, Strandness DE Jr: The accuracy of the supraorbital Doppler examination in the diagnosis of hemodynamically significant carotid occlusive. Surgery 79(1):42-45, Jan 1976.

Machleder HI: Evaluation of patients with cerebrovascular disease using the Doppler ophthalmic test. Angiology 24(6):374-381, Jun 1973.

Machleder HI, Barker WF: Stroke on the wrong side: use of the Doppler ophthalmic test in cerebral vascular screening. Arch Surg 105:943, 1972.

Machleder HI, Barker WF: Stroke on the wrong side: use of the Doppler ophtalmic test in cerebral vascular screening. Arch Surg 105(6):643-647, Dec 1972.

Maroon JC, Campbell RL Dyken ML: Internal carotid artery occlusion diagnosed by Doppler ultrasound. Stroke 1(2):122-127, Mar-Apr 1979.

Maroon JC, Pieroni DW, Campbell RL: Ophthalmosonometry. An ultrasonic method for assessing carotid blood flow. J Neurosurg 30(3):238-246, Mar 1969.

McDonald PT, Rich NM, Collins GJ, Andersen CA, Kozloff L: Doppler cerebrovascular examination, oculoplethysmography, and ocular pneumoplethysmography use in detection of carotid. Arch Surg 113(11):1341-1349, Nov 1978.

Moore S, Bean B, Burton R, Goldstone J: Use of the Doppler flowmeter in stroke prevention. Med Prog Technol 4(3):117-121, 1976.

Moore WS, Bean B, Burton R, Goldstone J: The use of ophthalmosonometry in the diagnosis of carotid artery stenosis. Surgery 82(1):107-115, Jul 1977.

Mrzyglod S, Warczynski A: Evaluation of the usefulness of measurement of blood flow by the Doppler method in retinal circulatory insufficiency. Klin Oczna 81(2):113-116, 1979.

Muller HR: The diagnosis of internal carotid artery occlusion by directional Doppler sonography of the ophthalmic artery. Neurology (Minneap) 22(8):816-823, Aug 1972.

Muller HR, Dunant JH, Waibel P: Reconstruction of the physiologic flow direction in the ophthalmic artery using endarterectomy in stenoses of the internal carotid artery. Vasa 1(3):196-200, 1972.

Muller HR: Directional Doppler sonography. A new technique to demonstrate flow reversal in the ophthalmic artery. Neuroradiology 5(2):91-94, Apr 1973.

Muller HR: Doppler sonography of the carotid vascular system. Internist (Berlin) 17(11):570-579, Nov 1976.

Mungas JE, Baker WH: Amaurosis fugax. Stroke 8(2):232-235, Mar-Apr 1977.

Nappi G, Bono G, Poloni M, Savoldi F: Comparative Doppler directional sonographic and ophthalmodynamographic study in the occlusion of the internal carotid. Eur Neurol 15(2):102-108, 1977.

Nappi G, Bono G, Poloni M, Sandrini G: Directional Doppler ultrasonography (DDS): theoretical bases and clinical methods. Boll Soc Ital Biol Sper 51(15-16):922-928, August 30, 1975.

Nuzzaci G, Briani S, Mennonna P, Evangelisti A: The Doppler ophthalmic test: report of a study on its value in diagnosis of internal carotid artery insufficiency. J Neurosurg Sci 19(3):129-138, Jul-Sep 1975.

Otis SM, Smith RA, Dalessio DJ, Kroll AD, Rush M, Dilley RB: Ineffectiveness of the Doppler ophthalmic test (DOT) in post-endarterectomy evaluation. Stroke 20(4):396-399, Jul-Aug 1979.

Pateisky D, Reisner H: The place of echoencephalography in neurology. Wien Klin Wochenschr 87(12):388-389, Jun 1975.

Prichard DR, Martin TR, Sheriff SB: Assessment of directional Doppler ultrasound techniques in the diagnosis of carotid artery diseases. J Neurol Neurosurg Psychiatry 42(6):563-468, June 1979.

Rendl KH, Paulowitz HP: Directional indirect Doppler-ultrasonography of the carotid artery. Wien Med Wochenschr 128(24):764-765, Dec 1978.

Rendle KH, Prenner K, Paulowitz HP: The diagnosis of carotid artery stenosis in medical practice. Wien Med Wochenschr 128(5):148-150, Mar 1978.

Rossazza C, Devlamynok S, Stecken M, Delplace MP: Doppler effect in isolated syndromes of central retinal artery occlusion. Bull Soc Ophthalmol Fr 78(12):941-945, Dec 1978.

Tada K, Nukada T, Yoneda S, Kuriyama Y, Abe H: Assessment of the capacity of cerebral collateral circulation using ultrasonic Doppler technique. J Neurol Neurosurg Psychiatry 38(11):1068-1075, Nov 1975.

Takaki HS, McNamara MF, Yao JS, Bergan JJ: Influence of noninvasive screening on care of patients with carotid stenosis. In: Noninvasive cardiovascular diagnosis, Diethrich EB (ed). Baltimore: Univ Park Press, Chap 1, 3-11, 1978.

Taniguchi H: A study on blood flow in the ophthalmic artery with an ultrasonic Doppler technique. The folia ophthalmologica Japonica 20(6):556-559, 1969.

Taniguchi H: Studies on the ocular circulation with an ultrasonic Doppler technique. Diagnosis and classification of Takayasu's. Acta Soc Ophthalmol Jpn 78(9):907-912, Sep 1974.

Taniguchi H, Moriyama H: Studies on the ocular circulation with an ultrasonic Doppler technique. Acta Soc Ophthalmol Jpn 75(8):1831-1836, 1971.

Towne JB, Bernhard VM, Salles-Cunha S, Ray LI: Supraorbital Doppler evaluation in vascular surgery. Med Instrum 13(2):92-94, Mar-Apr 1979.

Towne JB, Salles-Cunha S, Bernhard VM: Periorbital ultrasound findings. Hemodynamics in patients with cerebral vascular disease. Arch Surg 114(2):158-160, Feb 1979.

Warter G: Encephalic Doppler ultrasonography in everyday ophthalmology. Ophthalmologica 178(1-2):37-42, 1979.

Wise G, Parker J, Burkholder J: Supraorbital Doppler studies, carotid bruits, and arteriography in unilateral ocular or cerebral ischemic disorders. Neurology (Minneap) 29(1):34-37, Jan 1979.

Zannini G, Bracale GC, Cennamo G, Rocco P, Gangemi M: Correlations between Doppler, thermography and ophthalmodynamometry for instrumental d'epistage of cerebral vasculopath. J Cardiovasc Surg 19(6):647-654, Nov-Dec 1978.

HAND-HELD CAROTID DOPPLER

Ackerman RH: A perspective on noninvasive diagnosis of carotid disease. Neurology (Minneap) 29(5):615-622, May 1979.

Balzer K, Stoveken HJ, Bernert J, Carstensen G: Measuring technics in indications for supra-aortic reconstructions. Med Welt 29(43):1680-1682, Oct 1978.

Barnes RW, Rittgers SE, Thornhill B, Nix L, Putney W: Noninvasive determination of carotid artery operability by Doppler ultrasound. Va Med 106(11):804-808, Nov 1979.

Barnes RW, Wilson MR: Doppler ultrasonic evaluation of cerebrovascular disease. University of Iowa, 1975.

Barriga P, Spencer M, Turnipseed W, Zagzebski J, Martinson M: Correlation of a non-sounding area in the carotid Doppler ultrasound evaluation with zerography of the neck. In: Ultrasound in medicine, White D (ed). Plenum Press. Vol. 3B, p 1395, Aug 1976.

Barsotti J, Pourcelot L, Greco J, Planiol T, Kiniffo HY, Castellani L: Use of the Doppler effect in peripheral vascular pathology and surgery. Ann Chir Thorac Cardiovasc 11(4):387-393, Oct 1972.

Barsotti J, Pourcelot L, Greco J, Planiol T, Kiniffo HY, Castellani L: The Doppler effect. Its use in peripheral vascular pathology and surgery. Nouv Presse Med 1(40):2677-2681, Nov 1972.

Baskett JJ, Beasley MG, Gosling RG, Hyams DE: Proceedings: The assessment and management of carotid arterial disease using spectral analysis of the Doppler signal. Br J Radiol 49(584):731, Aug 1976.

Bernstein EF: The current place of noninvasive diagnostic techniques in evaluating cerebrovascular disease. J R Soc Med 71(10):709-710, Oct 1978.

Bes A, Guell A, Braak L, Geraud G, Jauzac P: Doppler sonography in the diagnosis of occlusion of stenosis of the internal carotid artery. Adv Neurol 25:211-222, 1979.

Boespflug O: The Doppler test: its practical importance in the study of lesions of the supra-aortic trunks. Phlebologie 31(4):343-353, Oct-Dec 1978.

Bohme G, Bohme H: Possibilities of assessing cerebrovascular disease by audiometry: comparison with Doppler ultrasound in the assessment of extracranial vascular occlusion (author's transl). Dtsch Med Wochenschr 104(41):1443-1447, Oct 1979.

Bouding G, Guillard A, Romion A: Comparison between Doppler findings and arteriography in cervical arterial pathology. Nouv Presse Med 6(27):2423-2426, Jul 1977.

Brewster DC, Schlaen HH, Raines JK, Abbott WM, Darling RC: Rational management of the asymptomatic carotid bruit. Arch Surg 113(8):927-930, Aug 1978.

Brinker RA, Landiss DJ, Croley TF: Detection of carotid artery bifurcation stenosis by Doppler ultrasound. J Neurosurg 29:143-148, 1968.

Budingen HJ, Von Reutern GM, Freund HJ: Diagnosis of cerebro-vascular lesions by ultrasonic methods. Int J of Neurology 11(2-3):206-218, 1977.

Budingen HJ, Gilsbach J, Von Reutern GM: Doppler-sonographic control of a carotid cavernous fistula occluded by balloon catheter (author's transl). Arch Psychiatr Nervenkr 226(1):19-27, Oct 1978.

Budingen HJ, Von Reutern GM, Freund HJ: The selective examination of the neck arteries by directional Doppler sonography. Arch Psychiatr Nervenkr 222(2-3):177-190, Oct 1976.

Bussee R, Sperling W, Korner H, Bauer RD, Pasch T: Usability of the ultrasound Doppler flow-velocity measurement for the diagnosis of carotid stenoses. Z Kardiol 63(8):755-767, Aug 1974.

Capon A, Lemaire P, Demeurisse G, Verhas M: Techniques for the diagnosis of cerebral ischemia (author's translation). Acta Chir Belg 78(2):67-72, Mar-Apr 1979.

Cole M, Kraehenbuhl G, Richard J: Differentiation of the dementias of old age by ultrasonic Doppler flowmetry: a pilot study. J Am Geriatr Soc 25(7):314-317, Jul 1977.

Colon EJ, de Weerd JP, Notermans SL, Vingerhoets HM: Reliability of Doppler sonography in extracranial cerebrovascular stenosis. Clin Neurol Neurosurg 81(2):108-113, 1979.

Courbier R, Reggi M, Jausseran JM: Exploration of carotid artery and vessels of the neck by Doppler techniques. In: Noninvasive cardiovascular diagnosis, Diethrich EB (ed). Baltimore: Univ Park Press, 1978, 61-73.

Cranley JJ, Mahalingam K, Ferris EB: Extending the vascular examination by non-invasive means. Am J Surg 134(2):179-182, Aug 1977.

Depresseux JC: Hemotachymetry by Doppler effect (author's transl). Acta Neurol Belg 78(6):341-353, 1978.

Dorogova EV, Florianovich NM: Application of ultrasound to the study of the carotid arteries. Nov Med Priborostr 1:89-94, 1967.

Felix RW Jr, Sigel B, Gibson RJ, Williams J, Popky GL, Edelstein AL, Justin JR: Pulsed Doppler ultrasound detection of flow disturbances in arteriosclerosis. J Clin Ultrasound 4(4):275-282, Aug 1976.

Franceschi C, Cormier JM, Lagneau P, Cassan JL: Doppler ultrasound studies in carotid prethrombosis (author's transl). Nouv Presse Med 8(36):2873-2876, Sep 1979.

Friedenberg MJ, Lake P, Landau S: Bilateral incomplete traumatic occlusion of internal carotid arteries. Am J Roentgenol Radium Ther Nucl Med 118(3):546-549, Jul 1973.

Ghilardi F, Liboni W, Morra A, Rivadossi G: Use of ultrasound in the study of vascular changes and cerebral circulatory dynamics. Minerva Med 65(66):3441-3457, Sep 1974.

Golek J, Berny W, Loboz K: Value of parallel ultrasound estimations of extracranial blood flow velocity and ophthalmodynamometry in disturbances of cerebral blood circulation. Acta Neurochir (Suppl) 2(28):531-535, 1979.

Handa H, Niimi H, Moritake K, Okumura A, Matsuda I: Analysis of sound spectrographic pattern for assessment of vascular occlusive disorders by continuous wave ultrasonic Doppler flowmeter. Arch Jpn Chir 46(3):214-225, 1977.

Horrocks M, Roberts VC, Cotton LT: Assessment of carotid artery stenosis using pulse wave transit time. Br J Surg 66(4):265-268, Apr 1979.

Itti R, Pottier JM, Pourcelot L: Examen Doppler de la circulation cerebrale. Exploration du système cardiovasculaire au moyen des radio-isotopes it interet de leur. Thèse pour le doctorate en médecine, 355-407, 1978.

Jacquy J, Jeanmart M, Urbain M, Piraux A, Noel G: Study of the cerebral circulatory resistance by the Doppler effect and rheography (author's transl). Acta Neurol Belg 76(1):5-9, Jan-Feb 1976.

Jonkman EJ, Mosmans PC: Doppler haematotachography: problems in interpretation and new applications. Clin Neurol Neurosurg 80(1):33-45, 1977.

Jonkman EJ, Tans JT, Mosmans PC: Doppler flow velocity measurements in patients with intracranial hypertension. J Neurol 218(3):157-169, Jun 1978.

Kaliman J, Zaunbauer G, Bardach G: Doppler ultrasound diagnosis of extracranial carotid stenoses (author's transl). Neurochirurgie 24(4):247-249, 1978.

Kaliman J, Deutsch M, Valencak E: Diagnosis of extracranial carotid stenoses using the Doppler sonography. Acta Med Austriaca 5(5-4):129-132, 1978.

Kanai N, Hayakawa T, Mogami H: Blood flow changes in carotid and vertebral arteries by hyperbaric oxygenation. Neurology (Minneap) 23(2):159-163, Feb 1973.

Kaneko J, Shiraishi J, Omizu H, Inaoka H, Ueshima T: Clinical application of a sonograph to the analysis of the blood rheogram. Brain Nerve (Tokyo) 17(12):1237-1245, Dec 1965.

230

Kaneko J: Diagnosis of cerebral vascular disturbances by ultrasonic rheography. Clin Neurol (Tokyo) 4(2):221-236, Mar 1974.

Kaneko Z, Shiraishi J, Omizo H, Kato K, Motomiya M, Izumi T, Okumura T: Analysing blood flow with a sonograph. Ultrasonics 4:22-23, Jan 1966.

Kaneko Z, Shiraishi J, Omizo H: Analysis of ultrasonic blood rheogram by a band pass filter. Angiology 19(1):10-24, 1968.

Keller H, Meier W, Yonekawa Y, Kumpe D: Noninvasive angiography for the diagnosis of carotid artery disease using Doppler ultrasound (carotid artery Doppler). Stroke 7(4):354-363, Jul-Aug 1976.

Keller H, Bollinger A, Baumgartner G: Doppler ultrasound sonography in the diagnosis of occlusions and stenoses of the carotid arteries with paradoxical. J Neurol 207(3):211-226, 1974.

Keller H, Baumgartner G: Doppler ultrasonography: a non-invasive examination method in the diagnosis and therapeutic control of carotid stenosis. Schweiz Med Wochenschr. 104(37):1281-91, Sep 1974.

Keller H, Meier W: Dopplersonography: supervision after endarterectomy: the carotid artery to detect rethrombosis (author's transl). Thoraxchirurgie 22(6):525-541, Dec 1974.

Keller HM, Meier WE, Anliker M, Kumpe DA: Noninvasive measurement of velocity profiles and blood flow in the common carotid artery by pulsed Doppler ultrasound. Stroke 7(4):370-377, Jul-Aug 1976.

Keller HM, Meier WE, Zumstein B: Cerebrovascular Doppler examination. A noninvasive diagnostic contribution in stroke prevention (author's transl). Praxis 67(20):748-759, May 1978.

Keller HM, Schubiger O, Krayenbuhl C, Zumstein B: Cerebrovascular Doppler examination and cerebral angiography — alternative or complementary. Neuroradiology 16:140-144, 1978.

Keller HM, Meier WE, Yonekawa Y: Pre- and postoperative Doppler-ultrasound measurements in carotid artery surgery (carotid artery Doppler). Thoraxchir Vask Chir 25(4):254-265, Aug 1977.

Klinger M: Comparative diagnosis of cerebrovascular diseases by using ophthalmodynamometry, Doppler ultrasonography and carotidography (author's transl). Lijec Vjesn 191(5):269-273, May 1979.

Kristensen JK: Carotid and vertebral blood-flow evaluation by means of ultrasound. Acta Neurol Scand 43 Suppl 31:116, 1967.

Liljeqvist L, Ekestrom S, Nordhus O: Doppler ultrasound technique compared to angiography, intraoperative pressure gradients and blood flow measurements. Thoraxchir Vask Chir 25(4):266-271, Aug 1977.

Lunt MJ, Reuben JR, de Boulay EP: Preliminary report on some ultrasonic methods for detecting carotid artery disease. J Med Eng Technol 2(6):289-297, Nov 1978.

Machleder HI: Strokes, transient ischemic attacks and asymptomatic bruits. West J Med 130(3):205-217, Mar 1979.

Manz F: Ultrasound-Doppler-sonography of carotid circulation. Munch Med Wochenschr 119(21):727-728, May 1977.

Maruta H, Hata H, Yamaoka I, Suzuki G: Ultrasonorheometry, a new method for measuring the cerebral blood flow. Brain Nerve (Tokyo) 18(6):637-643, Jun 1966.

Matsuo H, Nimura Y, Kitabatake A, Hayashi T: Analysis of flow patterns in blood vessels with the directional Doppler technique through a transcutaneous approach. Japanese Circul J 37(7):735-746, Jul 1973.

Meier WE, Keller H: Valve of intraoperative carotid Doppler sonography with regards to the prognosis of the postoperative course. Helv Chir Acta 43(1-2):107-110, Mar 1976.

Melis-Kisman E, Mol JMF: L'application de l'effet Doppler à l'exploration cerebro-vasculaire. R Neural 122:470-472, 1970.

Melis-Kisman E, Mol JM: Application of the Doppler effect in investigating the cerebral Circulation Electro Clin Neurophysiol 30(3):48, Mar 1971.

Miyazaki M, Kato K: Measurement of cerebral blood flow by ultrasonic Doppler technique. Japanese Circulation J 29:383-386, Apr 1965.

Miyazaki M: Measurement of cerebral blood flow by ultrasonic Doppler technique. Quantitative detection of cerebral arteriosclerosis. Jap Circ J 31(5):781-788, May 1967.

Miyazaki M: Measurement of cerebral blood flow by ultrasonic Doppler technique. Pulsatile variation of the vascular diameter of the human common carotid artery. Jap Circ J 32(7):1003-1009, Jul 1968.

Miyazaki M: Study on cerebral circulation using the ultrasonic Doppler method—with special reference to pulsatile change of the internal diameter of the common c. Naika 23(1):139-143, Jan 1969.

Miyazaki M: Quantitative detection of cerebral arteriosclerosis by means of the pressure-velocity hysteresis technique. Jap Circ J 40(7):739-745, Jul 1976.

Miyazaki M: Circulatory effect of respiratory maneuvers. Angiology 29(7):541-547, Jul 1978.

Miyazaki M: Measurement of cerebral blood flow by ultrasonic Doppler technique. Cerebral hemodynamics during voluntary hyperventilation and the valsalva maneuver. Jap Circ J 32(3):315-319, Mar 1968.

Miyazaki M: Study of cerebral circulation by Doppler ultrasonic method—with reference to the quantitative diagnosis of cerebral arteriosclerosis. Naika 19(4):733-738, Apr 1967.

Miyazaki M: Measurement of cerebral blood flow by ultrasonic Doppler technique. Hemodynamic correlation between cerebral and peripheral-ophthalmic artery. Jap Circ J 30(10):1353-1358, Oct 1966.

Miyazaki M: Measurement of cerebral blood flow by ultrasonic Doppler technique. Hemodynamic correlation of internal carotid artery and vertebral artery. Jap Circ J 30(8):981-985, Aug 1966.

Miyazaki M: Measurement of cerebral blood flow by ultrasonic Doppler technique. Effects of low temperature, induced hypertension and arrhythmia on cerebral circulation. Jap Circ J 30(7):863-867, Jul 1966.

Miyazaki M: Measurement of cerebral blood flow by ultrasonic Doppler technique. Effects of several vasodilators of cerebral circulation with special reference to aminophylline, nicotinic-acid and papaverine. Jap Circ J 30(9):1023-1029, Sep 1966.

Miyazaki M: Studies on cerebral circulation by ultrasonic Doppler technique—with special reference to clinical application of the technique. Prog Brain Res 35:1-23, 1972.

Miyazaki M: Multiple and simultaneous blood flow measurements by the ultrasonic Doppler technique in man—with special reference to the circulatory effects of ind. Jap Circ. J 35(4):405-412, Apr 1971.

Mol JMF, Rijcken WJ: Doppler haematotachographic investigation in cerebral circulation disturbances. In: Cardiovascular applications of ultrasound. Reneman RS (ed). Amsterdam-London-NY: North-Holland/American Elsevier. 1974, 305-314.

Muller HR: The place of computerized tomography and carotid Doppler sonography in CV episodes. Adv Neurol 25:181-197, 1979.

Nevrtal M, Kubak R, Zouhar A, Jehlicka K, Pucalka A: Ultrasonic assessment of changes occurring in the hemodynamics of carotid and vertebral circulation (author's transl). Cas Lek Cesk 115(52):1593-1601, Dec 1976.

Nimura Y, Matsuo H, Hayashi T, Nagata S, Miyatake K, Asao M, Terao Y, Senda S, Kitabatake A: Studies on flow patterns in the common carotid artery in cases of hypertrophic cardiomyopathy. In: Non-invasive cardiovascular diagnosis, Diethrich EB (ed). Baltimore: Univ Park Press, MD (Pub.), 417-427, 1978.

Nordby HK: Circulation in the common carotid artery and its branches. Some experiences with the percutaneous Doppler technic. Tidsskr Nor Laegeforen 99(2):89-90, Jan 1979.

Otis SM, Smith RA, Kroll AD, Krasny SE, Seltzer KA, Dalessio DJ: Vasospasm and vascular headaches: selective vasoconstriction in the carotid vascular system measured by Doppler. Headache 19(4):200-203, May 1979.

Peloponnisios P: Role of ultrasonography in the study of peripheral vascular disease and carotid diseases. Rev Med Suisse Romande 96(11):857-867, Nov 1976.

Perrin G, Goutelle A, Pierluca P, Chacornac R, Allegre GE: Reliability of the results of the ultrasonic hemodynamic recording (Doppler effect) in the diagnosis of cerebral ischemic ischemia of carotid origin. Neurochirurgie 23(3::215-225, May-Jun 1977.

Planiol T, Itti R, Pourcelot L, Groussin P: Study of carotid circulation by external physical methods. 2. Results in obstructions. Nouv Presse Med 2(45):3030-3036, Dec 1973.

Planiol T, Pourcelot L, Itti R: Radioisotopes, ultrasonics and thermography in the diagnosis of cerebral circulatory disorders. Rev Electroencephalogr Neurophysiol Clin 4(2):221-236, Apr-Jun 1974.

Planiol T, Pourcelot L: La circulation carotidienne et cerebrole. Nouv Presse Med 2(37):2451-2456, Oct 1973.

Planiol T, Pourcelot L, Pottier JM, Degiovanni E: Étude de la circulation carotidienne par les méthodes ultrasoniques et la thermographie. Revue Neurologique (Paris) 126(2):127-141, 1972.

Popoviciu L, Popa DP, Zakarias I, Corfariu O, Pascu I: Methods of investigation in the diagnosis of cerebral circulatory disorders caused by lesions of the carotid artery. Rev Med Intern (Neurol Psichiatr) 22(2):123-130, Apr-Jun 1977.

Pourcelot L: Clinical applications of transcutaneous Doppler examinations. In: Velocimetrie ultrasonore Doppler. Peronneau P (ed). Paris: INSERM, 213-240, 1975.

Pourcelot L: Indications of Doppler's ultrasonography in the study of peripheral vessels. Rev Prat 25(59):4671-4680, Dec 1975.

Rachdi M: Atraumatic methods in the diagnosis of a case of internal carotid artery occlusion. Tunis Med 56(1):45-61, 1978.

Reneman RS, Reid JM, Spencer MP: Doppler audio spectra in carotid stenosis in man. Federation Proceedings 37(3), Mar 1978.

Reneman RS, Spencer MP: Local Doppler audio spectra in normal and stenosed carotid arteries in man. In: Ultrasound in medicine and biology. Pergamon Press, Ltd (Pub) 5(1):1-11, 1979.

Risoe C, Wille SO: Blood velocity in human arteries measured by a bidirectional ultrasonic Doppler flowmeter. Acta Physiol Scand 103(4):370-378, Aug 1978.

Ruckert U, Altstaedt F, Schjeld M, Trede M: Results of reconstruction of the carotid artery (author's transl). Dtsch Med Wochenschr 104(12):428-431, Mar 1979.

Rushmer RF, Baker DW, Johnson WL, Strandness DE: Clinical applications of a transcutaneous ultrasonic flow detector. JAMA 199(5):326-328, Jan 1967.

Rutherford RB, Hiatt WR, Kreutzer EW: The use of velocity wave form analysis in the diagnosis of carotid artery occlusive disease. Surgery 82(5):695-702, Nov 1977.

Sandok BA: Noninvasive techniques for diagnosis of carotid artery disease. Stroke 9(5):427-429, 1978.

Shiraishi J: Ultrasonic blood rheography. Saishin Igaku 25(6):1332-1338, Jun 1970.

Spaan G, Dittrich J, Rexroth W, Stein U, Wagner E: Ultrasound in angiology. ZFA (Stuttgart) 55(11):673-680, Apr 1979.

Spence JD: Effects of antihypertensive drugs on blood velocity: implications for prevention of cerebral vascular disease. Can J Neurol Sci 4(2):93-97, May 1977.

Spencer MP, Reid JM: Quantification of carotid artery stenosis from spectral analysis of Doppler audio signals. Federation Proceedings 37(3), Mar 1978.

St Oveken HJ, Balzer K, Bernet J, Carstensen G: Experiences in 130 operations of carotid elongation (author's transl). Langenbecks Arch Chir 348(2):141-146, May 1979.

Thompson JE, Patman RD, Talkington CM: Carotid surgery for cerebrovascular insufficiency. Curr Probl Surg 15(12):1-68, Dec 1978.

Turnipseed WD, Berkoff H, Barriga P, Rouse M, Jarrett F: Echo Doppler scanning and spectral frequency analysis: a noninvasive test for carotid artery disease. Trans AM Neurol Assoc 102:28-32, 1977.

Van de Berg L: Ultrasonic vascular examination. Rev Med Liege 26(5):168-174, 1971.

Von Reutern GM, Budingen HJ, Ortega-Suhrkamp E, Voight K, Freund HJ: Differenzierungsmöglichkeiten der extrakraniel Hirngefabe mit der Ultraschall-Doppler-Sonographie. In: Ultraschal-Doppler-Diagnostik in der Angiologie. Stuttgart: Georg Thieme Verlag, 105-113, 1978.

Von Reutern GM, Ortega-Suhrkamp E, Spillner G: Is the non-invasive Doppler sonography alone sufficient to indicate carotid surgery. In: Cerebral Vascular Disease 2, Meyer JS (ed), Excerpta Medica 46-49, 1979.

Von Reutern GM, Budingen HJ, Hennerici M, Freund HJ: The diagnosis of stenoses and occlusions of the carotid arteries by means of directional Dopplersonography. Arch Psychiatr Nervenkr 222(2-3):191-207, Oct 1976.

Von Reutern GM, Voight K, Ortega-Suhrkamp E, Budingen HJ: Doppler findings in intracranial vascular disorders. Differential diagnosis of extracranial and intracranial vascular occlusions. Arch Psychiatr Nervenkr 223(3):181-196, May 1977.

Von Reutern GM, Budingen HJ, Hennerici M, Freund HJ: Diagnose und Differenzierung von Stenosen und Verschlüssen der arteria carotis mit der Doppler-Sonographie. Arch Psychiat Nervenkr 222:191-207, 1976.

Widder B: A simplified Doppler-angiography apparatus for noninvasive diagnosis of carotid stenosis (author's transl). Nervenarzt 48(7):397-399, Jul 1977.

Yao JS, Bergan JJ: Diagnosis of cerebral vascular disturbances by ultrasonic rheography. Clin Neurol (Tokyo) 14(3):215-225, Mar 1974.

Yoneda S, Nishimoto A, Nukada T, Kuriyama Y, Katsurada K: To-and-fro movement and external escape of carotid arterial blood in brain death cases. A Doppler ultrasonic study. Stroke 5(6):707-713, Nov-Dec 1974.

Yoshida S, Fujimoto J, Tone K, Sawami K: Comparative study of Xe133 washout method and ultrasonic blood rheography. Saishin Igaku 25(6):1339-1346, 1970.

CAROTID DOPPLER IMAGING

Barnes RW, Bone GE, Reinertson JE, Slaymaker EE, Hokanson DE, Strandness DE
Jr: Value of blood velocity analysis during pulsed Doppler ultrasonic imaging of
carotid artery disease. 29th ACEMB Meeting, Boston, Mass. Nov. 6-10, 1976.

Barnes RW, Bone GE, Reinertson J, Slaymaker EE, Hokanson DE, Strandness DE Jr:
Noninvasive ultrasonic carotid angiography: prospective validation by constrast
arteriography. Surgery 80(3):328-335, Sep 1976.

Blackshear WM Jr, Phillips DJ, Thiele BL, Hirsch JH, Chickos PM, Marinelli MR,
Ward KJ, Strandness DE Jr: Detection of carotid occlusive disease by ultrasonic
imaging and pulsed Doppler spectrum analysis. Surgery 86(5):698-706, 1979.

Blackwell E, Merory J, Toole JF, McKinney W: Doppler ultrasound scanning of the
carotid bifurcation. Arch Neurol 34:145-148, Mar 1977.

Blackwell E, Merory J, Toole JF, McKinney W: Evaluation of carotid and vertebro-
basilar insufficiency by Doppler ultrasound scanning. Joint Mtg on Stroke & Cerebral Circulation, Dallas, TX, Feb 1976.

Bohme H: Possibilities of early diagnosis of degenerative vascular disease (editorial).
Munch Med Wochenschr 120(1):7-8, Jan 1978.

Carson SN, Blaisdell FW: New techniques in the evaluation of cerebro-vascular
disease. West J Med 131:355-363, Nov 1979.

Crummy AB, Zwiebel WJ, Barriga P, Strother CM, Sackett JF, Turnipseed WD,
Jarrett F, Berkoff H: Doppler evaluation of extracranial cerebrovascular disease.
AJR 132(1):91-93, Jan 1979.

Curry GR, White DN: Colour coded differential velocity carotid bifurcation tomogra-
phic scanner. 11th Int Conf Med and Biol Engng, 1976.

Dalessio DJ, Otis SM, Smith RA: Detecting extracranial cerebrovascular disease with
noninvasive techniques. AM Fam Physician 17(1):118-125, Jan 1978.

Davis RC, Johnson WA, Gingery RO: Doppler sonographic imaging and carotid
phonoangiography in the evaluation of asymptomatic carotid bruits. (In Press). In:
Noninvasive cardiovascular diagnosis. Diethrich EB (ed). PSG Publishing Co, Inc,
Second Edition, Feb 1979.

Gosling RG: Doppler ultrasound assessment of occlusive arterial disease. Practitioner
220(1318):599-609, Apr 1978.

Hokanson DE: United States patent # 3. 777, 740, Issued December 11, 1973.

Hokanson DE, Mozersky DJ, Sumner DS, McLeod FD Jr, Strandness DE Jr: Ultrasonic arteriography. A noninvasive method of arterial visualization. Radiology
102(2):435-436, Feb 1972.

Jarrett F, Barriga PJ, Turnipseed W, Berkoff HA, Crummy AB: Comparison of carotid
echo Doppler scanning with arteriography. In: Noninvasive cardiovascular diagnosis,
Diethrich EB (ed). Baltimore: Univ Park Press, 39-50, 1978.

Lewis RR, Beasley MG, Hyams DE, Gosling RG: Imaging the carotid bifurcation
using continuous-wave Doppler-shift ultrasound and spectral analysis. Stroke
9(5):465-471, Sep-Oct 1978.

Lewis RR, Beasley MG, Gosling RG: Disease at the carotid bifurcation: diagnosis by
Doppler ultrasound imaging. Gerontology 25(5):291-298, 1979.

Mozersky DJ, Hokanson DE, Baker DW, Sumner DS, Strandness DE Jr: Ultrasonic
arteriography. Arch Surg 103(6):663-667, Dec 1971.

Mozersky DJ, Hokanson DE, Sumner DS, Strandness DE Jr: Ultrasonic visualization
of the arterial lumen. Surgery 72(2):253-259, Aug 1972.

O'Donnell TF Jr, Pauker SG, Callow AD, Kelly JJ, McBride KJ, Korwin S: The relative value of carotid noninvasive testing as determined by receiver operator characteristic curves. Surgery 87(1):9-19, Jan 1980.

Patel J, Lee KF, Goldberg B: The role of ultrasonography in the diagnosis of certain neurologic disorders. A preliminary report. Neuroradiology 16:583-586, 1978.

Reid JM, Spencer MP, Davis DL: Ultrasonic Doppler technique for imaging blood vessels. Science 176:1235-1236, 1972.

Reid JM, Davis DL, Phillips JB, Spencer MP: Transcutaneous flow mapping with continuous wave Doppler. In: Cardiovascular applications of ultrasound, Reneman RS (ed), North-Holland Pub 20:244, 1973.

Reid JM, Davis DL, Phillips JB, Spencer MP: Some recent advances in continuous wave Doppler instruments. International Congress, Series No. 309. Ultrasonics in Medicine 267, 1973.

Reid JM, Spencer MP, Davis DL: Ultrasonic Doppler imaging systems. In: Ultrasound in medicine, White D (ed), Plenum Press. Aug 1976.

Reneman RS, Hoeks A, Spencer MP: Doppler ultrasound in the evaluation of the peripheral arterial circulation. Angiology 30(8):526-538, Aug 1979.

Shoumaker RD, Bloch S: Cerebrovascular evaluation: assessment of Doppler scanning of carotid arteries, ophthalmic Doppler flow and bruits. Stroke 9(6):563-566, Nov-Dec 1978.

Siemens Aktiengesellschaft: English Patent (London) #1 356 671, issued June 12, 1974.

Spencer MP, Reid JM, Davis DL, Paulson PS: Cervical carotid imaging with a continuous-wave Doppler flowmeter. Stroke 5:145-154, Mar-Apr 1974.

Spencer MP, Li JW, Brockenbrough EC, Reid JM: Doppler detection of the atherosclerotic plaque. Circulation 52(2):80, Oct 1975.

Spencer MP, Brockenbrough EC, Davis DL, Reid JM: Cerebrovascular evaluation using Doppler C-W ultrasound. In: Ultrasound in Medicine, White D (ed), Plenum Press, 3B, Aug 1976.

Spencer MP, Reid JM, Paulson PS: Diagnosis of carotid artery disease and cerebral vascular insufficiency with Doppler angiography and ophthalmic artery sonography. In: Cardiovascular Applications of Ultrasound, Reneman RS (ed), North-Holland Pub 21:249, 1973.

Spencer MP: Non-invasive detection of carotid artery stenosis with Doppler ultrasonic angiography. Circulation Suppl IV: 7-8, Oct 1973.

Spencer MP: Non-invasive methods defended as valuable. Stroke 10:458-480, 1979.

Spencer MP: Doppler ultrasonic imaging and non-invasive cerebrovascular evaluation. Int J Neurol 11(2-3):223-242, 1977.

Spencer MP, Reid JM: Quantitation of carotid stenosis with continuous-wave (C-W) Doppler ultrasound. Stroke 10(3):326-330, May-Jun 1979.

Strandness DE Jr, Sumner DS: Clinical applications of continuous wave and pulsed Doppler velocity detectors. In: Velocimetrie ultrasonore Doppler, Peronneau P (ed). Paris, INSERM 147-190, 1975.

Strandness DE Jr: The use of ultrasound in the evaluation of peripheral vascular disease. Prog Cardiovasc Disc 20(6):403-422, May-Jun 1978.

Strandness DE Jr: Doppler ultrasound in vascular surgery. Aust NZ J Surg 47(1):115-118, Feb 1977.

Sumner DS, Russel JB, Ramsey DE, Hajjar, WM, Miles RD: Noninvasive diagnosis of extracranial carotid arterial disease: a prospective evaluation of pulsed-Doppler imaging and oculoplethysmography. Arch Surg 114(11):1222-1229, Nov 1979.

Thomas GI, Spencer MP, Jones TW, Edmark KW, Stavney LS: Noninvasive carotid bifurcation mapping. Its relation to carotid surgery. Am J Surg 128(2):168-174, Aug 1974.

Turnipseed W, Berkoff H, Barriga P: Doppler scanning and xerography: a screening procedure for high risk carotid lesions in surgical patients. J Surg Res 22(6):683-686, Jun 1977.

Turnipseed WD, Vasko JS, Lubow M: Surgical management of the totally occluded carotid artery. Surgery 82(5):689-694, Nov 1977.

Zwiebel W, Turski P, Strother C, Crummy A, Sackett J, Barriga P: Doppler ultrasound evaluation of extracranial cerebrovascular disease. Neuroradiology (Springer-Verlag), 16:145-146, 1978.

INTRACRANIAL DOPPLER

Despland PA, Regli F: Clinical and ultrasonographic diagnosis of cerebrovascular diseases. Nouv Presse Med 6(18):1570-1571, Apr 1977.

Hitchon PW, Kassell NF, Carlstrom TA, McDonnel DE: The Doppler ultrasonic flowmeter as an adjunct to operative management of cerebral arteriovenous malformations. Surg Neurol 11(5):345-347, May 1979.

Hopman H, Gratzl O, Schmiedek P, Schneider I: Dopplersonographic control of microvascular bypass function. In: Microsurgery for stroke, Schmiedek P (ed), New York: Springer Verlag, 230-232, 1977.

Hopman H, Gratzl O, Schmiedek P, Schneider I: Ultrasonic Doppler technique for microvascular bypass (author's transl). Neurochirurgia (Stuttg) 19(5):190-196, Sep 1976.

Nornes H, Grip A, Wikeby P: Intraoperative evaluation of cerebral hemo-dynamics using directional Doppler technique. Part 1: Arteriovenous malformations. J Neurosurg 50(2):145-151, Feb 1979.

Nornes H, Grip A, Wikeby P: Intraoperative evaluation of cerebral hemo-dynamics using directional Doppler technique. Part 2: Saccular aneurysms. J Neurosurg 50(5):570-577, May 1979.

CERVICAL VERTEBRAL AND SUBCLAVIAN DOPPLER

Ardouin M, Urvoy M, Sabouraud O, Herve C, Leboissetier E: Vertebro-basilar insufficiency and the Doppler effect. Bull Mem Soc Fr Ophthalmol (87):197-203, 1976.

Corson JD, Menzoian JO, LoGerfo FW: Reversal of vertebral artery blood flow demonstrated by Doppler ultrasound. Arch Surg 112(6):715-719, Jun 1977.

Courbier R, Jausseran JM, Reggi M: Surgical treatment of lesions of the supra-aortic trunks. Ann Chir Thorac Cardiovasc 15(2):143-150, Apr 1976.

Czajkowski J, Mazurek M, Berkan L: Ultrasound assessment of blood flow velocity based on Doppler's effect in subclavian steal syndrome (authors' transl). Klin Oczna 48(3):111-112, Mar 1978.

DeBray JM, Dauzat M, Teisseire-Girod F, Davinroy M, Emile J: The Doppler effect applied to the study of the vertebral arteries (author's transl). Nouv Presse Med 7(1):39-42, Jan 1978.

Grossman BL, Brisman R, Wood EH: Ultrasound and the subclavian steal syndrom. Radiology 94(1):1-6, Jan 1970.

Hauke P, Zeumer H: Doppler ultrasonic diagnosis of the subclavian-steal syndrome (author's transl). Dtsch Med Wochenschr 101(52):1912-1915, Dec 1976.

Kaneda H, Irino T, Minami T, Taneda M: Diagnostic reliability of the percutaneous ultrasonic Doppler technique for vertebral arterial occlusive diseases. Stroke 8(5):571-579, Sept-Oct 1977.

Keller H, Muller A, Meier W, Schonbeck M: Transoral Doppler ultrasound echography under local anaesthesia for the assessment of vertebral artery blood flow. Dtsch Med Wochenschr 100(17):937-938, 943-946, Apr 1975.

Lamis PA, Stanton PE, Hyland L: The axillo-axillary bypass graft: further experience. Arch Surg 111(12):1353-1356, Dec 1976.

Matsunaga T, Kawamoto H, Okumura S, Naito T: Ultrasonic blood rheography in vertebral artery of vertigo patients (Doppler method)—with the glass model experiments. Med J Osaka Univ 25(1-2):43-56, Dec 1974.

Mozersky DJ, Barnes RW, Sumner DS, Strandness DE Jr: Hemodynamics of innominate artery occlusion. Ann Surg 178(2):123-127, Aug 1973.

Mozersky DJ, Sumner DS, Hokanson DE, Strandness DE Jr: Subclavian revascularization by means of a subcutaneous axillary-axillary graft. Arch Surg 106(1):20-23, Jan 1973.

Platz M: A typical subclavian steal-syndrome. A case report (author's transl). Nervenarzt 50(5):317-319, 50(5):317-319, 1979.

Pourcelot L, Ribadeau-Dumas JL, Fagret D, Planiol T: Contribution of the Doppler examination to the diagnosis of subclavian steal syndrome. Rev Neurol (Paris) 133(5):309-323, May 1977.

Voight K, Kendel K, Sauer M: Subclavian steal syndrome. Bloodless diagnosis of the syndrome using ultrasonic pulse echo and vertebral artery compression. Fortschr Neurol Psychiatr 38(1):20-33, 1970.

Von Reutern GM, Budingen HJ, Freund HJ: The diagnosis of obstruction of the vertebral and subclavian arteries by means of directional Doppler sonography. Arch Psychiatr Nervenkr 222(2-3):209-222, Oct 1976.

Von Reutern GM, Pourcelot L: Cardiac cycle-dependent alternating flow in vertebral arteries with subclavian artery stenosis. Stroke 9(3):229-236, May-Jun 1978.

Von Reutern GM, Budingen HJ: Doppler sonographic study of the vertebral artery in subclavian steal syndrome (letter). Dtsch Med Wochenschr 102(4):140-141, Jan 1977.

Yeh HC, Mitty HA, Wolf BS, Jacobson JH: Ultrasonography of the brachiocephalic arteries. Radiology 132(2):403-408, Aug 1979.

Yoneda S, Nukada T, Tada K, Imaizumi M, Takano T: Subclavian steal in Takeyasu's arteritis. A hemodynamic study by means of ultrasonic Doppler flowmetry. Stroke 8(2):264-268, Mar-Apr 1977.

Zajgner J, Hain-Mazurkiewicz G: A trial of using Doppler's ultrasound effect for investigating vertebral arteries in degenerative cervical spine dis. Pol Przegl Radiol 42(1):1-2, Jan-Feb 1978.

CREDIT AND RECOGNITION LIST

The authors of this book wish to extent their appreciation and provide credit and recognition to the following publishing organizations for granting permission to use specific illustrations in order to enhance the contents of this book.

Chapter 1

Figures 3 and 13   Plenum Press, White C (ed), pp 1291-1310, Aug 1976. Ultrasound in medicine, vol 3B, cerebrovascular evaluation using C-W ultrasound. Authors: Spencer MP, Brockenbrough EC, Davis DL, Reid JM.

Figures 2, 5, 6 & 8   International Journal of Neurology, 11(2-3):228-242, 1977. Doppler ultrasonic imaging and non-invasive cerebrovascular evaluation. Author: Spencer MP.

Figure 4a   Angiology 30(8):526-538, Aug 1979. Doppler ultrasound in the evaluation of the peripheral arterial circulation. Authors: Reneman RS, Hoeks A, Spencer MP.

Chapter 2

Figure 3 and 11   Handbook of clinical ultrasound, 1978, (ed) by de Vlieger et al, pp 82.

Figure 7   Fundamentals of medical ultrasonography, 1973 (ed) by Gilber Baum, GP Putnam & Sons.

Chapter 3

Figure 1   Handbook of clinical ultrasound, 1978, (ed) by de Vlieger et al, pp 82.

Chapter 4

Figures 1, 2, 3 & 4   Ultrasound in medicine, 1977, vol 3B (ed) White ON and Brown RE. Authors: Reid JM, Spencer MP, Davis DL.

Chapter 6

Figure 12   Pergamon Press, Ltd. Ultrasound in medicine and biology, 51(1):1-11, 1979. Local Doppler audio spectra in normal and stenosed carotid arteries in man. Authors: Reneman RS, Spencer MP.

Chapter 8

Figure 2   Circulation Research Vol IV, No 4, July 1956. The aortic flow pulse as related to differential pressure. Authors: Spencer MP, Denison AB.

Figure 3	Circulation Research, Vol IV, No. 4, July 1958. Dynamics of the normal aorta, inertiance and 'compliance' of the arterial system which transforms the cardiac ejection pulse. Authors: Spencer MP, Johnson FR, Denison AB Jr.
Figure 4	Circulation Research, Vol X, No 3, March 1962 (Part 1) Dynamics of Ventricular Ejection. Authors: Spencer MP, Greiss FC.
Figure 5, 6 & 8	American Heart Association, Chapter 25, Handbook of physiology, Section 21 Circulation, II (Sect Ed Hamilton, Pub by American Physiology, Soc) 1963. Pulsatile blood flow in the vascular system. Authors: Spencer MP, Denison AB Jr.
Figure 7	American Heart Association American Journal Physiology, 125:45, 1939. An experimental study of standing waves in the pulse propogated through the aorta. Authors: Hamilton WF, Dow P.

Chapter 9

Figure 7	Bulletin of the Mason Clinic, Vol 20, Seattle, WA, No 1 March 1966, pp. 1-12. Evaluation of cardiovascular lesions by means of an impedence plot at the time of surgical correction. Authors: Spencer MP, Johnson DL, Lawrence GH, Tytus JS, Hill LD.
Figures 8, 9 & 15	Stroke 10(3):326-330, May-June 1979. Quantification of carotid stenosis with continuous-wave (C-W) Doppler ultrasound. Authors: Spencer MP, Reid JM.

Chapter 10

Figures 1, 2, 3, 4, 5 & 6	Ultrasound in Medicine and Biology. Journal of the World, Federation for Ultrasound in Medicine and Biology. (ed) DN White.

INDEX